New Haven's
Civil War Hospital

Best wishes,

New Haven's Civil War Hospital

A History of Knight U.S. General Hospital, 1862–1865

IRA SPAR, M.D.

McFarland & Company, Inc., Publishers
Jefferson, North Carolina, and London

ISBN 978-0-7864-7682-4

softcover : acid free paper ∞

LIBRARY OF CONGRESS CATALOGUING DATA ARE AVAILABLE

BRITISH LIBRARY CATALOGUING DATA ARE AVAILABLE

On the cover: Knight Army Hospital Grounds, New Haven, Connecticut
(The New Haven Museum & Historical Society)

Manufactured in the United States of America

*McFarland & Company, Inc., Publishers
Box 611, Jefferson, North Carolina 28640
www.mcfarlandpub.com*

Table of Contents

Preface

The impetus and initial research for this work began in September 1969 when a freshly minted hospital intern was assigned as surgeon for the 2nd/47th Battalion, 3rd Brigade, Ninth Infantry Division near the village of Bin Phouc, Mekong Delta, Republic of South Vietnam. An interest in photography and civil war history led to studies on the medical aspects of the Fifteenth Connecticut Volunteers, New Haven's regiment in the Civil War. With the acquisition of the six volumes *Medical and Surgical History of the War of the Rebellion* (*MSHWR*), I noticed the extraordinary similarity between monthly reports of regimental surgeons with the equivalent battalion surgeon over a century later. An honorary appointment as librarian for the Hartford Medical Society led to a perusal of its rare book section uncovering two copies of Vesalius prints, unopened since the 1920s. Also discovered lying flat on its side was a bound copy of the entire edition of the Knight U.S. Army General Hospital newspaper, the *Knight Hospital Record*. It contained fictional stories of romance and adventure, poems, national and local events, ads, politics, and descriptions of health care delivery, hospital statistics and lists of dead and wounded. Previous research had familiarized me with many of the participants. Experiencing the vicissitudes of war close up along with the trauma experience of an orthopedic surgeon provided insight and perspective others might lack. A book was conjured, to be completed in three months. That was seven years ago.

How can society in the worst of times, the calamitous Civil War, create a national hospital system virtually from scratch, staffed with competent medical personnel, appropriate drugs and equipment, along with an evacuation and social support system? A federally financed, single-payer universal health care system for sick and wounded returning soldiers was created, supplemented by doctors in private practice with state and individual citizen funding.

What was the science of the mid-nineteenth century and how was this taught in medical schools and apprenticeships? Who were these doctors whose personal sacrifices were essential for success? What was the ladder of professional advancement towards becoming regimental surgeon? What were their patient outcomes? Why was the military hospital placed in New Haven, how was it built and how did it function? What was the influence of politics on health care delivery and its providers?

1

Two narrative threads are woven in this tapestry. An independently wealthy governor with a stunning capacity to govern, administer and execute was magnified by remarkable personal generosity. The hospital chief of staff was an on-the-job trainee in building and administering a state-of-the-art thousand-bed health care facility. Stories of dealing with often hopelessly sick and wounded and their families, along with deserters, malcontents and those otherwise hiding from the battlefield are tempered by reports of front line reality from his volunteer nephew and namesake. The chapter on this young man's life resulted from the efforts of the late Sharon Steinberg of the Connecticut Historical Society who found a cache of his letters at the Virginia Historical Society.

This is not a rewrite of general Civil War medicine and for that Frank Freemon and Alfred Bollet are best. This is a metaphor on health care delivery in the nineteenth century through the lens of the twenty-first, described by the participants as it happened. The letters from Governor Buckingham, Washington officials, doctors, patients and families were culled from numerous archives. Period newspapers, medical manuals, textbooks and journals provided further insight. The interaction of the provost marshal with the health care system, including medical furloughs, desertions, exemptions and the draft, was distilled from the Draft Registration Records in the National Archives in Waltham, Massachusetts. Individual military and pension records from the National Archives in Washington helped determine patient outcomes. Archives at the Connecticut State Library, Connecticut Historical Society, Yale University and the U.S. Army at the Carlisle Barracks rounded out the collection. Gratitude for all the archivists' guidance and patience can't be overstated.

Since 1865 over 80,000 books about the Civil War have been published with over six thousand on Lincoln alone. His beliefs on slavery, emancipation, and even homosexuality, vampires and colonoscopy have been exhaustively studied. There is a sameness of ground traveled and material offered differing only by prose and viewpoint. Most of this book's material has not been previously reported and hopefully presents a fresh look at a problem that vexes us today, providing health care for all citizens.

Prologue

In the spring of 1861 America came of age, taking its place as a giant amongst nations. The eyes of the world were focused on whether the political experiment initiated with the American Revolution of 1776 would succeed or drown in blood and tears. Would the establishment of elective democracy, a republic of free men, continue as a workable political enterprise? Was the current crisis simply growing pains from unresolved contradictions, temporary and self-limiting? Here glowed the beacon of democracy, a source of light and warmth that would incubate the hopes and aspirations of humankind. Freedom of religion and speech was guaranteed by law, along with the rights of individuals to life, liberty, and the pursuit of happiness regardless of color, creed, or national origin. This supposed that all men were created equal, not just half or three-fifths' worth, but equal without exception. The American proposal was "one man, one vote," and equal representation by a government composed of its citizens for the benefits of all. Americans wrestled mightily over the truth of these core matters. Did guaranteed rights apply only to white men of property or did that include men of color? Would the biblical admonition that there shall be one law for all, whether sojourner or citizen, about to become a prophetic reality?

The abscess of slavery festered worldwide and for centuries, and particularly in this supposed land of the free and home of the brave. To preserve the Union and cure this illness, radical surgery seemed necessary. Fulfillment of the covenant made by the forefathers demanded one unified nation. The declarations America signed in 1776 would be forged for the ages in the blast furnace of civil war.

"These are the times that try men's souls." "Rally round the flag boys as victory is liberty." "We fight to preserve our way of life." "This war is to make men free and preserve democracy for all and for all times." "The people cry out for vengeance!" "The war will be quickly won as we are righteous, our soldiers brave and invincible and God is on our side." These were the sound bites of the 1860s, their familiarity echoing throughout time. American patriotism was rooted not in selfishness but for the sake of humanity, a war of justice against injustice, of holiness against sin. Both sides were certain of a quick victory, not realizing that both might lose. Like many other conflicts this War of Rebellion would exceed by far predictions of its length, embitterment, blood and financial losses. Amputated limbs and terminated lives can be measured and accounted for, but not so easily emotional and spiritual damages.

In 1860 the entire United States Army consisted of 14,000 men with 40 hospital beds and 113 doctors.[1] The unquenchable appetite of war would explode these numbers as the tranquility of peacetime garrison life gave way to the requirements of a modern medical department. By September 1864 there were 136,000 beds in the Union army alone, located in 202 hospitals, with a medical staff of over 10,000 doctors.[2] The eruptions of a cataclysmic war produced festering mountains of sick and wounded, requiring a level of medical care never before provided much less anticipated. How this society managed health care for its citizens, a service difficult to achieve under the best of circumstances, was a feat unmatched in its scope and might serve as a model for future generations to study and improve upon.

Success in wartime would be further complicated by the need to cover great distances in hostile environments while providing and transporting great quantities of men and materials. This required building an infrastructure of people, supplies, and facilities to store, service, and transport whatever, whenever and wherever it was needed.

The patients were millions of soldiers and civilians, black and white, rich and poor, trapped in a devastating modern war where thousands of wounded would be the norm rather than the exception. How to evacuate and treat, and in a timely manner, such a compressed mass of suffering humanity tested the limits of human capability both then and now.

Lessons from past wars would be relearned. New techniques and better judgment would result from hard experience, trial and error, and necessity born of desperation. Doctors would train anew and reeducate themselves while perfecting the artful product that is the best health care possible. This was the first "modern war," where the earth was scorched, producing endless rows of disease-ridden embattlements, and body and soul withered in a new form of madness called trench warfare. This would culminate fifty years later in the death of millions in World War I.

New technology in armaments produced mass casualties with devastating wounds for which state-of-the art medical treatments could offer uncertain results at best. Rifled gun barrels and artillery pieces produced greater accuracy at longer range. The Minié ball, named after the French lieutenant who designed it, was a conical, partially hollowed-out .58 caliber lead bullet with which a sharpshooter could hit a man at half a mile. If he could see it, he could hit it.[3] At one hundred yards, with a clear view not obscured by smoke and dust, certainty replaced chance in creating casualties. And then there were the cannons. The brilliant flash of explosions from artillery and mortar shells lit up the firmament while dispersing unforgiving sharp chunks of metal, functioning like a scythe cutting a field of hay. The blood of America's sons, the best in the land, flowed like a river from the destructiveness of war.

As terrifying as the new science of war had become, there was worse. The most common cause of death was disease, medical conditions for which the causes were mostly unknown and effectiveness of treatment anecdotal at best. Carrying the wounded off the battlefield in an efficient manner required ambulance units dedicated to that task, a capability devoutly to be wished for but not available until late in the war. Field hospitals with experienced personnel specifically assigned to the definitive treatment of those casualties needed to be trained and made ready to receive. Dealing with the impact of contagious and infectious diseases, especially on standing armies, demanded attention to sanitation. Each soldier's environment needed to be reexamined and improved. His shoes, clothing, and personal habits also played roles in health and disease. Sore, ulcerated feet from ill-fitting shoes, exposure to the elements, contaminated water, improper diet, and even venereal disease all contribute to a soldier who can't fight, much less march or dig a protective hole in the ground.

Nineteenth-century medical care was provided in the home and doctors made house calls by horse and buggy. The few existing hospitals were maintained for seamen, the homeless and destitute. The poor were relegated to the "pest house," or public hospital. In New York City, streetwalkers when arrested were offered the choice of serving time in jail, paying a fine, or working as a "nurse" at Bellevue Hospital. Surgery was done only in exceptional cases, and often at the patient's home. An assistant, using ether or chloroform, would provide anesthesia. So unusual was surgery that people often came to watch the spectacle. Some even sold tickets for the event.

War, however, brings with it a whole new set of medical conditions unique in its complexity and in large numbers. Conceive of a circumstance requiring 35,000 amputations, or the care of 1.1 million cases of malaria. These were the figures for the Union army over a four-year span. Medical diseases accounted for two of every three deaths, the most common being diarrhea/dysentery at 44,000. Next was typhoid fever at 29,000, and third was pneumonia with 20,000 victims. There were 620,000 deaths on both sides and millions of others sick and wounded, many cases going uncounted because of absence of support facilities.

This story is about the transformation of a small and antiquated medical workforce barely adequate for low-level demand, to a modern health care system able to deal with huge numbers of patients. This required skilled, dedicated, and caring people, for failure was not an option. The timid may someday inherit this earth, but not a surgical ward with the unbearable stench of gangrene and the cries from agonizing pain and suffering. This environment required tough-minded and stiff-necked individuals who would not flinch from the horrors of war. Only men and women of grit and undaunted courage needed apply. The qualifications to be a surgeon are said to be the eye of an eagle, the heart of a lion, and the hands of a woman. Also recommended are a spine of steel and an incorruptible soul with which to blunt the critics and deny the corrupt and incompetent entrance into the temple of medicine.

The Civil War would test the mettle of the American people. Some were crushed by the onslaught. Others buckled but gradually rose back to their full height and moved forward with even greater stature. Sacrifice, character, and honor were necessary ingredients for the successful management of so much suffering humanity.

Many of the techniques we take for granted were many years away. This is a look through the prism of history to medical practice at a time *before* bacteria were known to cause disease, *before* doctors wore masks and gloves, and *before* antibiotics. Antiseptic technique described by Joseph Lister was not reported until 1866 and took twenty years to be accepted worldwide. There were no intravenous fluids or blood transfusions to prepare a patient in shock for surgery or to treat simple dehydration. The first X-ray showing the small bones of the hand was not done until thirty years later. Penicillin was first used clinically during World War II. None of this was in the armamentarium of a nineteenth-century physician.

We do not criticize General Robert E. Lee for not calling in air strikes as there were no airplanes, nor do we chastise General Ulysses Grant for not thrusting forward mechanized armor as there were no tanks. That would be foolish and unfair. The same standards should apply to the surgeons of the time. Lessons of history are best learned, not by judging people from a different era by current standards in science and morals, but to understand the past through their eyes.

Just who were the men who met these fateful challenges while facing down their darkest fears? Who made the necessary sacrifices both personally and professionally on behalf of the millions of sons, fathers, and brothers whose lives and limbs were at stake? A hospital was built in New Haven to provide the best available treatment for returning soldiers of Connecticut suffering from disease or injury. For the first time in American history the federal government provided single-payer universal health care for its returning soldiers. For each hospital bed filled, the central government paid $3.50 per week. Additional sources of funding came from individual citizens and the state.

How this hospital came to be and who ran it is told in part by the *Knight Hospital Record*, the newspaper of this Civil War hospital.[4] Of the soldiers, by the soldiers and for the soldiers, it is unique in being the only complete Civil War hospital newspaper that exists. It offers an unparalleled eyewitness account of the period, written as it occurred, from inside the institution. Its writings illustrate patients, medical staff, local merchants, and civilian and military leaders. It reports local as well as national news. The weave of politics, economics, religion, philosophy, medical science, and human frailty make for an inspiring tale of how a society can provide state-of-the-art health care for millions of its citizens under the most difficult of circumstances.

CHAPTER ONE

Nineteenth-Century Medicine

In the absence of modern medical science and surgery, what was the basis for health care in the mid-nineteenth century? Every great general from Caesar to Napoleon and the giants of medicine relied on the sanitary laws expounded by Moses in Leviticus. In biblical eras it was priests who promoted hygiene and public health. Prevention was preeminent in an era absent effective remedies. Isolation or quarantine, fumigation and avoiding contagion were some features of this approach. An infection resulted from being unclean or defiled. Clean, uncontaminated water was essential for well-being. Rainwater had to be stored in covered cisterns. This prevented the contaminating properties of insects, rodents or fomites. "If any of those falls into an earthen vessel, everything inside it shall be impure and the vessel itself you shall break" (Leviticus 11:33). Water acted as a transportation system for poisonous elements and therefore was the source of disease.

Blood, human excreta, dead animals, and dead humans were to be buried with dispatch and beyond limits of camp. Both Union and Confederate manuals stress the importance of waste disposal. The eminent Philadelphia surgeon Dr. Samuel Gross had this to say:

> All offal's should be promptly removed from the camp and carried to a distance of several miles, or be well buried. The privies should be in the most favorable location as it respects ventilation, and be closed at least every three or four days. Every man should be compelled to bury his alvine excretions, as was the custom in time of war among the ancient Hebrews, each man being obliged to carry a paddle for that purpose. The emanations from these sources cannot receive too much attention especially when large masses of men are crowded together, as they are then extremely prone to induce disease.[1]

Sinners beware! Failure to follow the commandments "will wreak misery upon you: consumption and fever, which cause the eyes to pine and the body to languish. And you shall be smitten by the enemy that will surround you and be vanquished by this invisible foe" (Leviticus 26:16–20).

Besides holy living, what else offered protection against the vile fevers of the night? The Arc and Tabernacle were circumscribed by fire and pyres of smoke. This and quarantine was offered as a defense against returning soldiers carrying disease. To avoid the wrath of his Eternal in the form of a plague, Moses orders Aaron to "take the fire pan, and put on it fire from the altar. Add incense and take it quickly to the community. He stood between the dead and the living, until the plague was checked" (Numbers 16:11–13). Incense burning, deodorizing and fumigating were considered preventatives and treatments by nineteenth-century practitioners. Caesar and Napoleon surrounded their armies with smoke to avoid malarial fevers. It was common practice during nineteenth-century yellow fever epidemics to set fires with tar which produced billows of smoke while assaulting the atmosphere with periodic firing of cannon whose goal it was to chase away "pestiferous poisons" lurking in the abyss of disease-ridden cesspools.[2] In the Bible, soldiers returning from war were quarantined for seven days before being admitted into camp. Disinfection was by smoke and fire, bathing and washing their clothes. The goal was to prevent epidemics of fevers and contagion from exposure to the dead. Sick and unclean persons were prohibited from entering the tabernacle.

From antiquity came the teachings of Hippocrates and the separation of medicine from religion. Disease came from nature and was not due to superstition or God. Humors of the body, both good and ill, determined well-being. Galen was personal physician to several emperors who attributed the differences in human moods to imbalances of the four bodily fluids. There was either an excess or an insufficiency of blood, black bile, yellow bile or phlegm. When the heart was discovered as the center of a circulatory system, new theories emerged to coincide with the new science.

Poisons were called contagion, toxin or virus — a rogue element running rampant that needed to be flushed out of the system. This might require the creation of new energies to fuel the engine of health. By the nineteenth century, contagion was seen as the direct passage of some chemical or physical influence from the sick to a susceptible person, by direct contact, by fomites or through the atmosphere, and demanded quarantine. Local officials and businessmen argued that total cleansing of their seaports would not stop the epidemics since cities with state-of-the-art sanitation had the same or lower febrile illness rates and deaths as those where large hotels dumped the products of privies into their streets.

In the encyclopedic two-volume description of yellow fever by Philadelphia's prominent Professor La Roche, theories of disease etiology are explored. The morbid poison may be imported from without or from within, might spontaneously generate and be noncontagious. If the latter is the case, no quarantine would be necessary, a position supported by the British, whose mercantile activities were at stake. The poison could be gas, solid or liquid. The source of the poison would be filthy localities such as houses, ships, jails, hospitals, cities, marshes or ponds. Some poisons, such as malaria, were noted to not exist at high altitude or near ships. Knowing the life cycle and living habits of mosquitoes would provide reasons why this was so. La Roche's "doctrine of infection" rounded up the usual suspects popular for the era: animal or vegetable decomposition, wood decomposition in the soil, morbid miasma, pestilential effluvia, accelerated decomposition of bone or compost, altered atmospheric conditions, and rapid propagation and migration of animalcular or fungi. Fever was caused by morbid material that found admission into blood leading to peculiar changes, while those who survived generated immunity.[3]

James Paget was a surgeon and pathologist whose two volume treatise on surgical pathology offered a new look at disease. Bone, lung and other organ tissue was analyzed grossly and microscopically to shed new light on the cause and perhaps treatment of disease. Blood took part in healing of injuries but "large clots were not necessary or advantageous and were absorbed in reparative tissue but probably [retard] healing in this respect."[4] Inflammation was paramount in disease production. It was caused by changes in the blood supply, its composition, its nervous source, and the status of the condition of the inflamed part.

Dr. John Riddell was professor of chemistry of the Medical College of Louisiana who did research with the microscope and was a member of the New Orleans Sanitary Commission in 1853. Writing about a series of recent yellow fever epidemics he noted "myriads of microscopic motes" in air and described an atmosphere containing forms of organic life not visible with a naked eye. Poisonous matter came from maturing germs and spores while surrounded by impure air. He wrote: "Emanations from putrefying matter, gas liquid and solid particles and the presence of specific organisms whose perfected spores constitute the material cause of yellow fever."[5]

Fevers were described by when they appeared: continually, several times daily, once daily, every other day, or every four days. They were remittent, intermittent, tertian, and quotidian. Daniel Drake, who did the first research on the American continent on this subject, described several types of febrile diseases in 1850.[6] A symptom such as a fever was considered the disease itself. The descriptive line-up was ague, dumb ague, and autumnal, bilious, congestive, intermittent, marsh, malignant, malarial, miasmatic, and remittent fevers.

During the early part of the nineteenth century treatment was "heroic." Doctor Benjamin Rush, a signer of the Declaration of Independence, was a major advocate. If the fever was due to acceleration of circulation, irritation of regulator nerves, or inflammation, then treat by depletion. Dr. Rush proposed: "There are three causes why we cannot cure disease, namely: Want of knowledge of that disease; want of remedy, and want of efficacy in the remedy when applied." Some accused him of curing his patients' complaints by killing them with excess bleeding.

The most aggressive depletion was bloodletting: cut a large vein and collect pints of blood in pewter or enamel receptacles especially made for the purpose. A spring lancet armed with one or twelve blades would release a much smaller amount, as did leeches and wet or dry cupping. The Europeans were the first to abandon venesection partly from experience and also from introduction of statistical analysis by Professor Pierre Charles Alexander Louis of Paris. He demonstrated failure of this mode of treatment by detailed clinical research providing statistics as a means of evaluating medical therapeutics. By mid-century this practice was mostly abandoned, following Hippocrates' admonition, "Above all else do no harm."

Mercury in the form of "blue mass" or calomel causes diuresis (voiding) and was used to treat heart failure well into the second half of the twentieth century. (The author as an intern used the injectable form as treatment of choice for shortness of breath in cardiac disease.) It is also a laxative and causes salivation, the stopping point in treatment.

Cathartics were used to run the bowel and evacuate whatever toxins were lurking in the dark and dank passages. Castor oil and liquid or smoke enemas also filled the bill.

Emetics caused vomiting, running the bowel in the opposite direction, often to the extreme distress of the patient and observers. Tartar emetic or antimony was exquisitely effective in that regard and was considered one of the vilest poisons ever foisted on the public. More commonly used was ipecac, considered a valuable stand-by.

Diaphoretics caused increased sweating. This was considered treatment for fever, assisted by opiates, alcohol, or ipecac.

Diet was a key therapeutic agent and one could adjust the nutritive value with bland or mostly liquid intake. Juices were extracted from meat, fruits or vegetables in iron presses made specifically for that purpose.

Nervous sedatives avoided effecting cerebral functions while reducing excess circulation. Examples are foxglove or digitalis, tobacco or smoke enemas.

Depressants diminished the vital functions of all organs. Cold and warm baths, opium and alcohol were treatments of choice.

A second major classification was the stimulants, such as coffee, tea, pepper, strychnine and spirits of turpentine. A subset was tonics designated to increase the vital actions. For low muscle tone, general weakness, poor appetite, indigestion and generally feeling low, fuel would be added to the dwindling fire. Some of the old reliable tonics included special diets, cod liver oil, opium, iron, ginger, cinchona (Peruvian) bark or quinine and alcohol (also considered a depressant and good for everything).

A doctor might recommend depletion with lancet, mercury to salivation, free and profuse purging and large doses of Peruvian bark or sulfate of quinine. La Roche reflected the enlightened European view to let nature take its course and avoid heroic therapy.

> The idea of curing the disease or greatly abridging its course is entitled to little confidence. To nature must be left chief management. Time allows for the elimination of poison. The physician keeps his hands off as much as possible. In all instances more damage is to be apprehended from too great than too little interference on the part of the medical attendant.[7]

Inflammation was treated as a form of disease with sedatives, evacuates, and purgatives. Diseases with congestion required external stimulation such as rubefacients, hot baths, and blistering agents. Internal stimulation was by tonic, mercury, mustard, ginger root, pepper and turpentine. Blistering was accomplished with croton oil, Spanish fly, creosote and hot pepper. To quiet the skin, emollients such as bread and milk, flaxseed, or olive oil served well.

If the treatment was worse than the disease, then therapeutic reevaluation was required. Plants and minerals were available, reasonably priced and thus prescribed freely. There were textbooks written for the laymen allowing them to self-diagnose and treat. William Buchan's *Domestic Medicine* went through 15 editions. The New Haven text published in 1816 was endlessly entitled "Every man his own Doctor; or a Treatise on the Prevention and Cure of Diseases, by Regimen and Simple Medicines. To which is added, a Treatise on the Materia Medica; in which Medicinal Qualities of Indigenous Plants are given and Adapted to Common Practice. Also information on Horses, Cattle, Sheep and Swine and the Art of Farrier."

The fierceness of traditional medical therapy encouraged the development of competing health care providers. The medical botanist goal was to assist nature in exterminating disease and hence act in accordance with natural laws. The Thomsonian movement challenged heroic medical therapeutics and replaced it with various herbs and teas, allowing the gentleness of nature to take its course and permit the common man to treat himself.[8] No less an authority than the dean of Harvard Medical School, Oliver Wendell Holmes, had similar views while wary of nontraditionalist groups encroaching on medical doctors and perhaps justifiably so.

> A noxious agent should never be employed in sickness unless there is ample evidence in the particular case to overcome the presumption against all such agents. Drugs should always be regarded as evils. The miserable delusions of homeopathy builds on the axiom opposed to the notion that sick are to be cured by poisons.
>
> Throw out opium, throw out a few specifics, throw out wine, and the vapors which produce the miracle of anesthesia, and I firmly believe that if the whole materia medica, as now used, could be sunk to the bottom of the sea, it would be all the better for mankind, and all the worse for the fishes.[9]

Voltaire described medicine as the art of keeping the patient amused while nature takes its course. While most diseases are self-limiting and patients get better sometimes in spite of rather than because of treatment, there were drugs with great therapeutic effect. The *United States Pharmacopeias* listed just a handful of agents that were disease-specific. Mercury was used for syphilis, heart failure, intestinal disorders, and numerous other ailments. Foxglove or digitalis was a proven remedy for heart disease, quinine for malaria, colchicine for gout and opium for pain. Botanical potions were being replaced by mineral drugs. Turpentine and mercury taken orally will kill intestinal parasites. Cold remedies and intestinal sedatives have not changed much over the years. Bicarbonate of soda is today's Alka-Seltzer, and bicarbonate antacids are Rolaids. Surgery consisted of bleeding, cupping, pulling teeth, lancing boils, pumping stomachs, reducing fractures and dislocations, and finally amputations. A quarter of hospital admissions were for trauma, but surgery was rarely done. The diagnosis of fever and inflammation accounted for half the hospital admissions.

Physiological responses to drugs such as perspiration, movements of the bowel, and urination were considered positive events for the patient and were supported by accepted tradition in both medical and religious texts. In the Talmud, for example, six things are said to augur well for the sick: sneezing, sweating, looseness of bowels, nocturnal pollutions, sleeping, and dreaming. The patient and his family could see the doctor causing an effect, heroic, perhaps, and beneficial for the patient, maybe. Trying to cure the disease by making things happen or at least assist the patient in getting through a health crisis was considered a positive outcome. This offered some assurance that disease was under the control or influence of a physician.

Proprietary medicines were affordable, available and widely advertised at a time when there was no government regulation of drugs or much else. Because no state or federal organizations existed to enforce standards and thus protect the public, the quality and composition of drugs were unknown. The medications' main effect was improving the sellers' bank account rather than the health of their customers. These were cure-alls for cancer to consumption and from lack of virility to excessive "female complaints." Cocaine was legally purchased from apothecaries without a doctor's prescription to treat backaches, malaise, or teething babies. One hundred proof alcohol, opium, and cocaine were frequent ingredients in over-the-counter products. There were some 1,500 proprietary medicines in the 1860s. Lotions, liniments, and beverages were available for whatever ailed you.

Hochstetler's Bitters was forty-four percent alcohol and was the only patent medicine known to have been government-issued. It was cheaper than others because no alcohol excise tax was levied due to its "medicinal value." Additional ingredients included pepper, chewing tobacco, quinine, and a wide variety of herbs thought to have medicinal value. The "chill tonics" and cold medicines often contained alcohol and opium, both of which are cough suppressants and thus effective in treating upper respiratory infections.

A food source for the soldier was the ubiquitous sutler who ran a store on hospital or regimental grounds that supplied tobacco, pies, candy, whiskey, and other items that might not otherwise be readily available. A study by the United States Sanitary Commission on "drunkenness" found that 31 of 200 regiments allowed sutlers to sell liquor.[10] In 177 regiments men got liquor from sutlers with or without approval. Intoxication was reported as common in only six regiments, occasionally occurred but not deemed a serious evil in 31, and rare in 163. In the majority of regiments there was little reported dram-drinking, except shortly after pay. Most of the liquor drunk by the volunteers was attributed to the "pie peddlers." In regiments with large numbers of Germans, lager beer had been freely used, for "its use was beneficial and disorders of the bowels were less frequent in companies regularly supplied with it in moderation than in other companies of the same regiment."

The Sanitary Commission made recommendations for the health and welfare of each soldier: "Each soldier should be provided with a clothes brush, shoe brush, tooth brush, comb and towel adapted to be carried snugly in the knapsack, and for which he should be required to account weekly." The provider would be state or federal government, or an individual might purchase directly from the sutler. The commission expressed reservations as to who had the soldier's interests at heart, being an organization favoring temperance and eventually prohibition.

> Evil comes to the men from the sutler's shop. Corrupt bargains have been formed between sutler and officers; officers receive wine and sutlers use influence and power over men to prevent them from saving from their pay for the sake of their families engaging in secret sale of spirits. Sutlers in actual practice are an unmitigated curse. Some of the men throw their rations away and literally live on sutler's trash. Others will eat a full ration and then go straight to the sutlers and eat three or four villainous pies. Many of these have been fried in condemned lard a week before the soldier eats them. The result is camp diarrhea, dysentery and all their concomitant evils. To keep a soldier healthy you must confine him to plain and regular rations.[11]

Twenty-two-year-old Captain Henry Peck of the 15th Connecticut Volunteers had definite views on the subject of alcohol consumption, which he confided to his sister and mother.

> 1 April 1862
> Every one admits that the influence of alcohol to excess is the most demoralizing and degrading influence in the world. The only safe ground for a man to stand on is total abstinence. The sot of today was the moderate drinker of yesterday and I will in no way or shape use tobacco or alcohol. While it may please my God to let me in, I as a Christian shall throw my influence on the scale against social drinking. If ever I have men in my employ I will not allow liquor to be taken into my house or field
>
> 29 Sept. 1862
> I am still not well. No sign of chill. The prayer is better than whiskey. We all go on together some shaking and some not. I have two men very sick indeed. One a fine fellow I fear may not live. Dave is not well. I am and so is Billy. I think we are the healthiest men in the Fifteenth allowing to our cleanliness. We bathe four times per week, change our garments often and keep our diet simple but bountiful at any expense.[12]

Peck died of typhoid fever in January 1863.

Chronic alcoholism was cause for rejection and considered distinct from habitual drunkenness, which was a disqualifier for military service. But there was no exemption unless there were also lesions of liver, kidney, brain, or digestive apparatus. Neither was cause for discharge from service unless structural changes were present. In a text on medical evaluation of recruits diagnostic details were revealed.

> Drunkenness is the principal cause of most of the military offences of which soldiers are guilty and for which they are punished, and is the source of many physical disqualifications disabling them from duty and rendering a discharge from the army ultimately necessary. Look for obvious signs: watery eyes, acne rosacea, coated tremulous tongue, tumid belly, unsteady gait, trembling hands, atrophy of lower extremities, gastro-intestinal disorders, piles, weakened intellect, limited power of attention, spasmodic modes of utterance and expression.[13]

Many doctors and the public as well considered alcohol a tonic or health-producing drug, even a gift from God: "Wine cheers the heart of men" (Psalms 104:14–15). "For the only good a man can have under the sun is to eat and drink and enjoy himself" (Ecclesiastes 8:13). The temperance movement warned of alcoholic excess, recommending religious conversion for treatment of the "fallen." They quoted a different part of the same Bible. "The vine for them is from Sodom, from the vineyards of Gomorrah; the grapes for them are poison, A bitter growth their clusters. Their wine is the venom of asps, the pitiless poison of vipers" (Deuteronomy 32:32–33).

Sermons on the subject could be heard from the pulpit and read in newspapers and periodicals. A pamphlet issued by southern prohibitionists entitled *Liquor and Lincoln,* authored by an anonymous physician, attributes the losing war effort to sinners with "groveling passions, depraved appetites, gambling in obscenity and profane jocularity, and the evil of distilled damnation. They have forsaken the Lord God and he hath brought all this evil upon them." The "shame of foul degrading moral affliction" could not be overcome by state pride and patriotism alone. It was "no wonder the bones of thousands of our brave defenders have been left to bleach on their native hills, when drunken ignoramuses, under the appellation of "Surgeon," have dealt them more numerous and deadly blows than the missiles of the enemy."[14]

Alcoholism during the entire war is covered in just two short paragraphs in the 6,000 pages of the *MSHWR* and is summarized below.

Inebriation	589 cases	110 fatal
Delirium tremens	3,744 cases	450 fatal
Chronic alcoholism	920 cases	45 fatal

Delirium tremens occurs only after many years of chronic alcoholism and is clearly underreported. Troops located near cities and a ready supply of alcohol had higher rates of alcohol-related complications. The Medical Department's position was succinct: "Preventive measures belong to the government and discipline of camps rather than to their sanitation and to the military more than to the medical officer." Alcoholism and its side effects were a moral and disciplinary problem, not a disease. It would be handled through administrative and judicial channels, not medical.[15]

Alcohol withdrawal, or the DTs, was discussed by the chief of surgery at Yale, Dr. Jonathan Knight, in medical student lectures in 1843.

> During the last 25 years I have not had a death from the disease in the New Haven jail. Give emetic of zinc sulfate and ipecac or ipecac with mustard and then cathartic. If there was a soft pulse and perspiration on the face and pallor give opium six grains every two hours. Opium is the remedy here, alcohol will not do. If urine is scanty and fever is present, use ipecac and then opium, followed by digitalis if needed. Also use irritant to spine as adjuvant and try to calm the patient from his hallucination.[16]

Doctors of the Hartford Medical Society came to different conclusions in the 1860s. At the House of Correction in Hartford all those treated with opium died. The drug treatment advocated by Knight was abandoned when subsequent clinical experience failed to reproduce his results, a not uncommon event in medicine.[17] Those treated with digitalis initially showed marked improvement, although at three weeks at some died with "affection of the heart." Patients were instead placed in isolation rooms, with attendants present to prevent self-inflicted harm. Nonviolent patients were freed of restraints. Decoction of wormwood (an herb) up to six quarts was made available. The next one hundred cases with the diagnosis ranging from delirium tremens to raving mania were thus treated, resulting in just one death and that from erysipelas. They basically forced fluids. (Intravenous fluid

replacement, sedation, and electrolyte control is the treatment of choice for alcohol withdrawal.)

The government purchased an ocean of whiskey, sherry, and wine: three million bottles
of ingestible alcohol. Derivatives of the grape were listed in the pharmacopoeia as having
medicinal value.[18] Their popularity with the troops, officers and enlisted men alike, was
undeniable. In the commodity market, spirits were of considerable monetary value. Taxes
and the soaring cost of grain drove the price of whiskey to new heights, providing speculators,
politicians, and still operators an economic opportunity. "Medicinal" alcohol avoided the
omnipresent tax man, thus creating an additional margin for profit. Those in possession
stood to profit mightily as the price of alcohol went from 20 cents a gallon to $2.20.

Opinion was divided among surgeons as to the value or necessity of including alcoholic
beverages in the soldiers' daily diet and of its efficacy in treating disease. Prophylactic use
of quinine for malaria, notoriously endemic in the South, became routine. To encourage
soldiers to take the bitter medicine on a daily basis, a shot of whiskey was added. Sergeants
supervised the procedure as some "forgot" to take the medicine and just swallowed the shot.
During the war, the Union army consumed 595,544 ounces of quinine sulfate and 518,957
ounces of cinchona extract.[19]

A study in the *MSHWR* indicated mixed reviews on the medical use of alcohol. Most
thought it injurious rather than useful, but on occasion advantageous. Responses of regimental surgeons are listed below.

> Evil and moral influences overbalances any good effect. Diarrhea and dysentery was not in
> the least prevented nor was the physical strength of the men perceptibly sustained.
> Whiskey should only be given in hospital setting.
> Does not promote the ability of soldier to endure physical exertion and […] it diminishes
> the ability to resist diseases.
> Using just whiskey alone had no influence in incidence of malaria, quinine not readily avail-
> able.
> If a man felt cold he got "a horn" to warm him; if he felt hot or feverish he got the same to
> make him "throw off the fever." Consequently the surgeons of those regiments were lauded to
> the sky, while those of the other commands (no whiskey) were abused both by officers and
> men.
> I would prefer instead the issue of good vegetables such as potatoes and onions, etc.
> The habitual issue of whiskey is useless, mischievous and demoralizing. I use it occasionally
> during severe fatigue duty or great exposure it is salutary.
> I used after unusual fatigue or exposure and to constitutionally feeble after ordinary duties,
> and after repeated attacks of cachectic or febrile diseases.
> It increases endurance and promotes health.
> It doubtless proved beneficial. It acted as an adjuvant to the digestive functions. The men
> would eat better, work better, and if they did not indulge to excess, they endured sickness bet-
> ter for it.
> Although a temperance man I have always used whiskey liberally with my men using a barrel
> in my regiment during a march. My testimony is unequivocally in favor of its judicious use —
> say an ounce daily to the weariest on a march.
> In bad weather or when exhausting duties were required. Not daily.
> In every instance the whiskey ration has done more harm than good.

Surgeon Robert Ware of 44th Massachusetts Volunteers described his medical therapy
for malaria prophylaxis in the Carolinas.

> We take our quinine regularly in a jovial company and laugh at each other's wry faces over the
> bitterness.[20]

Private Lewis Nettleton of the 15th Connecticut Volunteers was dubious about doctors in general and pessimistic about their drugs, as he wrote from Portsmouth, Virginia, in 1863.

> I have just been for my dose, quinine, water and whiskey. I have but little faith in the medicine they give us here, but we must take it, kill or cure. [21]

Judson Abernathy was of the same regiment. He became a church deacon after the War and abstained from alcohol. Here he writes from New Bern, North Carolina, during the oppressive summer of 1864:

> 11 July
> Doctor gave me an emetic with pills and quinine. A little bitter must be mixed in with the sweet in this life. I am at bed rest and having chills.
>
> 17 July
> I feel well today. Anticipate a bad day today as fever and ague is a constant visitor on the seventh day after a preceding one. But I was up sometime this morning and had a dose of quinine pills down me as a preventative. They worked well and though I felt somewhat sick from the affects [*sic*], the feeling was nothing compared with the chills and fever.[22]

His commanding officer was Major Henry Osborne, who described his experience to his mother in August 1864:

> It is hard to write in this infernally hot country. I have had chills and fever and pretty severe shook too. It took ten or twelve pounds of meat off from me without much trouble. The chill lasts one hour and the fever about four hours. The chill is the worst part of it. If you escape from the seventh day and to the twenty first day then you should be all right. I have enough quinine to drive away all sorts of fever from my immediate vicinity for a year to come.[23]

An honest assessment to his parents came from twenty-year-old Private Alfred Holcomb of the 27th Massachusetts Volunteers in April 1862. He sustained two minor injuries later in the war: burns of both hands from premature discharge of a cannon during a siege in North Carolina in April 1863 and a slight leg wound at the siege in Petersburg in June 1864. He mustering out of service two months later.[24]

> I take this opportunity to let you know that I am well and enjoying myself first rate. I have been sick about as much as well, since I have been here. We draw one ration of whiskey every day. I do not drink more than half of mine. I sell it to George. He can have as much as half a dozen rations if he can get it as the Doctor orders it. We had quinine in it at first for the ague. The doctor gave me quinine and he said that I had the ague. He gave me so much that it made my teeth sore so that I could hardly eat. They have got me well now have got a good appetite so that I can eat most everything. I am not very strong yet and my hand trembles as you see from writing. I have fret away a good deal since I been here. George is pretty tight and has bought a bottle of whiskey where I saw it in his pocket. Drew a big ration and got another fellow to give him his. It made him crazy far more.[25]

Going on sick call just to get one's whistle wet was not unknown and was considered patriotic if it got men back on full duty. Henry J. Thompson of New Haven's 15th Volunteers was the drum squad leader whose duties included sounding all calls promptly. He was also a stretcher bearer, and reported sick men to the orderly. Stationed in New Bern, North Carolina, in August 1864, he described being treated with the combination of quinine and alcohol for the dumb ague with dysentery.

> Cold streaks run down and up the back, then hot streaks then full fever and stomach sick, you have to lie down, then numb all over, goes on generally just at night. Next morning, feels as if

cart load of stone had been tipped up on you and been pounded all but to death, every bone in the body will ache — feel as if every cord had been pulled out of you, so you can judge it was no pleasant feeling.

It rains here every day. I have got a bottle of bitters made of wormwood and it is bitter too: part honey, part water, part whiskey, half wormwood. The Doctor give me an order to get all the whiskey I want and told me to use it till I got over being nervous so I guess I shall stand it a few days longer. They give all the sick 3 horns of whiskey a day. I guess they begin to find that having so many sick don't pay.[26]

Addiction to drugs, whether narcotics or alcohol, has been referred to as the "soldier's disease." Whether the stress of war causes drug addictions or uncovers and exacerbates pre-existing disease is open to question. (Studies of Vietnam War soldiers showed that 96 percent of drug- or alcohol-addicted soldiers were so afflicted *prior* to entering the army.) The motto "Help yourself and God will help you" represents the bootstrap approach towards the self-destructive behavior of alcoholism. Support services for the mind and soul of patients played an important role and comprise some of the material found in the hospital newspaper.

Lessons from previous wars often need to be relearned as the key issues remain the same. In the Crimean War of 1853, eighty percent of the deaths were from medical diseases rather than battle wounds, whereas the ratio of medical to traumatic deaths was two to one in this conflict. Leading the hit parade then were diarrhea and dysentery, followed by cholera, typhoid fever, malaria, typhus, pneumonia, and scurvy. Had they continued without major changes, the armies on both sides would have been totally wiped out just from disease. The efforts of Florence Nightingale and the British army to implement basic sanitary practices were reported internationally.[27]

In 1861 the United States Sanitary Commission published *Rules for Preserving the Health of the Soldier* as a guide for all Union soldiers.[28] All soldiers, without exception, if ordered, should be vaccinated for smallpox. Whether in camp or barracks, officers must inspect kitchen and kettles daily. "There is no more frequent source of disease, in camp life, than in-attention to the calls of nature," it said. Trenches and privies were to be built away from camp and covered with lime and dirt. Sleeping upon the damp ground was considered a cause of dysentery. Fevers could be prevented by using rubberized blankets, straw or hay. Underclothing should be washed and thoroughly dried once a week and soldiers the same. As for the feet, a daily bath would do.[29]

In his concise military surgery handbook of 1861, Dr. Samuel Gross recommended avoiding "badly kept sinks and its contagion," isolating the sick, providing good ventilation, maintaining bodily cleanliness, avoiding crowding, procuring fresh vegetables, and offering "careful and tender nursing." As for heroic medicines, he cautioned that "more men have been killed in this manner in the armies and navies of the world than by the sword and the cannon. Let medicines be used sparingly. Let the secretions be well seen to; but purge little, and use depressants with all possible wariness. Support with quinine grains three to five daily.[30]

For the army, field sanitation and hygiene were based on physical and chemical concepts of cleanliness. Camps were inspected for health measures by field officers and doctors alike. Some camps were neat but disease-ridden, as large numbers of susceptible men were thrown together, aggravated by fleas, flies, lice, mosquitoes, poor personal hygiene and improper camp sanitation. Contaminated food sources, malnutrition and preexisting disease compounded the problems.

Carrying heavy equipment on long marches was thought to be a cause of deformity of the chest and hypertrophy of the heart which contributed to various camp diseases. Another theorem held the pressure of the belt loaded with a full cartridge box injured the stomach and liver, causing functional derangement of these organs. Morbid states, scorbutic taint, malaria, lowered vitality of the blood, and special cachexia all contributed to diminished resistance to disease and delayed or prevented healing, which in turn allowed the spread of infection. Moral causes of disease such as cowardice, malingering, homesickness, mania, and melancholia were also considered factors affecting the physical stamina of the soldier. Gross wrote:

> Some derangement of the health in the man preceded the mental phenomena. According to my observation deranged sexual functions were more frequently precedent to the mental changes than any other single physical condition. Masturbation and spermatorrhea produced a mental state more favorable to nostalgia than any other cause. A cure can only be wrought by sending the patient to his home.[31]

Young men and those married and middle-aged who were given to these solitary vices were risking dementia, imbecility, feebleness and even death! Performing these ruinous acts was grounds for discharge but not exemption to serve. Of course, providing evidence in front of a consenting witness might prove awkward.

The admixture of farm boys not exposed to the infectious diseases found in crowded cities encouraged spread of disease. The consequences of exposing large numbers of men with no prior immunity were illustrated in letters from twenty-one-year-old farm laborer Oliver Case of the Eighth Connecticut Volunteer Regiment to his sister while on the schooner *Recruit*. Upper respiratory infections, measles, typhoid fever, cholera and a host of other infections spread quickly.

> 3 Jan 1862
> There are all kinds of cough here from the common cold cough to the consumptive and from the whooping cough to the crazy hack. It is amusing to be awake and here [*sic*] the different kinds of hack and to count them.[32]

He was killed at Antietam eight months later.

In his manual for field medical officers, Dr. Tripler wrote, "The water men drink is of great consequence, and should be selected with as much care as possible. Certain kinds of water seem to cause diarrhea. If so then boil it." As for disease in general, he surmised that the etiology might be self-inflicted: "Poor blankets, swampy locations for camps, heavy details of labor in the field, picket duty, and the citizen soldier's ignorance," were the five primary causes of disease. The greatest amount of sickness resulted from the laziness and stupidity of officers, for theirs was the power to check "bad cooking, bad police, bad ventilation of tents, inattention to personal cleanliness, and unnecessarily irregular habits."[33]

Flannel cloth was used to treat abdominal pain, diarrhea, and even appendicitis as late as the twentieth century. The comfort of a heating pad in alleviating pain has long been observed. The heat might be from a hot water bottle, a skin irritant such as mustard plaster or turpentine, or an old-fashioned blanket warmer with coals. This New Haven newspaper ad of 1862 appeals to the average soldier who was bound to have suffered at some point with abdominal pain and diarrhea.

A STARTLING FACT!
HIGHLY IMPORTANT TO SOLDIERS
Statistics show (and figures can-not lie) that four times as many men die from sickness contracted in camp as are killed in battle. Bowel complaint, malaria, dysentery and diarrhea are

the great scourges of a soldier's life. Dr. D. Evans Medicated Flannel Abdominal Supporter is the great safeguard against camp sickness, and should be worn by all persons exposed to malarias disease. As a health protector it has proved itself the best invention of the war." Its peculiar effects are to give strength and vigor to drooping muscular action and protect the system against colds, dysentery, and diarrhea. They are a vast improvement over the homemade belts. The highest medical and scientific authorities endorse them.[34]

In 1866 Fred Dibble won the Jewett Award for his presentation at the Connecticut Medical Society (CMS) meeting entitled "Hygienic Teachings of the Late War."[35] This was based on two tours of duty over four years as a regimental surgeon, tempered by a Yale education and applied understanding of sanitary laws of the day. He begins his presentation by asserting that "by 1861 the greater part of the literature was altogether worthless, not to say ridiculous." He supported the teachings of Dr. Benjamin Rush that "those officers and soldiers who wore flannel shirts and waistcoats were less liable to disease than those who did not take this precaution." Dibble understood that thirsty soldiers will drink anything regardless of color, smell, or consistency as long as it is wet. Diarrhea, dysentery, typhoid, and cholera could flourish as water purification meant removing sticks, stones, and other visible objects sometimes with a canvas bag as a gross filter. If you could see through it, the water was considered drinkable. If you could not see through it, it was down the hatch just the same. The ninety-two-year-old granddaughter of Private Benjamin Ross of the 15th Connecticut Volunteers recollected remarks about his evening drink from the nearby stream. "It would be our ration of meat also, as the water was full of pollywogs [frogs]."[36]

Dietary deficiencies such as scurvy prevented wound healing. Many of the substitutes used for prevention, such as dried potatoes or potash, were ineffective remedies. Getting fresh fruits and vegetables during active campaigning was difficult to impossible.

> The lack of proper foods was thought to be the cause of debility of the digestive organs, the scorbutic cachexia [scurvy] and diarrhea in particular. Those troops near supply stations lacked these diseases. Those troops called on for hard fighting and hard digging with severe picket duty and far from base with diminished ration suffered mostly from this malady.[37]

Dibble declared "pure air dilutes, dispels and destroys in some ways the virulence of the contagious principle and there is no disinfectant, no deodorizer, which can be compared to it in efficiency." Sunlight would be the sword to vanquish the deadly poisons of typhoid and malaria. Soldiers in open-air medical facilities seemed to fare better than those in tents. The latter did better than those in barns who fared better than those in fixed buildings. Soldiers on the move seemed healthier than those in fixed installations. The physical environment was considered critical and controlling it would lessen disease.

Following sanitary laws and these hygienic teachings "would render the taking of medicine, either for the cure or prophylaxis of disease, entirely unnecessary." "Men who came into the hospitals with pleurisy and rheumatism soon lost the types of original disease and suffered or died by fevers. Hospitals are the sinks of human life in an army and should war continue to be the absurd and unchristian mode of settling national disputes, it is hoped that it will produce an abolition of hospitals for acute diseases." Hospital-acquired infections and the pestilence of war were a nettlesome fact of life. Blaming the hospital for its contents, namely terribly ill patients, repellent, stifling odors, and moans and shrieks of suffering, is blaming tigers for their stripes. Transmitting infection from patient to patient in the absence of modern sterile techniques was endemic for the times. That the "animalcules" seen under the microscope for two hundred years were bacteria, fungi and other living organisms came to light post war with the germ theory of infection. Effective remedies were many years away.

Dr. Dibble could say with pride that he served in the "army best fed, best clothed and best cared for in every respect of any that ever took the field against an enemy." This was a time when the government was considered "benevolent and not ruled by economics but by what was best."

CHAPTER TWO

The Early Lives of Pliny Adams Jewett and Jonathan Knight

Dr. Jonathan Knight was part of the original faculty of the Medical Institution of Yale College. He taught anatomy and then surgery over half a century.[1] He came from distinguished roots as both of his grandfathers were medical doctors. His father was regimental surgeon under Colonel Durkee of Norwich, Connecticut, and served at Valley Forge under George Washington during America's darkest hours, continuing through 1780. His mother was Ann Fitch, the daughter of Dr. Asabel Fitch of Redding, Connecticut. He was born 1789 in Norwalk and initially was educated at home. The local pastor provided advanced study in preparation for college, which was customary for young men trying to advance in society, and focused on religious studies, bible and catechism. Following admission to Yale College at age fifteen, his studies began with Dr. Nathan Smith, the first professor of surgery at Yale, and Dr. Sillman in chemistry. His mentors encouraged further study in anatomy and medical botany, which entailed sessions at the University of Pennsylvania, thus exposing him to some of America's finest doctors of the period, including Benjamin Rush of Philadelphia.

After four years of study he returned to New Haven and the practice of physic and surgery. As professor of anatomy in the new medical school, he would deliver lectures for a quarter century and continue teaching medical students until his death fifty-two years later. As a budding surgeon, Knight was well served by this lab work, which gave him invaluable dissecting experience and a profound knowledge of anatomy that others lacked. He allowed his students to pay fees in part, with the remainder to be paid in the indeterminate future. He was known for his generosity both financial and personal. He advanced matriculation and tuition fees, a practice that offered good will to young medical students, many of whom stayed in Connecticut and provided a referral base for his growing surgical practice. His work was statewide and consultation often required traveling to outlying towns. He married Elizabeth Lockwood, the daughter of James Lockwood, a graduate of

Yale (1766), but had no children. In 1838 following the death of his predecessor Dr. Thomas Hubbard, he became Yale's second professor of surgery, a position he held until his death in 1864. He was not an originator and published few papers. His treatment of a case of popliteal aneurysm (ballooning of the artery behind the knee, which can be limb threatening) seemed unique. He had relays of students compress the artery for forty continuous hours. The treatment may have worked, as the patient survived with no clinically apparent aneurysm on follow-up. His colleagues referred to him as "the beloved physician." His experience and knowledge was exceptional and seasoned with justified modesty, considering the reality of treatment outcomes in the nineteenth century. He read widely, had a uniquely large library and used this material for his lectures. When a visitor entered his classroom Knight might sit down, more than willing to listen to another professional discuss the subject at hand, and allow the guest the honor and attention of the audience. He was not bold, authoritative, imposing or inspirational but was considered "a finished and effective lecturer having a handsome appearance and a finished diction."[2] Perhaps more telling are the traits he found exemplary in other surgeons that others saw in him: "For the performance of surgical operations he was peculiarly fitted as he had a mind that was never flustered or disconcerted and a hand that never trembled during any operation. He had a happy dexterity in the use of instruments which gave him the power of operating with great accuracy, neatness and rapidity. He amputated the thigh in forty seconds."[3]

After Nathan Smith he was considered the foremost surgeon in Connecticut until his death. Dr. Knight was described as thoughtful, gentlemanly and experienced. "In all that time he never did an unnecessary or premature operation. His surgery was described as showing "conscientious attention to every detail. Surgery was well considered, guided by thorough anatomical knowledge and special dexterity or nimbleness of manipulation." On one occasion, he had arrived in the operating theater and was greeted by an unexpected crowd who had come to see the exalted professor at work. He declined to perform for the public and returned the next day to perform the surgery without an audience.[4]

He was the first president of the American Medical Association and continued on for a second term because "of the admirable way in which he at its first meeting guided the somewhat unwieldy body on its way."[5] Until his death he was president of the Connecticut Hospital Society, an organization combining the resources of both Yale College and the Connecticut Medical Society. This led to building the New Haven Hospital that was later renamed Knight Army General Hospital. The secretary of the Connecticut Hospital Society was Dr. E. H. Bishop, who left his post in 1847. Knight

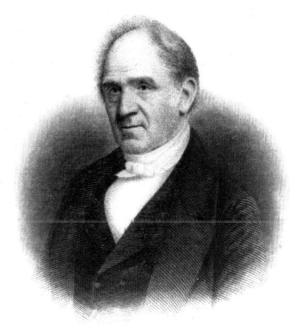

Jonathan Knight, M.D., 1789–1864, Yale College Professor of Anatomy and Physiology, 1814–38, Professor of Surgery 1838–64, Department of Medicine Yale College (circa 1860s) (author's collection).

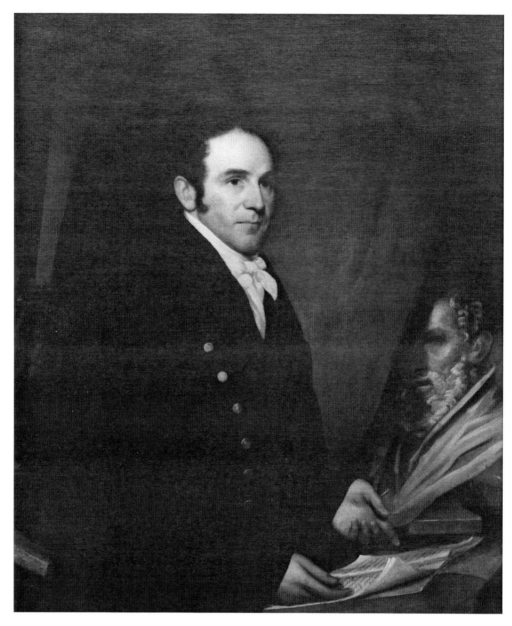

Jonathan Knight, M.D., oil on canvas, 112.4 × 39.5 cm by Nathaniel Jocelyn, 1827 (courtesy Yale University Art Gallery, gift of the Medical Class of 1828 to the School of Medicine).

filled it with his junior partner and protégé Pliny Jewett. He was also president and medical examiner of the American Mutual Life Insurance Company and board member and incorporator of Townsend Savings Bank of New Haven.[6]

Knight was a man with multiple revenue sources, including banking, insurance companies, private practice, and university duties. By 1833 he was receiving $125 a year and in 1837 $200 yearly for his teaching services, which included anatomy dissections. His annual income in 1817 was $789; in 1825 $1,743; and in 1859 $3,613. By the 1850s, the average doctor earned less than $500 annually. Political acuity and financial acumen are traits not always found in doctors. The senior surgeon was well placed in society, well-heeled, and both he and the institution he represented stood to benefit.

The Yale library has early issues of the *Medical and Surgical Reporter*, which bear his signature as original owner. His lectures reflected medical thinking of the day. Burns were treated by excluding air. Animal or vegetable oil, molasses, soft soap, gum Arabic, wet cloths, and limewater were used as wound covers. Indolent ulcers were treated with corrosive sublimate (a potent mercurial compound), silver nitrate, nitric, or sulfuric acid. Venereal ulcerations also received the strongest acid solutions or mercurial ointments.[7] A fingertip abscess was treated by "plunging the finger into hot lye, as strong and hot as can be born [*sic*]. Vessication [blistering] was needed. Soak finger in alkali and scrape cuticle off. Narcotic and poultices are helpful." For chronic wounds, he recommended friction, cantharides, a splint, and bandages.

The prodigal son he mentored was equally talented, though less reserved and a more imposing figure. At six feet and 230 pounds, outspoken and certain of his views, Pliny Adams Jewett, MD, made an indelible impression. Autocratic, self-assured, and at times explosive, he was not one who tolerated fools gladly, and not a polished politician was he. For most of his life, there was no need to compromise.[8] He was the son of a well-heeled Episcopal minister with a promising professional career his for the asking.

The Jewetts were English, arriving from Yorkshire in 1638, and settling in Rowley, Massachusetts. The original Joseph Jewett became a large landowner, and the family grew, prospered, and dispersed across New England, one serving as a sergeant in the Revolutionary War and another in the War of 1812.[9]

Stephen Jewett, Pliny's father, was born in 1783 in the town of Lanesboro in the Berkshire Mountains of Massachusetts. He was fond of reading and taught himself the rudiments of an English education. His parents were Congregationalists and he was a student at the Episcopal Academy in Cheshire for four years. Then he taught in Dalton, Massachusetts, preparing young men for college. He was ordained as an Episcopal minister in 1811 at Trinity Church in New Haven and became church rector in Hampton, New York, while still living in his parents' house. On one occasion, he traveled forty miles to attend a funeral, and on another, received a child who traveled 100 miles just to be baptized. He thus served as a "missionary" for over eighty communicants. He married Elizabeth Backus of

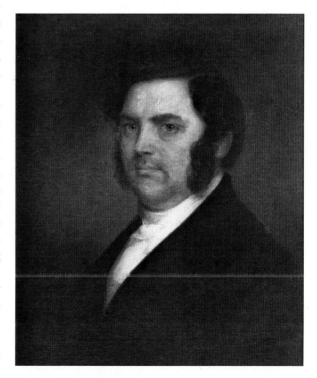

Pliny Adams Jewett, M.D., 1816–84. Chief of Staff, Knight U.S. Army General Hospital, artist unknown, circa 1840–1850, oil on canvas, 38.1 × 30.5 cm (courtesy Yale University Art Gallery, gift of Dr. Charles A. Lindsley to the School of Medicine).

Norwich, Connecticut, in September 1813 and assumed the rectorship at St. James Church in Derby, Connecticut, in 1821. His salary was $500 per year plus firewood. Along with his church duties he conducted a private prep school, a job for which he had previous experience.[10]

The Reverend Jewett had three sons. The first was Thomas Backus Jewett, born in 1814. Pliny Adams Jewett was born in 1816, and the third, Henry Hatch Jewett, in 1821. All married and had children. The joy of having three healthy sons was magnified with a fourth blessing, another great delivery from his wife Elizabeth in the form of her wealthy brother's bequest. If the truth be known, the Jewett family was not well off until this considerate brother-in-law's sudden death left a learned but financially challenged minister in clover. Since a woman could not own property or vote, all monies were deposited under her husband's name. The Jewetts waved farewell to the small but faithful congregation on the border of New York and Connecticut and moved back to New Haven, where Jewett had been ordained. He was retired until his death forty-three years later. He elected to forgo the final two years of salary in Derby and gave the largest single gift that Trinity College had ever received. He also paid off half the debt of Trinity Church with another gift and served thereafter in a voluntary capacity.[11]

The Jewetts were thus nouveau riche and sharing the wealth. Years later, at Jewett's funeral, the Reverend E. Beardsley described the "feeble health, excessive nervous debility and many infirmities" that limited the working life of the Reverend Jewett. His life seemed filled with reading and philanthropic concerns rather than stocks, bonds, or other investments that might have added to the family fortune. The accumulation of wealth did not interest or occupy his time. He was described as "frank, and outspoken in his opinions." He lacked patience for any "Jesuitical, Romanizing influence, or departure from old scriptural lines."[12]

He seemed grateful to be able to retire from gainful employment so early in life, and thus aid the work of his Almighty. Fixed in his ways and beliefs, he "forgot nobody or anything." "The Reverend Stephen Jewett is reputed to have been something of an autocrat in his profession, holding sway over the then feeble parishes of the lower Naugatuck valley. The son seems to have inherited somewhat of his father's disposition." His strongly held manners and codes of behavior would be passed on to his son Pliny.[13] He died in 1861 at age seventy-eight.

Duty to country was not new to this family. A man grounded in such solid foundations would not be easily swayed or compromised. Education, religious teachings, and family traditions were their pillars. The Reverend Jewett was a member of the Trinity University Board from 1836 through 1861. Pliny graduated from Trinity in 1837 and from the Medical Institution of Yale College in 1839. From the beginning, his excellence in scholarship was magnified by personal attributes of hard work, intellectual curiosity, and honesty.

Dr. Jewett's strength lay not in his pen but in his surgical sword. His skill in use of the blade proved far more influential than his writings. He wrote few medical papers, but each was to the point, modest in tone, and clear-headed. This surgeon was able to declare "I do not know," a trait not often seen in those with authority and quite praiseworthy for any physician, particularly for a surgeon in a teaching position. It requires broad knowledge and background, honesty and confidence.

His graduation thesis, "Contraction of the Chest Consequent to Pleurisy," was on a complex and difficult subject in an era before X-ray, pulmonary physiology, or discovery of the tubercle bacillus. His presentation occurred in September 1839 before a committee of experienced physicians in a public ritual reported in a New Haven newspaper: "Examination in the Medical Institution of Yale College."[14] He starts out by declaring nothing was known. "The anatomical characters of this deformity have, until quite recently, been but little understood: indeed we find nothing of any account written upon the subject, or any attempt at an explanation of the anatomical changes which had taken place to produce it until the time of Laennec."[15]

Jewett separates the acute from the chronic forms of pleurisy and discusses the different types of serum that might account for contracture: thin serous versus the thick "fibro-cartilaginous or semi concrete" variety. He differentiates between true membranes versus false, secondary to a process called "inflammation." The contraction is owing to the formation of the "false membrane," the consequent adhesion of the opposite surfaces of the pleura, and finally the effusion of serum. One side is stuck down and the other is lubricated, so with growth a curve develops regardless of painful, unnecessary and ineffective "medical" bracing. "Many persons, laboring under this affection have without doubt been induced to allow their bodies to be encased in machinery and to undergo useless torture and expense, which might have been avoided by a proper knowledge of the difficulty."[16]

Atelectasis, or lung collapse, is common with tuberculosis (pulmonary phthisis). Authorities believed (incorrectly) that acute pleurisy was not caused by tuberculosis and that chronic pleurisy did not become tubercular.[17] Jewett surmised correctly that pneumonia and atelectasis coexist with phthisis. He admits being stumped as to why, in the absence of paralysis, contracture still appears, and concludes, "As I am unable to find anything written on the subject, I shall be content to leave it for the present, trusting that at some subsequent period a wiser and a clearer head may be induced to take the matter into consideration, and offer some solution of the difficulty."

In the nineteenth century, the centers of medical education were in Europe. Children of the wealthy were sent to Paris, Edinburgh, and London for the best education available. Pliny Jewett spent two years traveling the Continent and learning from the best medical and surgical minds of the day. In Paris at La Charité hospital was the remarkable head of medicine Professor Louis. Tall, elegant, soft-spoken, and enormously popular with patients, students and colleagues, he approached all with the same caring manner. He had done extensive research on the causes of tuberculosis, abandoning his private practice "at an age when physicians in general cease their attendance at hospitals, and forego the collecting of cases in order to devote them-selves exclusively to practice."[18] From 1821 through 1832 he evaluated each of the 1,960 patients admitted to his hospital, of which 358 died and of those 123 from phthisis. His collection of observations at bedside and correlation with anatomical autopsy was reported to the Royal Academy of Medicine and then published in book form.

He specifically looked at the effects of climate, dress, occupation, heredity, poverty, bad food, exposure to animal emanations, dust, age, wet or dry atmosphere, sedentary versus active lifestyles and could find no correlations with the disease.

As for the efficacy of various treatments, he could show no scientific evidence any worked. This included venesection (bleeding), leeches, changing environment, counter-irritation, tartar emetic, mercurial compounds, digitalis, prussic acid, iodine, and quinine. Despite these findings, the standard thinking on this subject continued as restated dogma. The book's translator agreed, noting, "On no subject has more been written or less satisfactory information obtained. It is better to admit ignorance than excite unnecessary fears and give useless if not dangerous advice." According to this new wave of medical thinking, considered opinions based on repetition, superstition, prejudice and authority should be replaced by truth and facts determined by research. Today we call this evidence-based medicine.

Laennec, a friend and colleague, had discovered the use of the stethoscope, allowing specific evaluations of lung and heart ailments. Professor Louis became an expert, spending hours performing bedside auscultation and trying to correlate this with anatomic studies from autopsy. He gathered numerous statistics and combined them with rigorous observation to elicit the truth and called this the Numerical Method. Deduction after analyzing symptoms, pathology and effects of drugs was his technique. Blistering and bloodletting were rejected as useless and probably harmful. The laws of nature were not invented by man but only discovered to work with nature rather than against it. A legion of American doctors returned home from Paris with enthusiasm, faith in the future and the profession, along with a new method of scientific exploration and respect for the truth.[19]

Tuberculosis was the leading cause of death in Connecticut and medical discharge from the army during the war. A summary of this disease was reported in the Yale Medical School graduation thesis of Samuel Wheat in 1858. Heredity played a factor. The typical patient had a long neck, prominent shoulders, narrow and flat chest, light hair, and delicate complexion. Exposure to cold was the most frequent exciting cause. Alternative causes were temperature and climate change, dust, tight corsets, occupations such as tailor, contaminated air, stoppage of menses, and chronic digestive organ disease. He accurately describes the signs and symptoms as well as the pathological findings seen in the lungs. The "tubercle was a morbid deposit, of gray or yellow cheesy material, [which] often forms cavities, with lymph fluid deposits." The treatment was to improve nutrition. Animal diet would invigorate the system: cod liver oil would enhance the appetite and evacuate undigested animal food in the stomach and thus run the bowel. Tonics such as iron, quinine, and alcohol were recommended to stimulate a depleted system. Narcotics and hycosomines worked as cough suppressants. The use of calcium magnesia and ammonia (Pepto-Bismol) to calm the stomach was recommended only early in the disease. Fresh air, away from the congested cities and towns, perhaps in the mountains, preferably in another state, was essential. This recommendation is known as "getting a bad case out of town before it further damages the reputations of those who are treating it." All of these treatments had been studied by Professor Louis and found ineffective.

Paget and other pathologists of the period were undecided as to whether tuberculosis and cancer were the same or two different entities. He correctly believed that tuberculosis granulomas were unique and tumor-like but not the same as a malignancy. Others believed it was a "seat of inflammation."

Shotgun therapy (essentially wishful thinking) prevailed, depending on the spectrum of symptoms and their intensity. Moving to a better climate was popular but not possible for most. For the army it was cod liver oil, whiskey half an ounce three times daily, and the usual tonics, including iron and quinine or cinchona bark. For hemoptysis (coughing blood), extract of hellebore, dilute sulphuric acid or persulphate of iron were used. Cupping, blistering and botanical preparations were other therapeutic possibilities.[20] Medical botanists weighed in with red raspberry leaves, agrimony, barberry bark, clovers, ground ivy, horehound, and cayenne pepper as a tea.

Samuel Morton's text listed thirty-two different treatments, including diet and exercise, which included daily and long horseback rides or carriages over rough roads. For a lung abscess a sea voyage was recommended, probably one way. For hemoptysis, bleeding up to twelve ounces taken rapidly from a large vein to decrease congestion in the lung was prescribed. For cough there was morphine. For ulcerated upper respiratory organs, iodine or sarsaparilla. Fumigation and inhalation was consummated by burning tar, resin, myrrh and other substances in chambers of the sick. For inhalation, vapor of ether saturated with coca leaves. Dressing warmly was essential, especially for the children, with flannel to the neck and furs for the feet.[21]

The Hartford Medical Society meeting of June 1860 discussed this disease as being usually but not always fatal. Treatment must be started early to be effective. Some were for exercise and alcohol and some not. Change of locale and occupation were beneficial. Some used cod liver oil and no other medications. Some used a host of drugs. Because the disease was considered contagious it was "exceedingly imprudent for a person suffering from it to sleep with any other person." Hereditary predisposition and intermarriage in rural areas accounted for the disease rates being the same as the city despite the fresh air.

Carl Ives of New Haven reported to the Connecticut State Medical Society (CSMS) in 1866 on prophylaxis of phthisis pulmonalis. He pointed out that one in seven deaths in Connecticut for the years 1863 through 1865 was from tuberculosis and concluded that "nearly all these might have been saved. Proper watchfulness, care and management, would have warded off the malady in the vast majority of these cases, for there is scarce a disease whose prevention is so much in our power as this. Prophylaxis resolves one simple rule: raise the physical condition of the whole system to the highest vigor possible." The disease was curable with deep breathing, gymnastics for weak lungs, pure fresh air, long, continued horseback riding, nutritious diet, clean skin, outdoor cold sponge baths even in winter, woolen clothing next to skin, no alcohol, and no excesses of any kind. Lack of education and training was the cause, not heredity. With complete physical training and full development of every part of the body, health would triumph over disease.[22]

Others also believed the disease was treatable with basic sanitary laws and fresh air.[23] The "White Death," along with other infectious diseases, was among the worries of many, including departing soldiers susceptible to a sales pitch offering medical certainty and safety at a low, low price. Thank heaven Dr. Trues came to the rescue, at least according to this ad in the *Palladium* from November 1864.

> THE GREAT CONSUMPTIVE REMEDY
> The lord hath created Medicines out of the
> Earth and he that are wise will not abhor them.
> With such doeth life heal men and take away
> Their pain
>
> DR. TRUES
> Tis one, cures all diseases of the Lungs, Throat,
> And Chest, Croup and Whooping Cough
> This syrup acts at the secretion to work in a natural
> Way. It acts particularly on the lungs, reduces
> Inflammation, restores healthy action, and produces
> Free and easy expectorations. All coughs benefited
> By it. Consumption cured when taken in season.[24]

In Paris reigned the greatest surgeon of the era, Guillaume Dupuytren, at the thousand-bed hospital D'hôtel Dieu. He combined a difficult personality with an unattractive physical appearance and was described by a colleague as "the first of surgeons and the least of men." He lived in the suburbs and walked to work each morning, leaving home at 4:30 A.M.

Patient rounds started at 5 A.M. After running clinics for the poor and performing their surgery, Dupuytren spent the afternoon with his private patients, who came from all over Europe, such was his fame. He had saved the life of a Rothschild, and for years afterward benefited mightily from the family's investing advice, which afforded him economic independence. Many in high places expressed gratitude for his services rendered to lower and upper classes alike, a popular sentiment that would help insulate him from political conflicts in the future. He left a significant volume of medical writings and is still remembered today for the hand contracture and ankle fracture, both of which bear his name.[25] Each morning young Pliny Jewett awaited the great professor.

Jewett's professors at Yale were Drs. Benjamin Silliman, Eli Ives, William Tully, Timothy Beers, Charles Hooker, and Jonathan Knight. Each was prominent and influential in his respective area. Jewett graduated from medical school in 1840 and, following his European experience, joined Dr. Knight as his junior partner while boarding with his parents. On November 10, 1847, he married twenty-year-old Juliet Mitchell Carrington of Bristol, Connecticut, whose father and brother were apothecaries. Their marriage produced three children. Thomas Backus (the namesake of Pliny Jewett's older brother) was born in 1851 and would later graduate from Yale Medical School. His sister Mary (born 1857) later moved to Montana. The third child William (born 1861) became an architect.

Pliny's younger brother Henry and his wife died in 1849 and 1850, respectively, leaving their daughter Elizabeth and son — also named Pliny Adams Jewett — to be raised by the surviving members of the Jewett clan. The Jewett house was a two-story white wooden building, large enough to accommodate the family and two Irish servants. Twenty-three-year-old Mary McCusker was born in Connecticut of parents from Ireland and thirty-year-old Kate O'Neil was born in Ireland.[26] His mother continued living there, the father having died in 1861.

By 1841, Dr. Jewett had become a fellow of the Connecticut Medical Society (CMS), and three years later he became a representative of New Haven County for both state and national medical conferences. Shortly thereafter he became secretary of New Haven Hospital, which, alongside the Connecticut Retreat for the Insane in Hartford, was the only hospital in the state. The state hospital was a creature of both the CSMS and Yale College under the auspices of the state government. By 1850, he added the Committee of Honorary Degrees and membership in the New York State Medical Society to his growing list of credits. Dr. Knight was then sixty-one years of age. Young Jewett was his right-hand man, assisting him on virtually all his surgery. Knight would not tackle any difficult case without the presence of his junior assistant.

In the summer of 1850, an epidemic of dysentery struck West Haven. Entire families were sickened and the disease was restricted to a specific neighborhood. The symptoms were bloody, frequent, often painful episodes of diarrhea with fever. Distinguishing one cause of diarrhea from another was neither possible nor even a consideration in those days, and the term was both symptom and diagnosis. Treatment was on even murkier grounds. Jewett tried the standard remedy of both mercury and opium, but with little success:

> Whether the dysentery was checked or not in a few days, collapse would set in with rice water evacuations and death soon following, in the large proportion of cases. In the territory named not one family escaped and in many instances whole families were down with the disease. There was not a single case in any other portion of West Haven. The disease prevailed to such an extent that there were not others well enough to take care of the sick. I sent relays of medical students over to act as nurses. At last I called in one of the clergymen and stated the case

to him. This way late in the week on Sunday he preached to his flock, and by Monday, I had more nurses than I could employ. I did not hear the sermon; but judging from the effect, I have no doubt he said something that touched their pride or their hearts.[27]

The epidemic ran from July through August and then ceased for want of more victims. In many epidemics, those with financial resources left the scene with family in tow. Doctors who stayed did so at great personal risk. Cholera epidemics are spread by contaminated water and result in a high mortality rate. The rice water evacuations described by Jewett are typical of that disease, but cholera was rarely seen in Connecticut and was not thought to be the culprit.

Regimental Surgeon Dibble wrote his medical school graduating paper on dysentery, declaring mucus and blood its hallmark. Most patients recovered, but some had ulcers that perforated with fatal consequences. Poor people in cities, as well as soldiers and sailors, were thought more susceptible due to deficiencies of pure air, water, food, or clothing, but it was thought that the disease was not contagious. The books of the time claimed "bleeding was favorable," but the clinical results did not support that conclusion. Remedies were many and equally ineffective.[28] Dysentery was the leading cause of death and the second leading cause of medical discharge from the army. One-fourth of all diseases reported in the Union army were in this category, amounting to 1,739,135 cases.

Regular Army Surgeon Tripler believed that epidemics of dysentery were "principally violations of the laws of hygiene. Remote causes are heat combined with moisture; immoderate and indiscriminate use of fruits, abuse of spirituous liquors; exposure to currents of wind, and night dews. The soldier tends to strip off his shirt and sleep in bare chest and legs which is prejudicial to the health. I believe it to be the exciting cause of a great many of these cases of camp dysentery."[29] Others wrote that sleeping outdoors was actually beneficial for the soldier.

Blaming patients for their diseases is a common theme in medical history. The poor and indigent suffer from disease because they are lazy, ignorant, dirty, immoral and blasphemous. Proclamations from the pulpit offer self-fulfilling prophecies: Failure to follow the teachings of the scriptures can lead to wrath from on high as punishment for sins. The newest immigrant classes were especially blamed for their disease. The notion that poverty, crowding, contaminated water, and malnutrition were the real culprits was not then generally accepted.

Medical Inspector Vollum expressed his views on the causes of diarrhea and dysentery in the six-volume opus the *Medical and Surgical History of the War of the Rebellion (MSHWR)*: "Quinine, fresh vegetables, and fruits relieve many cases and seem to point to a constitutional condition on which disease may be based. The frying pan causes the disease frequently and many cases are attributable to green fruits and stale hard bread." Scurvy was considered another cause, its curability and prevention with fresh fruits known by the British navy for many years. The existence of vitamin and other nutritional deficiencies were unknown.

The army's treatment was emetics and purgatives to rid the body of impurities and deplete excessive tone. Dr. E. Cowles took a week-long written and oral exam for admission as assistant surgeon in the regular army administered under the auspices of the surgeon general's office in Philadelphia in 1863. Among the many questions was one on the treatment of dysentery. His written answer to a panel of regular army doctors was "apply leeches to anus, use ice water injections and castor oil." He passed the exam but how his patients responded to his treatment is doubtful.

From the records of monthly meetings of the Hartford Medical Society, we know that for "pure dysentery," calomel and opium were the drugs of choice in 1864. A thirty-five-year-old male was thus treated and due to failure to improve received quinine, castor oil, Dover's powder, and lead acetate, but the outcome was not reported. When things do not go well, the contents of the kitchen sink may be thrown into the fray. This is called the shotgun approach, or polypharmacy, where wishful thinking endeavors to overcome reality. Some have observed that when a sick person appears to be dying, the physician uses the most doubtful and dangerous medicines. Desperate times call for desperate measures.

In 1854 Dr. Jewett was appointed to fill a vacancy on the committee to nominate a physician for the Retreat for the Insane. This was the first psychiatric hospital in the United States to use humane treatment instead of chaining patients under lock and key in a cellar or prison facility. In 1856 he was appointed professor of obstetrics of Yale School of Medicine. His predecessor Dr. Beers had begun his career with Dr. Knight and retired. He was the uncle of the young man destined to become Jewett's junior partner, Timothy Beers Townsend.

In 1857, he was placed on the Committee on Publications along with Gurdon Russell, a prominent Hartford doctor with whom he served on other committees and who would contribute mightily in the war years in selecting regimental surgeons for Connecticut. By 1861 Dr. Pliny Jewett was on a career path to the most prestigious medical job in New England, the Chief of Surgery at Yale College. He held a number of administrative posts in the Connecticut Medical Society and was secretary of New Haven Hospital from 1844 through 1864. But what is past is not always prologue.

CHAPTER THREE

Dr. Timothy Beers Townsend

By 1860 Dr. Knight was seventy years old and doing little surgery, leaving that to his protégé. Jewett needed his own assistant, as surgical practice required being on duty every day and at all hours. He too was becoming longer in tooth, shorter in stamina, and his heavy frame less buoyant in step.

Timothy Beers Townsend was the sixth of eight children. His father, William Kneeland Townsend, was born 1796 in New Haven. His Anglo-Saxon ancestor, Thomas Townsend, landed in Lynn, Massachusetts, in the late sixteenth century. The father of this budding physician was the director of a New Haven bank, president of other businesses, a lieutenant in the Governor's Horse Guard, and a state representative. In 1820 he married Elizabeth Ann Mulford, a society figure with old family roots who lived to be eighty-two.[1] Timothy Townsend retired due to ill health in 1830 at age thirty-four and died 1849 at age fifty-three.

Timothy Beers Townsend, known as Beers, was born November 21, 1835, and attended Farmington English and Classical School for boys in 1847 and 1848. He then prepared for college at the General Russell Collegiate and Commercial Institute, and graduated from Yale Medical School in 1858 with his final thesis "On Indirect Inguinal Hernia." Like other offspring of a wealthy family, he was sent to Europe for medical finishing school, studying in London, Dublin, Edinburgh, and Paris. In Paris, he "acquired exceptionally fine equipment for his future career," a surgical instrument set with leather carrying case made by the finest French instrument maker of the era, Luér of Paris. Craftsmen who made cutlery or swords often ventured into the medical field, some specializing and innovating as a sideline. His was a top-of-the-line set with "T. B. Townsend" engraved in brass on the cover as well as on a neatly configured leather carrying case. In the case lay maroon velvet-lined boxes with exact fitting compartments for a wide variety of ebony-handled knives, long and short saws for the long and short bone, skull trephine, tourniquet, bone clamps, bone rongeur, bone brush, retractors, forceps, needles and cotton sutures. This was a fine assortment of instruments that any surgeon would be proud to own.[2]

Avoiding the risks of starting their own ventures, Townsend's five brothers entered the network of family businesses. Young Townsend chose the path of surgeon, a more challenging and sometimes life-consuming work, admirable in one born with the silver spoon. Townsend practiced medicine under the considerable wing of New Haven's leading surgeon, Pliny A. Jewett, becoming his junior partner in June of 1860. The accounts of this association were from its very beginnings meticulously recorded by young Townsend, who documented to the halfpenny their charges, expenses, and types of cases. The front page of their ledger book proclaims, "Pliny A. Jewett M.D. and T. B. Townsend associated themselves in the practice of surgery and medicine June 19, 1860." Their office was located in the Tontine Building, in the center of town, where, as Townsend put it, "they remained in the fear and service of God."

For any doctor, there is anxious concern about earning a living. Although he had the full support of New Haven's premier surgeon and his extensive, wealthy and influential family, his fears and self-doubt were not easily overcome. His brother James, who was twelve years older, was quite optimistic about his prospects.

> Dr. T. B. is doing splendidly. He has about all the practice he can attend to. His name has been in the newspapers a number of times in connection with accidents. Ellen Gibber has been ill and Beers attends her and has done well. Both Thomas and Ellen think he is the greatest doctor in the world. Beers introduced some new treatment which worked admirably. [The patient] had neuralgia in the head and had not slept for a number days and nights. Beers introduced some instrument under the scalp and injected some narcotic which relieved her almost immediately whereupon she went to sleep and awoke refreshed.[3]

Subcutaneous injections of morphine had been just introduced as treatment for various pain syndromes. As with many innovations, an initial burst of enthusiasm was followed by more restrictive use. Dr. Ben Catlin published an article in the *Proceedings of the Connecticut Medical Society* in 1861 entitled "Hypodermic Injections under Abdominal Skin." He injected one grain of acetate morphine dissolved in rainwater. This new treatment for pain was announced by this peer-review organization but no long-term results were available. Young Townsend seemed enthusiastic about this new procedure and billed for it over twenty times in the first few months following its description in the medical literature. He stopped billing for it because he stopped doing it. The public often clamors for the latest medication or procedure before it is proven beneficial. Greybeards of medicine have always admonished "Above all else do no harm" and "Don't be the first and don't be the last."

A young woman named A. Townsend, a distant cousin, was chronically and persistently in need of medical attention. Most of Beers' calls in November of 1860 and fifty-five of seventy-four calls in December of 1860 were on her account. He was charging $1 per house visit while Dr. Jewett charged $2. In March of 1861, the lady in distress required visits every other day. In October of 1861, there were forty-five visits, and the following month twenty-one. So "ill" must she have been that the famous Dr. Jewett came twice. As other patients who were not friends or relatives began appearing in the new doctor's office, her visits began to disappear. She was cured, discouraged, or found another prospect.

Townsend's types of cases and their charges can be gathered from his records that begin on his first day in practice and continue through 1863. (See Appendix I.) At a time when soldier's pay was $13 a month, a routine office visit was $1, hip fracture $15, and visits for syphilis, buboes, or gonorrhea $2. For the last condition Hartford doctors charged $5, "always in advance." Only one ethnic group was described in his billings: "Irishman (clap)," "dressing Irishman's hand," "Bill Mitchells Irishman," and "John York's Irish girl."

The treatment of gonorrhea consisted of irrigating the urethra with a "penile syringe" filled with either silver nitrate or potassium permanganate over a period of sixty seconds.

The former made it turn black, the latter purple. Hot sitz baths could be used for the afflicted anatomy, as could leeches, hot water bottle to the pubic area, and warm saline enemas. Calomel (mercury) was the mainstay for the treatment of syphilis for centuries. This could be taken orally or as ointment applied to the skin lesions or ulcerations.[4] Fumigation with mercury in closed spaces was no longer in fashion. For the routine cases, rest in recumbent position, no sexual excitement, dim light, no alcohol or coffee, and testicular support was ideal. Bowels were opened with cathartic pills. For the more recalcitrant cases, the penis

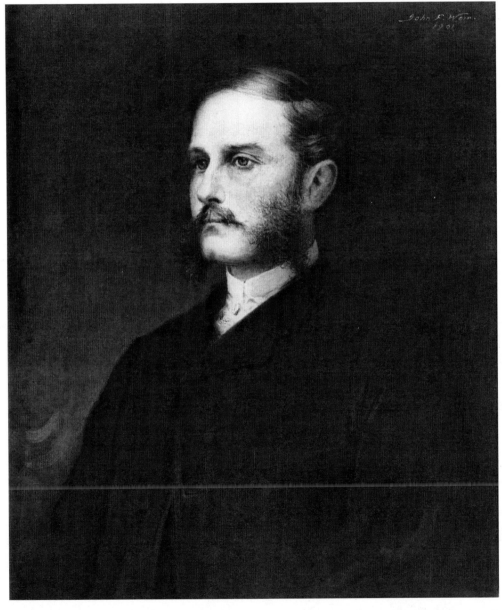

Timothy Beers Townsend, M.D., 1835–93. Junior partner of Pliny A. Jewett, 1860–62. Medical Staff, Knight U.S. Army General Hospital, by John Ferguson Weir, 1901, oil on canvas, 76.5 × 63.8 cm (courtesy Yale University Art Gallery, gift of the Townsend family to the School of Medicine).

was immersed several times daily in hot solution of lead and opium, then washed with hot saline and boric acid for 10 minutes each. It was felt this was done best by the surgeon.[5]

The rates of venereal disease were higher at the beginning and end of the war and especially in or near cities. The 109,397 cases of gonorrhea reported in the Union army amounted to 82 per thousand white troops. Syphilis, a more debilitating disease, numbered 73,382.

Assistant Surgeon R. Stratton of the 11th Illinois Cavalry reported in June 1862: "It was impossible to cure gonorrhea while the patients were exposed to the rain and had to sleep on the damp ground and live on a salt and stimulating ration."

Surgeon W. Blakeslee of the 115th Pennsylvania noted in October 1862: "Gonorrhea was greatly modified and in most cases completely subdued by injection of a solution of chlorate of potash, every hour for twelve hours and then gradually ceasing its use over three days. Rest and saline laxatives also were helpful."

Surgeon Isaac Galloupe of the 17th Massachusetts Volunteers noted in February 1863: "Syphilis and gonorrhea prevailed extensively in regiment during its stay in Baltimore. Rapid and complete recovery was secured in all cases treated as follows: inject weak solution of sulfate of zinc every hour and provide a light diet."[6]

For the soldier, marching with one's instrument stuck to the pants is at best inconvenient and at worst painful. The added urge to stop and void, which was a burning experience, rendered "claptrap" an ailment to be avoided. Medical texts of the period considered gonorrhea a mild disorder that "always heals without unfavorable symptoms." Primary heroic treatment of urethral discharges was considered a "most unjustifiable interference with nature." This was not the case. Urethral strictures and swollen testicles were often the long-term consequences. S. C. Gordon reminisced from a surgeon's point of view years later: "'Ladies fever' broke out and ran its course, leaving as a result strictures and bladder troubles from which many a poor fellow suffers to this day, with the only consolation that he can have a pension. Applicant is required only to state what he finds and the rate for it, not how or why it occurred."[7]

A systematized effort at prevention was instituted in Nashville and Memphis, Tennessee, "to rid city of diseased prostitutes infesting it." The police force placed on a steamer all women of the city publicly known to be of "vile" character and dispatched them to Louisville, Kentucky. Officials there refused to allow the ship to unload, and the boat elicited the same response from Cincinnati. The boat returned from whence it came where "the passengers resumed their former modes of life." Colonel Spalding suggested a system of licensing with frequent inspection for removal to hospital of those diseased. There were weekly medical exams, hospital care in a specialty facility if needed, a thirty-day jail term for those practicing without a license, and a weekly tax on the workers to defray expenses. The results were aptly described by Surgeon R. Fletcher in charge of the Female Venereal Hospital on August 15, 1864.

> We now have a support system that protects their health and delivers them from the extortion of quacks and charlatans. They gladly exhibit to their visitors the "certificate" when asked for which happens frequently as word spreads. Most of the hospital patients are voluntarily admitted as they expect to get disease and are not sent from the inspection room. When a soldier of the post force is infected it is not uncommon for his captain to report the case with the name of the suspected woman who is immediately arrested and examined.[8]

Townsend and Jewett's office expenses were ubiquitous but a necessary constant, as young Townsend meticulously recorded in July of 1862: plaster, forceps, splints, scissor and rent to the penny. Dr. Jewett now had an eager associate to assist him in surgery and perform the necessary menial chores, just as he had for Dr. Knight. The apprentice system provided on-the-job training for which no textbook can substitute. Both men stood to benefit from this relationship.

By June 1862, the partnership was over because Dr. Jewett gave up his practice to become chief of staff of the army hospital in New Haven at a monthly salary of $160. Townsend inherited the considerable practice of Drs. Knight and Jewett while joining the hospital staff in 1863 as acting assistant surgeon, or contract surgeon at $100 a month. With two sources of income, Townsend thus became a "double-dipper," as opposed to his senior partner who was paid solely as a federal employee and with a modest salary at that. The junior surgeon benefited both financially and professionally as he gained clinical experience destined to offer great dividends as a surgeon. His earnings would become extraordinary for any practicing physician. He made twice what Dr. Knight had earned in his peak years and three to four times what Dr. Jewett made as army surgeon. From the beginning there was equal distribution of income, with Townshend doing all the house calls, for which he was paid extra. His office income averaged $36 a month for 1860, $64 for 1861, $200 for 1862, $298 for 1863, $451 for 1864 and $363 for 1865. [9]

In March of 1862, office rates were raised from $1 to $1.50. In November 1864 the fee for a doctor's office visit was raised to $2, where it stayed until just after World War II. Railroad accidents resulted in several amputations generating steep medical bills, fees that ordinary patients without means could not remotely pay. Those with deep pockets tend to pay for the health care of those with empty or no pockets.

The question of fees and billing has always stirred up controversy. The American Medical Association was founded in 1847 over the attempt of insurance companies and other organizations to make doctors salaried employees. Fee-for-service was threatened with extinction. The practice of capitation had been used in parts of the antebellum South where a physician would be paid per slave per year. Plantation owners, their wives, and overseers often undertook the region's medical care. Because of lack of transportation in this agrarian society, local illness had to be treated with local resources and remedies.

Some doctors earn more money than others for a variety of reasons. The stark facts of medical economic reality were stated in the *Boston Medical and Surgical Journal* of that time:

> The fact is there are dozens of doctors in all great towns, who scarcely see a patient from Christmas time to Christmas time. There are prodigious Ramadams in the receipts of every physician engaged in city practice. As a general rule, there is not a broken bone a piece in a 12-month period. If it requires a long and thorough drilling to succeed at all in the country a man is compelled to labor patiently many years in a city before he can command his daily bread in exchange for prescriptions.[10]

Another medical grumbler sighed about lack of appreciation. "It appears that we are too often looked upon as necessary evils rather than benefactors." Dr. Josiah Beckwith of Litchfield addressed these issues as president of the CSMS on May 29, 1862.

> The ablest in the profession have given their services without pecuniary compensation. It is conceded that at least one-third of all professional services rendered by physicians in the city, and in the country perhaps much more, is gratuitous with no compensation than the consciousness of doing good and contributing to the relieve the mass of suffering and misery which meets us on every hand. No other profession renders to all men such an amount of service for the same pecuniary compensation. He is called upon in midnight darkness, and in tempestuous storms as well as in the glad sunlight. He renders the same cheerful services to the poor as the rich.[11]

The war brought with it rising prices and consequently higher medical fees to keep pace. In 1864, the *Boston Medical and Surgical Journal* editorialized that "we have always been far too modest in our own estimate of the value of our services and in order to obtain anything like the competency needed have been obliged to do at least twice the amount of work as the law does. Hence, there is the necessity of continuing active practice far into old age. Office visits in Boston are now $3, and capital operations [amputations] $100 to $1000."

Spearheaded by Dr. Gurdon Russell, Hartford doctors composed a booklet entitled *Fees for Professional Services, as Established by the Physicians and Surgeons of Hartford*, which was published in August 1863. Russell's thoughts on the subject were exact: "It is only just to the public that it should be acquainted with our fees. This is after all a detail of business. The buyer and the seller, the one who gives and the one who receives should understand fully the grounds upon which they are dealing. Common sense alone demands it." The document advises doctors to charge for every visit made on the same day regardless of the number. The charges could be altered up or down depending on the discretion of the physician. More or less difficult treatments could be charged differently. If the patient cannot not afford to pay full price, alteration of the fee was permissible. It warned, however, that "it shall be considered unprofessional to diminish the standard fees with a view to mercenary competition." Price cutting to get more patients was discouraged.

For Hartford doctors, a visiting fee was $1.50, and prescriptions for additional family members were fifty cents each. Traveling fees were fifty cents per mile, with $2 minimum. Visits from 10 P.M. to sunrise were $3 and an additional $1 per mile.

Townsend was sent by the state to visit Connecticut troops after the Battle of Fredericksburg, in December 1862. He saw the residuals of Union defeat following a series of futile, poorly planned and executed charges against entrenched and experienced Confederate troops. Among the 11,000 Union casualties were many of Connecticut's finest. Some medical school classmates had enlisted for tours of duty ranging from three months to three years in duration, exposing themselves to the notorious often fatal "fevers" as well as the inherent dangers of battlefield exposure.

Being an army surgeon meant hardship, with associated risks of injury, disease, or worse. Death from malaria, typhoid fever, or dysentery had the same finality as that of grapeshot or the Minié ball. Townsend stayed home, wore civilian clothes, and made a few government dollars less than his equivalent in the field, but he had the luxury and safety of sleeping in his own bed at the end of each day. From April 1863 through June 1865, he treated sick and wounded soldiers at Knight U.S. Army General Hospital.

It is an unfortunate truth that wars provide experiences not present in civilian life and thereby allow the medical community to develop new ideas and techniques. Necessity often becomes the mother of invention. Doctors received on-the-job training, learning new skills and techniques that benefited subsequent patients. Young Townsend observed and performed surgical procedures for which he would not otherwise have had the opportunity. Specialization in both medical and surgical fields was introduced for the first time. Large numbers of peripheral nerve, spinal cord, and head injuries gave impetus to the founding of Turner's Lane Military Hospital in Philadelphia, where Silas Muir Mitchell became the first neurologist in America in a specialized hospital dedicated to such injuries.

Seven of his army hospital surgeries were published in the *Medical and Surgical History of the War of the Rebellion*. The surgical descriptions were unembellished, unvarnished, and sometimes painfully honest. The surgeon's name, patient's name and unit, cause of injury, description of the operation, and results of the surgery were reported for thousands of cases, and some were illustrated with drawings and photographs. Privacy and liability issues did not exist. (See Appendix II.)

One of Townsend's cases concerned J. Jackson, a private in Company K of the 9th Massachusetts Volunteers. He sustained a severe injury to his left leg following derailment of a train filled with soldiers that had departed from Knight U.S. Army General Hospital en route to Massachusetts to make room for more patients. Jackson was one of many critically wounded on October 15, 1864. He had a flap amputation of the left leg two days later and died on October 19, 1864.

The *New Haven Daily Palladium* had a reporter and member of the hospital on the site of the accident.

> October 17, 1864
> Terrible Railroad Accident
> Train on shoreline smashed
> 12 men killed, 9 men dangerously wounded, 40 or 50 slightly injured.
> Saturday morning a special shore line train of six cars left at 8 A.M. with 400 soldiers on board. They were heading for Readville, Massachusetts, and were one mile south of East Lyme. They were thrown from the track at Rocky Neck. Three cars were dashed into atoms and two badly smashed. Seven soldiers and one brakeman were killed instantly. Nine soldiers and two brakemen were severely mutilated. Fifty soldiers are with bruises and contusions. The dead, the mangled and the slightly wounded were brought back to the hospital. The accident occurred in a deep rock cut that was 400 feet long and about 15 feet deep. The rock on each side of the cars seemed to crush in on them like an anvil. The bodies were terribly crushed and hardly recognizable. The locomotive was not badly damaged but the other cars were pretty much destroyed. Surgeons from New London were called and placed wounded on train to head south. A special train with laborers and tools with Surgeon Townsend and Assistant Surgeon Hill left at 3 P.M. Surgeon T. H. Bishop and lady were on the front car and avoided any injury. Both returned with Townsend.

A returning railroad car was filled with the dead and mangled bodies. A patient with a battlefield gunshot wound of his arm suffering just soft tissue injuries now had a fracture as well. He and others were reportedly of good cheer, and replied they "learned to bear hardships in the Virginia battlefield and were not going to knock under now."

As part of the rescue effort, an extra train had been sent to the scene carrying surgeon Townsend and workmen with tools. The soldiers "manifested much satisfaction" when their previous treating physician, Dr. Townsend, appeared in their midst in the dead of night, illuminated by lantern, to render medical assistance. The train slowly returned to New Haven, and all possible efforts were made to relieve the injured. The accident might have been due to the buckling of a rail, a rockslide, or breakage of the flange of a wheel. "No human foresight could have prevented the accident," said officials at the scene. The *Palladium* reporter later visited the ward full of train casualties and wrote that "they were receiving every attention possible. Most critical was Daniel Sergeant of the First Massachusetts Cavalry who had a skull fracture. He was wandering in mind, and sometimes required four men to hold him down and keep him in bed. A large gang of laborers was sent to repair the track. The trains were running in 48 hours."

The *Knight Hospital Record* reported that seven of the nine soldiers had died instantly and that thirty-two were seriously injured; moreover, "the cars were completely smashed up and it was a miracle that many escaped injury." The cause of the accident was "a rail breaking in two," and the names of the dead and wounded were dutifully listed. Townsend billed the railroad $100 for his efforts.

There were 603 miles of railroad track in Connecticut carrying four million passengers a year. Trains traveled at an average speed of twenty-four miles an hour. Adults and children falling out of moving trains and other train accidents were reported in the local newspapers weekly. In 1866 there were 117 recorded railroad injuries with fifty-two killed. Townsend treated four such accident victims in January 1863, billing $1, $3, $5, and $16 respectively. The following month there were nine such patients, including an arm amputation at $25 and the setting of a femur fracture at $50. In November 1863 yet another accident led to amputation of an arm and both legs, operations which were soon followed by death and the doctor's bill for $100. No lawsuits were filed. It was safer to be a soldier on the battlefield at Waterloo or Gettysburg than a patient in a civilian hospital with an open long bone fracture. Mortality rates ranged from 75 percent for the thigh to 50 percent for the leg.

Townsend took over a practice long in standing that allowed him to become a leading figure in the field of surgery. Professional advancement while absorbing medical and surgical skills was not likely doing no more than treating gonorrhea, colds, and sprained ankles in a regiment stationed in the boondocks. At a thousand-bed convalescent hospital, unmatched clinical experience awaited the eager and willing young doctor.

Townsend's office records indicate that he saw patients virtually every day from his first day of practice in 1860 through the Civil War years. He seemed to be always on call and routinely worked Christmas, New Year's Day, and Thanksgiving. His first vacation was in August of 1865, five years after he started his practice. He traveled with his family to Europe. The three A's for a doctor to be successful are be available, be affable, and lastly be able. Except for his vacation, this doctor was, if nothing else, available day and night, weekdays, weekends, and holidays.

After the war was over he continued as lecturer for surgery at Yale School of Medicine through the 1867-68 academic year. At age thirty he successfully performed a Caesarian section on a sixteen-year-old black woman, Mrs. R. A. Dudley, that produced an eight pound, three ounce healthy boy. The patient had been referred by his classmate and veteran Dr. Frederick Dibble and by consultant Dr. Charles Lindsley, the new dean of the Yale School of Medicine. This was one of the first Caesarian sections done in Connecticut and was duly reported in the medical literature and lay media of the time. His biographer wrote that the success was "on account of his great surgical skills and his carefulness and rapidity in operating," and that by "performing this difficult surgery he became famous." Mortality at that time was between forty and eighty percent. Fifteen years later the same operation was repeated on Mrs. Dudley by another surgeon with a fatal result.

Dr. Lindsley described his colleague to a newspaper reporter as "a very rapid and exact operator. Rapidity was essential in the days of unclean hands. Not one case of amputation in a whole year was not done by Dr. Townsend. He had a large medical and surgical practice, which may have led to his invalid years. He was always sympathetic, and ready to drive many miles into the country for calls, besides having a large city practice. He was genial, sociable, and entertaining, and was instructor at Yale for a number of years."[12]

The last entry in his office register is in January 1872, a month during which he saw 208 patients and billed $406. His career as an active surgeon ended at age thirty-seven. Perhaps this solo surgeon had too large a workload, combined with virtually no vacation time and not much personal family life. Was this a recipe for burnout early in a career? He remained unmarried except to his profession, a passion not always sustainable. His father had died at a young age, a cautionary fact of family history.

A colleague believed that "owing to over work and sun stroke suffered while attending an accident case on Canal railroad he had to give up practice as a young man." This was in reference to the train wreck Townsend so ably responded to during the war and from which he was unlikely to have sustained disability. He was chief consultant for the New Haven Railroad in his later years, doing primarily administrative work, and adopted a retired lifestyle towards the end. This pattern of early retirement was not unusual for the well-off, for his father had done the same. Arriving at the age when inheritance began to flow led many well-to-do students and "gentlemen" to avoid the stresses of business or medical practice. Townsend lived his last decade in New York City and traveled to Europe and especially Dublin, Edinburgh, Paris and London, usually with family members, revisiting the places of his early medical studies to satisfy both nostalgia and the search of treatments for his maladies. In his final years, he lived as an invalid at the Townsend estate. By March 1893, he resided in the Buckingham Hotel in New York City where he died at 57 from pneumonia. He had five surviving brothers, a nephew, and an uncle who was a federal judge. He remained a bachelor, and was still a relatively young man at his death, close to his father's lifespan of fifty-three. He was born to the upper class but chose the difficult path of surgeon as a career choice when others might have chosen leisure.

CHAPTER FOUR

Doctor's Apprentice

The making of a physician is a complex process that continuously mixes art, science, and the humanities. Physicians are prepped in apprenticeship, then baked in the oven of practice. Reality brings to fruition hours spent in lecture halls memorizing isolated and often unrelated facts. The foundation of medical education begins with the full complement of basic sciences which permit basic understanding of the more practical subjects. The medical student watches how something is done by the experienced and then repeats it. The expression "See one, do one and teach one" is the hallmark of this tradition.

As the Civil War began, there were two basic types of medical school: doctor-owned (or proprietary) and university-based. Castleton Medical School in Castleton, Vermont, was an example of the former. It was founded by a grocer from Farmington, Connecticut, and managed to graduate most of the doctors in New England from 1818 through 1862. It was financed strictly from the fees collected from its students, which proved not to be a particularly steady source of income since some paid none or only part of their fees. The more prominent professors often traveled to other medical schools that were eager to land a celebrity physician in order to draw more students to their classrooms.[1] It became clear that hands-on teaching on live patients was essential and that simply listening to lectures and reciting text books aloud would no longer suffice. This approach required a hospital environment and clinics with large numbers of patients. This, along with insufficient financial support, doomed the doctor-owned schools. State and local governments in partnership with universities became the new model for success. Cities and not rural towns, universities and not store-front shops would train doctors, as large population centers were required to provide modern medical education.

Albany Medical College touted its "large and commodious Hospital opposite the college with lecture room, dispensary and every requisite for the study of clinical medicine and surgery to which students are admitted free of charge." The University of Nashville Medical College advertised free access to the Tennessee State Hospital. "This Hospital is no make-shift or make believe. It is a fine pile of substantial stone buildings surmounted by a dome It presents a center building three stories high, two wings with two stories the entire front being 206 feet. The Hospital is capable of accommodating 150 patients in well ventilated wards." It was described as a "model" and "in every respect a First Class" hospital run by the Sisters of Charity. Their catalogue listed eighteen operative procedures done in just one week: four amputations, four cataract excisions, two abscesses drained, two bone excisions, three lacerations, one elbow fracture, one contused ankle, and one circumcision. Vermont Medical College offered a "Medical and Surgical Clinique" on each Saturday at a "Dispensary" where patients were treated without charge.[2]

The Connecticut Medical Society and Yale College conceived of the Medical Institution of Yale College in 1810. Opening its doors in 1812, it would become the eighth oldest university medical school in the United States. The founding entities were two separate private organizations, the former made up of practicing and dues-paying physicians in the Nutmeg State. The medical society retained the right to pass upon candidates for graduation. Certificates were signed by the president of the medical society and countersigned by at least a majority of the committee. The same agreement also provided that each candidate "shall have graduated at some college, shall be required to have studied three years with some respectable physician or surgeon; and if not a graduate, four years, and to have attended one full course of lectures on the several branches of Medical Science, and to have arrived at the age of twenty-one years."[3] Three members of the medical society were chosen annually to form the Committee on Examination and in 1834 this number increased to six. This voluntary joining of the "towns and gowns" was effective and promising for future cooperation. The requirements for a degree of doctor of medicine at Yale included presenting a medical dissertation, passing exams on all medical subjects, and paying all fees. The medical degree was considered a license. Licensing was honorific or an expression of favor rather than competence.

Pennsylvania had no licensing at all and most states abandoned the process entirely by the 1830s. In 1763 eleven doctors in Norwich, Connecticut, applied to the legislature for the power "to distinguish between the Honest and Ingenious Physician and the Quack or Empirical Pretender" so as to avoid "great injury of the People as well as the Disparagement of the Profession."[4] It did not exclude others from practicing medicine, but their petition was rejected as restraint of trade.

By 1792 a charter for the Connecticut State Medical Society (CSMS) authorized the appointment of committees to examine candidates and license those found qualified for practice of "physic" or surgery. Some origins of the committees were countywide and some were statewide. There were no standards set and no formal licensing exams, no platform to revoke licenses issued, and the only penalty was not being able to recover debt or fees in court. This was a minor advantage, as doctors rarely sued since juries predictably found for the defendant. Exempted from this were apothecaries, midwives and those practicing botanic medicine. In 1834 a clause was added that to be licensed required being a member of the medical society. Upon pressure from what are now described as nontraditional health care providers, this was revoked in 1842.[5]

For the next half century there were no restrictions, licensing or regulations for the practice of medicine in Connecticut. The one significant exception occurred during the Civil War when a panel of three doctors representing the state gave formal exams to applicants for the post of regimental surgeon. The Botanical Medical Society was chartered in 1848 and allowed to grant licenses, the Eclectic Medical Society in 1855, and the Homeopathic Medical Society in 1864. The absence of effective licensing laws was pointed out by the New Haven Medical Association in 1878. It called Connecticut the "happy hunting ground of the medical tramp." "Certification" was accomplished by simply hanging out a sign or shingle and thus ply one's trade.

Medical students, or cadets, were a diverse group, including lawyers, ministers, and southern plantation owners hoping to absorb the latest in medical science in order to serve their parochial concerns. Southerners sent their sons or plantation managers to northern schools to improve medical treatment of slaves and local citizens. As an added benefit, they avoided the often-fatal fevers brought on by the summer heat by spending that time in New England.

After medical school, apprenticeship with an established doctor usually but not always followed. The experience was dependent on the skills, personality, and library of the teaching doctors, who charged $100 to $200 yearly for this training. House calls, which occurred on any day at any time and in any weather, were made by horse and buggy. This was an example of hands-on experience, seeing unfiltered humanity at its best and worst, albeit perhaps not at a convenient time or place. The time of day when an important teaching patient appears is unpredictable. More times than not, they are seen in the late hours of the night when sensible people are in bed. Peaceful sleep on a cold and rainy night might be a small blessing for the fatigued practitioner, made drowsy by the drone of the horses' hoofbeats and his apprentice's erudite pronouncements on anatomy, physiology, medical minutiae, or local gossip.[6]

By the 1850s, the annual enrollment of Yale's school of medicine was fifty students, of whom fewer than seventeen graduated. The average student had some college education and was about twenty years old. Over 50 percent of college graduates entered the law or clergy, with 8 percent entering medicine. Of the latter students, 44 percent had fathers who were doctors; thus continuing the tradition of the family business. A student's youthful appearance might not inspire confidence in his patients regarding their doctor's experience and judgment. To present a more mature façade, many students grew full beards, which were fashionable at the time. Older doctors seem wiser and more reassuring. While gray hair and a receding hairline may to some promise better health care, this correlation has never been demonstrated to be the case.

Medical students did not always have the public's confidence because of grave robbing. Bodies were required for anatomical dissection, the fresher the better, as preservatives were expensive, unavailable, or ineffective. For centuries several religious and political groups forbade dissection of the human body. Both in the United States and in Europe, it was not uncommon for public demonstrations over grave desecration. In 1788 a New York City mob rioted over bodies dug up from graves; seven people were killed and many wounded. Similar events occurred over the years in other towns and cities. To prevent grave robbing, in 1784 Massachusetts decreed that those killed in duels or executed for killing could be used for dissection; in 1831 unclaimed bodies were added, and in 1835 Missouri made deceased slaves available for the same purpose.

Dissection was usually carried out on the second floor where a skylight for illumination was located and where foul odors more easily dissipated through an open window. The 1861 catalogue of Cincinnati Medical College emphasizes practical anatomy and the availability of fresh specimens presented in a "dissecting amphitheater at the top of the main building well lighted and healthily ventilated." Bodies decompose with an unforgettable stench, and were best handled by speedy dissection, prompt parts removal, and working in cold months. Embalming with arsenic or sulfuric salt solutions could prolong cadaver usefulness, but eventually rot always followed. If police investigation was a possibility, since obtaining cadavers could be difficult or even illegal, dissection might be done in the evening by candlelight. For some schools, human cadavers were not part of the curriculum.

The most significant improvement in clinical teaching in the first half of the nineteenth century was the use of textbooks, which came first from Europe. In America hospital patients were first used for teaching in the mid–nineteenth century. Prior to 1850, fewer than 10 percent of doctors had hospital training, and very few medical schools required any hospital work at all. After 1850, medical school faculty began writing books, editing journals, and leading in community consultation.

The library at Yale Medical College in 1865 contained 1,200 volumes. (Castleton Medical School had 3,000.) Dr. B. H. Catlin advised medical students at the January 1865 Yale graduation that the well-to-do were fortunate in being able to procure a large library, for reference collections are "one of those helpers which are so important to a young physician." For the starting physicians with no patients and time on their hands, books should be available because "reading without practice is neither as agreeable nor profitable still it should not at this time be neglected." For the busy practitioner, "a part of every-day should be devoted to professional reading. The urgency of calls will sometimes prevent this, but see that it is the exception not the rule." Students were expected to "read, write, and cipher." Some differed from this point of view. In the late 1850s, the eighty-two-year-old surgeon general of the United States felt that book learning was a waste of time and money and therefore declined to fund medical education for the army's doctors. His particular time on earth and his views on medical education ended just as the war began.[7]

Yale's library had solid representation in all areas of study. Subjects studied included anatomy, chemistry, physiology, materia medica, theory and practice of medicine, astronomy, obstetrics, and surgery. Added later were botany, medical jurisprudence, mineralogy, pharmacy, zoology, pathology, microscopic anatomy, toxicology, and dentistry. As new areas of science opened up, new techniques became part of the doctor's armamentarium, such as urine analysis, auscultation and percussion of the chest and abdomen, and speculum exams of the uterine cervix. Urinalysis and use of the microscope were first added to the curriculum in the 1850s at Harvard Medical School under Oliver Wendell Holmes. For him lectures were a subsidiary as half of his students had faculty preceptorships.

> The great purpose of lectures should be to teach students how to learn by himself. They are not to take the place of private individual study but to inform the pupil how that duty may be pursued to advantage. Learning is a thing which no man can do for another, the weight of education must fall upon the learner.[8]

Medical students have always been taught that the first step in evaluating a patient is a proper history and physical examination. Listening to the patient requires no equipment besides patience and some understanding. After all, he is trying to tell you his diagnosis and paying for the privilege. Early in the nineteenth century, Laennec introduced the practice of listening to chest sounds through a hollow tube or stethoscope. There was elegance in a wooden tube that allows better clinical examination of the lungs and heart and enough distance from the actual patient to maintain civility. Better still, doctors could bill an extra dollar for this new procedure. The detailed analysis of the sounds of the heart and the lungs, such as murmurs in rheumatic heart disease and rales and rhonchi in tuberculosis, were remarkable for the descriptive terms used and their reproducible accuracy. An 1854 textbook on this subject by Professor Austin Flint of Harvard is strikingly accurate even by modern standards.[9]

Advances in technology do not always result in better patient outcomes. An exception was the work of Henry Ingraham Bowditch, a fervid abolitionist and physician specializing in pulmonary diseases in Boston. His expertise with auscultation allowed him to make exquisite diagnoses about the lungs. Tumor, abscess, pneumonia, or pleural effusion (fluid on the lungs) could be differentiated and localized with relative certainty. Fluid could then be safely drained by needle and syringe, resulting in significant clinical improvement. His text *The Young Stethoscopist* was first published in 1846 and went through many editions, serving as primer for student and practitioner alike.[10] His mentor in Paris was Professor Louis, who spent half an hour just listening to the patient and the same listening to his chest.

There were four rules to follow. First, look at the patient, or *observe*. Next, *palpate*, feel for abnormal rubs or bruits. Third, *measure* the chest movements and structure. Finally *auscultate*, or listen carefully for as long as is required.

Physical examination placed much reliance on the pulse. The rate, strength, and regularity were noted, whereas the temperature and blood pressure were not measured or recorded. Encyclopedic examination of the tongue seemed central to the work-up. Its turgor, color, grooves, size, feel, direction, mobility, and strength seemed endlessly fascinating for many practitioners. Wondrous deductions were made on the basis of the patient sticking out the tongue and saying "ah." After the history and physical come the laboratory studies, which at that time were nil. Laboratory work consisted of looking at the urine and its sediment under a microscope, testing for albumin, and tasting for sugar with one's finger as dipstick.

The diagnosis was made empirically and often solely on the basis of symptoms. Much of the medical field was descriptive and deductive in nature rather than based on hard scientific facts. The patient was hot or febrile, the severity and frequency confirmed by the doctor's touch, known as the laying-on of hands.

Core principles for the practice of medicine concerned the art of physical diagnosis: using wet and dry preparations, and plates which demonstrated morbid changes in various diseases. Specimens of plants, minerals, and other items needed for concocting drugs were meticulously studied. Medications and their mechanical and chemical modes of action, physical appearance, preparation, adulteration, dose and mode of administration, and therapeutic actions were stressed. The physician compounded prescriptions, made powder into pills, and provided patients with medications as an essential ingredient in patient care. As is the case today, the real need and effectiveness of drugs were in dispute.

Students practiced delivering babies on mannequins. Surgery was practiced on cadavers and was assisted with models of organs made of wood, wax, plaster, and papier-mâché. Slaves in southern states created lifelike reproductions of human organs for students to study and practice. Splints, surgical instruments, and "modern surgical appliances" were applied on inanimate objects created for that purpose. The University of Vermont claimed that its models for successful and scientific midwifery were so lifelike that "no student is excusable who fails to master it properly."[11]

There were four terms of sixteen weeks each over a two-year period. Lectures ran either five or six days a week, with five or six sessions of lectures daily starting at 8 A.M. and ending at 6 P.M. Saturdays were sometimes spent in a clinic setting where charity cases were evaluated. Some semesters were spent with students reading aloud from medical texts and monitored by an assistant to the professor. Rote learning and recitation were considered highly educational. Memorizing books, however, did not necessarily transfer into successful patient care. Some doctors prided themselves on having a small to nonexistent library and relying on experience to do what purportedly "worked." A treatment "working" might mean that the patient had a clear-cut reaction to treatment and survived.

Lectures were delivered in tiered lecture halls, didactic in nature and without practical hands-on experience or patient contact. To make class more interactive, in 1855 quizzing and lab studies were instituted. The cost of medical education was about $750, at a time when the average skilled craftsman earned $1 a day and a bushel of wheat cost forty cents. After two years and four separate semesters basically repeating the same lectures and reading sessions, a graduation ceremony was performed but not required. An additional expense for the student, it involved an oral and sometimes written exam. As late as 1890 in the state of Vermont, 30 percent of practicing physicians had no medical degree. The mandate requiring medical licensure with a uniform and formal testing program awaited the Flexner Commission in the next century.

After each course was completed, its professor issued signed tickets that served as proof of attendance. This certificate gave young doctors the cachet of academic excellence. Some of the professors lectured at several schools, as school terms often overlapped. (Professor Jewett, for example, also taught surgery and obstetrics at Castleton Medical School in Vermont.) Tickets cost about $15 each, $10 in rural areas and up to $20 in large city schools. At Yale, this meant $100 to $150 tuition per fourteen-week session, held twice annually. Yale also gave one "meritorious and necessitous student" from any county free schooling. A summation of costs is listed in Table 1.

To save expenses some students boarded with farmers. Among other chores they would chop wood and tallow candles at ten cents per dozen. Some students paid half or a third of their fees in cash and signed a note to pay them later (if they paid them at all). The University of Nashville Medical School charged $145 a session, Geneva Medical School in New York $103 and Bellevue Hospital Medical College in New York $150, with room and board $3.50 to $5 per week. The University of Vermont described in its 1864 catalogue the "comfort and convenience" of its medical college building overlooking Lake Champlain where "the scenery is unsurpassed in beauty and grandeur by any other locality in the country." It also had the lowest fees at $71 a session.[12]

TABLE 1. MEDICAL SCHOOL EXPENSES

Item	Fee
Matriculation fee	$5
Ticket fees	$100–$150, @$15 each
Practical anatomy and dissection	$5–$10
Hospital or clinical fee	$10
Exam or graduation fee	$10–$40
Apprenticeship	$100
Room and board	$1.50–$2.50 per week

Medical student letters to the deans of the Yale School of Medicine, Hooker and his replacement Lindsley, reflect the general anxiety, financial concerns, and mind-set of students. The absence of adequate funds seems a common denominator in the life of medical students throughout the ages. The vicissitudes of life do not change, as the following excerpts indicate.[13]

September 1863
Could I pay the required fees half at middle term, and the remainder at the close? Other professors agreed to the same, such as Dr. Hooker. My preceptor Dr. Perkins kindly offered to guarantee payment.
Gratefully yours,
John Brundage

June 1864

At no time since its reception has it been convenient to remit the amount until now. With deep feeling of gratitude for your great accommodations to me in time of need.

Your obedient servant

David Ainey

14 July 1864

When is the exam for M.D. this month as I would like to appear before the board though I have but little hopes of succeeding this time? My circumstances were such that I have been obliged to practice my profession since last January. I have done a good business consequently I have not read as I ought to have done for this examination. I have read only "Theory and Lectures of Surgery" since I left Yale lectures and rely on them only as I read up on cases I had. I have had a good variety of diseases to treat and made during February and March from 12 to 18 calls per day. I cut a tumor from a woman's head, reduced a dislocated wrist and mended up broken bones but I can't pass as good an examination by great ordeals as I could last Christmas for fear that I shall never be better prepared. I think I will try my hand this month if possible for me to raise the requisite number of greenbacks! Will you be kind enough to write me and oblige?

Yours respectfully

John D. Brundage

Litchfield

October 1864

I am ashamed at the long interval which has elapsed since I left New Haven and with my bill with you unsettled. I have no desire to cheat you of what is honestly due. I have been in debt and it has been the bane of my existence. I will pay with interest soon.

A. H. Abernathy

August 18, 1866.

I would like to attend the winter course. Which is the better way? Take a room and look out for one-self or board and let someone else do the looking out. What qualities should a student have or doesn't he want to know anything? I don't is the reason of my asking. My life for the past six years has not been calculated to improve mental organization. I am willing and able to learn though not as fast as others. The local doctor said, "I guess you'll make a good surgeon but I don't know how it will be about physic." I am not afraid of scratches. Please give me a lot of wholesome advice and I shall very much be obliged.

Very respectfully,

Byron W. Munson

This timid and self-effacing young man in just three years underwent a transformation of mind and heart. No longer doubting but self-assured and expert in his field, he is more than willing to share his wisdom and critiques with the professional pillars of his day. Expertise for some medical students comes after staying awake through one forty-five-minute lecture.

July 69

I hear Professor Steel is lecturing on medical Electricity. He is both ignorant and stupid. Many have suffered from his quackery. I will furnish names and dates. He has been arrested for fraud. He is ignorant, unscrupulous, stupid, and totally unfit. His lectures are soft soap doggerel. I appeal to the Dean of the faculty to save New Haven from suffering what surely will come upon them if they trust this consummate fool and rascal.

Very respectfully your obedient servant,

Byron Munson

A term paper published at the student's expense was required in order to graduate and obtain a degree at Yale. At first papers were presented in Latin and in later years in English.

The dissertation was presented in a public forum and defended from probing questions from the medical staff. Often they were summations of existing reports in the medical literature and as such offer us a window into the medical practice of the day. This was not a time so much of inquiry and research but of dogma and authority. In 1858 there were seven student papers, some of which follow.[14]

Daniel Armstrong Deforest's thesis was titled "On Typhoid Fever" and offered seemingly contradictory advice. He correctly warns against using a cathartic to start treatment. Despite a 25 percent mortality rate due to bowel ulcerations with or without treatment, the recommendation of the time was "the bowels need be evacuated fully." Magnesium sulfate or castor oil and a drop or two of laudanum "worked well." In the later stages, oil of turpentine seemed effective. Turpentine could be applied in rollers or flannel topically or be taken orally in pill form and thus end the life cycle of worms or other parasites lurking in the depths of the bowel. For abdominal pains, warm fomentations, rubefacients, poultices, and mustard would do well. Ice was for headaches, and tonics were for the depleted systems. Large blisters to the scalp were advised for delirium or coma. In the case of hemorrhages, acetate of lead with opium and vegetable astringents worked best.

Timothy Beers Townsend, who would be teaching surgery at Yale just a few years later, defended his paper on inguinal hernia. He describes treating a strangulated bowel from an incarcerated hernia by putting the patient face up, placing a hand between the thighs, and turning the affected knee inward to relax muscles, emptying the contents of the hernia sac into the abdomen, and then applying abdominal pressure no longer than fifteen minutes to avoid producing "inflammation." If this failed, cold water, ice, opium, retention tobacco enemas, tartar emetic, ether, chloroform, or warm baths should follow. The last option might be a surgical approach: open the hernia sac and return the bowel to its rightful place. His deductive reasoning was innovative and correct, but the procedure had yet to be successfully performed. Bowel surgery was not done in this era, though his remarks were prescient for future treatment of this condition. A case report doing exactly what young Townsend recommended would first appear in the medical literature five years later (1863) in the *Proceedings of the Connecticut Medical Society*.

James Havirott discussed bilious remittent fever. He notes its quotidian character and geographical characteristics. Malaria had been endemic across America but had become mostly a southern disease by wartime. Mercury was considered best in small doses and quinine the treatment of choice when the disease was acute or in remission. In the seventeenth century missionary Jesuit priests in the Andes of South America noted the natives used bark of the Cinchona tree to treat fevers. This contained quinine in varying concentrations and was the principal drug used for fevers until the chemical was synthesized by French chemists in the 1830s.

John William Lawton discussed fractures: "It seems easy, but when one does the case, there may be great anxiety for the surgeon and the patient." His paper is quite short, but shows wisdom beyond his age in appreciating the difficulty and skill required in orthopedics.

From 1861 through 1870, 125 students graduated from Yale Medical School. About one in four had a liberal arts degree from college. The graduates' names and thesis titles were routinely published in the New Haven papers. The *Palladium* declared on its front page of August 26, 1862, that "the Medical Institution of Yale College was commencing 18 September a seventeen week course" and listed the names of the professors of surgery, anatomy, medicine, obstetrics, pharmacy and chemistry, materia medica, and therapeutics. In 1863, out of forty students, thirteen graduating papers were presented in public. The subjects included peritonitis, colitis, quinine, pneumonia, rheumatism, measles, aneurysm, gunshot wounds and yellow fever.

In January 1865, a large attendance of the public witnessed eleven students graduating with papers on variola, croup, cholera, malaria, albuminuria, typhoid fever, enteric fever, and gonorrhea. How the public reacted to the last subject was not recorded. The Jewett prize of $30 was divided between students Van Wyek and Rodman but, feeling it did not adequately recompense him for his effort, Rodman declined to accept. His letter to Professor Sanford of the Anatomy Department stated he was "perfectly satisfied if none allotted. I consider my preparation worth to me $30, the amount offered as a prize." Half a loaf is better than no loaf in some neighborhoods, but not apparently in Mr. Rodman's.

From the medical school's inception, rules and regulations were emphasized both in the written curriculum and in unwritten social mores. Students were expected to heed a strict code of conformity wherein inquiry and challenging of existing theorems were not encouraged. By 1815 a series of specific commandments would regulate the universe of Yale medical students. A listing of these follows.

1. Students shall have satisfactory evidence of a blameless life and conversation.
2. There will be no profanity or indecent noise on the Sabbath. Students shall attend some place of public worship. Any student denying the Holy Scriptures or any part thereof to be of divine authority or propagate among the students any error or heresy subverting the foundation of the Christian religion shall be dismissed.
3. Medical Professors may visit rooms of students or any of faculty and break open any room closet or study where admittance is refused.
4. All damages to any part of medical College shall be charged to all those who inhabit building.
5. Every medical student shall be subject to laws and government of medical institution and show in speech and behavior all proper tokens of reverence and obedience to faculty of college as well as of the medical institution.
6. Any student guilty of blasphemy, robbery, fornication, theft, forgery, assault on Professors, dueling or any other crime shall be expelled.
7. Any student guilty of challenging, being turbulent, wearing women's apparel, fraud, lying, or defamation shall be punished by admonition or other collegiate punishment suited to the nature and demerit of the crime.
8. Every student in studying time shall abstain from hallooing, singing, loud talking, and playing a musical instrument and other noise around medical college.
9. There shall be no firearms, gunpowder or gambling on the premises.[15]

Instances of inebriated medical students or those incapacitated from laughing gas were not unknown. Compared to body-snatching, such behavior was considered trifling, hardly worthy of mention in the local newspapers. Fornication on Yale property was grounds for dismissal. Men wearing women's clothing was worthy of admonition only. Committing a crime, blasphemy and not being Christian was conduct totally unacceptable. (*Christian* meant white, Anglo-Saxon and Protestant.)

In 1847 the American Medical Association assembled 250 delegates from twenty-two states to discuss, among other issues, the state of medical education. Physician compensation topped the list of concerns. Another issue was doctors who spoke ill of each other in public for economic, personal, and professional reasons. The new national policy was "Thou shall not speak ill of thy brethren." The AMA recommended "a good English education, knowledge of natural philosophy and elementary mathematics, enough knowledge of Greek and Latin to write prescriptions and understand scientific language." Preceptors would certify passage of a three-year experience, and the examiner of the highest standing. Subjects should be standardized, attendance records kept, and hospital exposure with bedside experience considered essential.

From 1851 through 1860, the average yearly medical school attendance at Yale was 36, with a total of 119 actually graduating. Out-of-state students might not want the expense nor have a need to get a degree. Medical students made up 8.2 percent of the student body.

As the war progressed, enthusiasm waned and the pool of willing volunteers evaporated due to death and disease. An exception was medical students whose numbers serving in hospitals and elsewhere increased. Different standards and expectations always exist for the medical community, and most served in some capacity after graduation. For the war period Albany Medical College graduated 159 students, of whom only sixty-six did not join the military. Two died in service.[16]

Five hundred forty students graduated from Yale College during the Civil War of whom 133 served, most entering right after graduation. From 1863 through 1865, out of 76 Yale men drafted only twelve served; thirty-four obtained exemptions and the rest bought a substitute. One hundred seventy-four Yale graduates died in service, 49 of whom were Confederates. (In contrast, during the Vietnam War, the number of Yale graduates who died in service was zero.) A total of 1,100 Yale graduates served in the Civil War, 113 participating as army surgeons. Six Yale medical school graduates died in service, all from medical conditions contracted while serving in the South. Five of the six deaths occurred in Louisiana and North Carolina. (See Appendix III.)

What kind of doctor was produced by this educational system? Dr. Josiah Beckwith of Litchfield delivered a paper to the Connecticut State Medical Society (CSMS) in May 1863 entitled "The Medical Profession — its dignity and grandeur." His remarks are characteristic of similar discourses of that period congratulating fellow men of science unparalleled in achieving the pinnacle of knowledge, science, and ability to solve the mystery of life and disease. Science alone keeps advancing for the betterment of all men. Doctors are hardworking, morally courageous, passionate, brainy, kind, considerate, and unfailingly polite.

> With learning, must be combined strong common sense, a retentive memory, and sound discriminating judgment. This requires intense labor, study, and observation. He must be a man of large brains and broad sympathies, broad enough to embrace the whole human family. He should be strong for toil, and capable of enduring the inspiration of the individual. The physician of this age must be eminently practical as well as liberal in his view. He must be a patient man, a gentleman, kind and courteous, obliging, modest, generous and genial, conceding, forbearing, not stubborn but maintaining a manly independence. He must have elements of moral greatness, inspire confidence, and nurture hope.[17]

What are the guidelines for appropriate behavior of the doctor? Where are the pitfalls, and how does one avoid them? The following extracts are from the commencement address of Geneva Medical College in upstate New York by Professor of Materia Medica and General Pathology Charles A. Lee, MD, in June 1852. It appears the answers to these questions and the reality of a medical career do not change.

> Scientific medicine of our day, is not the medicine of former ages, a strange medley of false facts, wild vagaries, gross credulity and superstition; but casting all these aside as belonging to the infancy of our race of the dark ages, it seeks to subject everything to the infallible test of reason, experiment and observation. The useful and practical are to be carefully separated from the speculative and fanciful.

There is a canker at the root of every flower. Success in our profession entails such labor that few who know its real nature can envy it for it is bought with the sacrifice of all healthy recreation both of body and mind. As the world esteems the practitioner, it deprives him of most of the social pleasures of life. He acquires property, loses his health, and leaves his estate to be squandered by his children whom it demoralizes. Of the very prosperous, envy and detraction follow him through life. Happiness and professional success do not necessarily go together — the former is nearer the domestic altar.

Once fairly upon the professional treadmill; there is no letting up without the danger of being carried under. The physician must be ever increasing in knowledge, experience, and skill. You cannot stand isolated, taking no interest in the great questions and movements of our age and country; as you share the benefits and partake of the blessings of our admirable institutions you must also contribute to their support.

Gentleman, do not regard your profession merely in the light of a money making business; a trade to be pursued like other trades, simply with a view to its profits. You are not to neglect the poor, nor be exorbitant in your charges. You are not to make the accumulation of wealth, the only object of life.

A medical grumbler is a sad character, eternally talking and complaining of the hardships of a physician's life, loss of sleep and rest, anxiety, exposure to heat and cold, fatigue, of poor pay, ingratitude, and quackery. He knew beforehand that he had all these to encounter, what right has he then to complain, they are the inevitable lot of all physicians who faithfully discharge their duty.[18]

In 1864, Dr. John Andrew addressed the graduating class of the University of Cambridge Medical School (Harvard).

A faithful and painstaking medical adviser, well instructed in his duties, an expert in his own calling, is what the sick and anxious patient covets by his bedside. One who can hope for him when he is himself discouraged, who can seem to clear away the mists which disease gathers about him. But the jaded, frightened, anxious patient, struggling for a straw of promise, clinging to any hope, however flimsy and foundationless, regards your profession as a mystery and not a science. You must promote the sciences, make war on ignorance, and take plain and simple men into your confidence

Dr. Frank Hamilton was a prominent surgeon in Buffalo and New York City who served as an army surgeon and later medical inspector. He wrote two well-received textbooks during the war years, *A Practical Treatise on Military Surgery and Hygiene* and *A Treatise on Fractures and Dislocations*. Both were designed to help young and inexperienced doctors perform their duty in an exemplary fashion. He gave his unreserved seal of approval to medical graduates:

They are trained in a Spartan school, under a law of ethics, which allows no man to turn his back upon danger. Whatever the peril, they are expected to go wherever their services are needed. They make no great ado about it, nor are their names often mentioned in the official reports. They go wherever they are called, quietly about their business, alone or in small detachments, in rain and in snow, by night and by day, on the march and on the bivouac, through watchfulness and fasting and fatigue into the midst of malaria, contagion and battle. The men, who can remain cool and self-possessed in the midst of deadly contagions, ought to stand well the fire of musketry.[19]

In 1860 in Italy, Professor Pelizzari injected medical students with the blood of syphilitics, thus demonstrating that in some instances the disease is transmitted through the blood. Less severe studies were done in America with yellow fever patients, using gastric fluids, blood, and saliva in an attempt to transmit the disease. In New Haven, the students were not guinea pigs but rather assisted in providing general health care in hospital wards, including wound dressing and assuring proper medications were prescribed.

The United States Sanitary Commission report *Hospital Transports* was a frank description of medical conditions by embedded doctors early in the war. It is here that we first see the efforts of students and nurses justifiably praised.

> Here were one hundred miserably sick and dying men, forced upon us before we had been one hour on board; and tug after tug swarming round the great ship, before we had a nail out of a box, and when there were but ten pounds of meal and two spoons to feed them with. No account could do justice to the faithful industry of the medical students and young men: how we all got through with it, I hardly know. The wound dressers (two year medical students) are generally ready for whatever may be required, and work heroically.[20]

The Satterlee Hospital in Philadelphia provided care for a daily census of 1,960 patients in thirty-six wards, with thirty-five medical officers, and forty-one medical cadets. Each ward had a surgeon, a sister of charity, a ward master and three nurses. A cadet was attached to each ward along with a resident assistant surgeon and an acting assistant surgeon.[21] New Haven's hospital worked the same way. Eight medical cadets, along with hospital stewards, cooks, and male and female nurses were all under contract to the General Hospital Society of Connecticut. The students were without salary but given room and board. Their school was on York Street, a five-minute walk to the new military hospital.

CHAPTER FIVE

The War Governor and His Agents

The "great man" theory holds that by dint of personality, knowledge, and skill an individual can profoundly affect history. William Alfred Buckingham was born on May 28, 1804, the descendant of Puritan stock who landed in Boston in 1637 among the original settlers of New Haven and founders of Yale College. His father, known as an "enterprising and thrifty farmer and Christian gentleman," and mother, said to be skilled at bedside nursing, settled in Lebanon, a small town unique in having spawned five Connecticut governors.[1]

He was educated locally, spending three years of his adolescence at the Bacon Academy in nearby Colchester. This school was founded by a $35,000 grant from Pierpont Bacon, a local farmer, upon the suggestion of his family physician, Dr. Watrous. Pierpont Bacon was tall, dark, and coarse-featured, and would be dead at age fifty-five. He was the antithesis of everything the Buckingham family held dear. He was a misanthropic, miserly, antisocial draft dodger who sent his slave to represent him in the Revolutionary War and later married his housekeeper just to save money. She left him childless, but he was unwilling to leave his fortune to family or town.

The academy opened in 1803 and emphasized writing, Greek, Latin, mathematics, philosophy, logic and rhetoric. The school bell rang at 5:30 A.M. and the day started with morning prayers followed by the headmaster's discussion on morals. This was a strict life where proper behavior and dress was demanded and punishment was by "reproof, correction, admonition or expulsion." Two students each day practiced public speaking before an audience of instructors and fellow aspirants. The first graduate was Stephen Austin, founder of Texas.

As a deacon of the Second Congregational Church, Buckingham was familiar with the doctrine of catechisms and the last judgment of mankind in which the "willful and impenitent sinners" would be punished and lead unhappy and unproductive lives ending in abject misery. The wages of sin was death, and redemption, the work of God, alone could change unwilling hearts from rebellion to eager obedience. The righteous, penitent, and dutiful Christian lived a bounteous, productive and joyous life. Buckingham and fellow benefactors spread the truth by teaching Sunday school and generously endowing libraries, schools, temperance societies, and missionary work.[2]

He was a teacher at eighteen and a year later a clerk in his family's dry goods business. At twenty-three he opened his own store in Norwich, later expanding into woolen goods and manufacturing ingrain carpeting. He began investing in businesses where he could exercise oversight, developing financial acumen and manufacturing experience. His prudent judgment became as valued as his purse.

His devotion and love for wife Elizabeth and two children was boundless. His only surviving child, Eliza, married in 1857. She received from her father heartfelt news about the death of her two-year-old brother from scarlet fever which haunted and grieved twenty years later: "Our cup of joy was overflowing. But He, who had given us such superabundance of happiness for reasons which made it seem right in his sight, soon visited us with his chastising hand…. No language can convey a proper idea of the strength of our love for you or of the comfort which we have not already experienced nor of the happiness which we trust will continue to flow into our hearts through you. Our love has been incessant and increasing. You have never caused our cheeks to crimson with shame but have been the joy of our lives."[3] In the same letter Buckingham then gives instructions on how to succeed in business. Ever the micromanager, he delves into the proper use of property as a value and blessing which demanded accurate accounts of receipts and expenditures. Stock worth $5,000 was Eliza's wedding gift for, he wrote, "wise improvement of your privileges and a judicious use of every means of influence." He reminded her, "The great end of life is to secure the highest good of ourselves and others. Know its value and use it to do goodness while providing for you. The future is unknown but its darkened path can be illuminated by prayer and reading the words of the Lord."

By 1848 Buckingham was ready to move on to the new technology, such as railroads, steamships, telegraph, and the development of the rubber industry. Two of Connecticut's own would play a key role. Nathaniel Hayward was an inventor who, by adding sulfa to India rubber, produced a substance that was stable, elastic, and durable. It would neither melt in the summer nor break into pieces in the winter. His patent, received in 1838, was sold a few years later to Charles Goodyear of Naugatuck for $2000. Hayward started a company in Lisbon for the manufacture of rubber shoes and moved it to Colchester in 1847 as the Hayward Rubber Company. In consideration of royalties paid to Charles Macintosh and Company, he was granted sole right to sell its footwear on the British market. This fledgling company was on the cutting edge of making rubberized boots, shoes and blankets, features that would be of great interest to an army at war. The company was financially unstable and poorly run. Buckingham remedied this in 1848 by becoming managing director and treasurer. Patent infringement lawsuits were common and expensive. To avoid them, the Goodyear Shoe Association was formed in 1848 by six licensed manufacturers, including the Hayward Rubber Company, so that prices could be regulated and quotas maintained. Men's boots were $4.50 a pair, and ladies' long boots $2.75 a pair. "Rubbers, rubbers, rubbers" read a newspaper ad from a shop in New Haven promising men, women and children feet kept dry with rubber shoes. By 1851 shops advertised, "We have the Hayward Rubber Company and the Goodyear Company both contributing their boots, and shoes, cloaks and capes, hats and caps, leggings and gaiters, belts and gloves and other water resisting armaments."[4]

The company was the main pillar for the borough of Colchester which by 1863 employed 243 men and women, mainly Irish immigrants. A Catholic church was built to accommodate them as business boomed "with untold prosperity," especially during the war years. The company owned the largest plant of its kind in the country, which at its peak made 10,000 pairs of rubbers a day.[5] The Civil War afforded the company a unique position to reap the benefits of government contracts. That Buckingham was the manager until 1858 and secretary-treasurer for life was not considered a fiduciary conflict at the time. He had expertise in many areas, especially footwear, and complained to the War Department of "shoes worn through in less than a week and soldiers under the necessity of drawing four, five and six pairs before the year is one-half or three-quarters gone."[6]

By 1860 there were 27 rubber establishments in the U.S., nine in Connecticut. By 1865 this number increased fivefold. Some companies sold military-specific items, including a portable boat, air mattress, haversack, knapsack, canteen, and leggings. Over four years, the Union army bought 2.7 million rubberized blankets ranging from $2.50 to $5 each and spent over $27 million for rubber goods.[7] Medical applications included tourniquets, crutches, air cushions for bedsores, ambulance shock absorbers, stretchers, bed covers, canteens, jars, surgeons' instruments, syringes, artificial limbs, catheters, bandages, rubber gloves, and stethoscopes. Hard rubber was used for reconstructive surgery of the mouth and face from traumatic wounds or mercury-induced gangrene.

Having conquered the world of business and manufacturing, Buckingham turned to politics as a Whig. He was mayor of Norwich in 1849, 1850, 1856, and 1857. He was a John Charles Frémont presidential elector in 1856 and was first elected governor in 1858, serving seven more year-long terms with ever-increasing plurality at the polls.

His was an Old Testament God who demanded stern justice and an unwavering faith of the Lord's chosen who would set the oppressed free. This man of faultless and stubborn character viewed the terrible instrument of war as necessity and not choice. Secession and the rebellion was a sin to be punished in a holy war. Buckingham's Proclamation of March 1861 declared, "Security is to be found under a government with laws based upon divine statutes properly administered. Look unto the God of Israel for help." He urged that Good Friday be a statewide day of "Fasting, Humiliation and Prayer" so that the Lord would give "wisdom" while "saving us from further strife and contention," to preserve the union.[8]

Twice a year as governor he issued proclamations corresponding to Easter in March and Thanksgiving in November. This Sunday-school teacher and deacon had deep religious convictions on the origin of all that is good and its relationship to society. In 1858, he wrote, "Thanks giving and praise to almighty God who has caused the earth to bring forth its fruits in their season. He has averted from us the pestilence and the sword; he has saved us from civil commotion and the supremacy of evil passions." In October 1862: "Let us be grateful for the blessed memory of the honored dead, who in camp and on the battlefield have cheerfully, heroically and religiously offered their lives upon the altar of patriotism. Let us rejoice and praise God that he holds the destinies of this nation in his hands, confirms and changes the purposes of man at his pleasure and overrules all human doings to establish righteousness, truth and justice in the earth." In March 1863: "The evils now extending over our country and calamities which weigh so heavily are God's righteous judgments for our sins." By March 1865 neither was "righteousness established nor Slavery abolished." Admission of sin, seeking truth and justice, repentance, hard work, sacrifice and faithful performance of good deeds would pave the road to salvation for individuals and the nation.[9]

In his address to the state legislature in May 1860, he defined their purpose: "The duty of state is justice, to aid the cause of education, make provision for those who by reason of afflictions of Divine Providence are unable to provide for their own necessities, shield morality and virtue from the open assaults of vice and crime, and protect every citizen in the enjoyment of his civil rights and religious liberty." As commander-in-chief of the armed forces of Connecticut he saw that these principles would be practiced and enforced for the health and welfare of his soldiers and their families. Commingled with this spirit was a loving and giving side exemplified in Isaiah 1:17: "Learn to do good. Devote yourselves to justice; aid the wronged. Uphold the rights of the orphan; defend the cause of the widow." Aggressive capitalism and charity would coexist and all would profit.

He proposed that "heavy burdens of war should not cut into care for the needy." Institutions of education and humanity would be funded with "enlightened philanthropy." Money was set aside in Connecticut for public education, schools for the blind, the deaf and dumb, the insane, health care for the indigent, and soldiers' benefits. In other states this was not the case. Fifteen percent of his budget supported families of soldiers. Seventy-eight percent paid state bounties and other purposes connected with volunteers and militia.[10] He wrote:

> The Institutions of humanity and education required our constant and forceful consideration. We should not be influenced by parsimony, neither should the heavy burdens of war be permitted to incline us to withhold such support as is essential to their usefulness. They are the fruits and evidences of an enlightened philanthropy, the barometer by which we can judge whether our country is advancing in the sunlight of intelligence, civilization and Christianity or whether is it so darkened and desolated by the storm of ignorance, depravity and selfishness.

In 1862 the Retreat for the Insane had 397 admissions. One hundred patients from 33 different towns in the state had been supported in whole or in part by the Connecticut Hospital Society with state appropriation, of which 6 died, 83 were discharged and 11 remained. One hundred eleven patients were admitted at Hartford Hospital, of which 13 died, 64 were discharged, and 34 remained. Buckingham wrote, "Both of these institutions have been invaluable to our volunteers by furnishing them with the comforts of a home while sick and rendering such necessary care and medical aid as could have been secured in no other way."[11]

By May 1863 Connecticut's prisons held 159 mostly white men who mostly committed burglary, thought to be due to high unemployment rates. However, this number was on the decline. The Retreat for the Insane had thirteen inpatients, each costing $1.50 a week for support; Hartford Hospital had 164 patients; the General Hospital Society 178 patients from 17 towns. The Connecticut School for Imbeciles had fifteen unfortunates, costing $100 a year per student; the School for the Blind seven. The American Asylum for the Deaf and Dumb had 224 students from all the New England states with only 45 from Connecticut.[12] Maintained fully funded were public schools with 76,207 students taught by 2,037 mostly male teachers who in Hartford received $70 per month (some three times the salary of females) and in New Haven $100 (four times). The governor's salary was $91 per month, and judges earned $166.

The ability to pay for the Civil War was critical. Buckingham outlined how this could be achieved led by the deft hand of an experienced and inspired financier and businessman. He was not elected governor based on personal charisma, ability as an orator, or being one of the common folk. Within days of the attack on Fort Sumter the banks of Connecticut telegraphed promissory notes to the governor totaling $460,000 with approval for another half million and more if needed. Willingness to give was based on the flames of patriotism that warmed the cockles of even New England bankers. The proposed expenditures were not authorized by the legislature, meaning the loans were backed solely by Buckingham's extraordinary character and personal financial status. The interest rates charged would be based on his credit rating, not the states' or federal government's, a savings of great importance. The degree of his financial acuity was well known to the treasurer of Yale College,

H. Kingsley, who asked his opinion on school investments in January 1865: "The college owns stocks of banks in New Haven, Hartford, Boston and New York. What is the propriety of that for this institution? Are they personally liable in addition to the stock value to another value equal to the stock itself?"[13] He answered that no impropriety existed but that investment means taking risks which are appropriate as long as they "are managed by judicious men."

Money would be raised by taxes on profits from business, property, bonds, stocks and even licenses for doctors at $10 per year. "Government is endeavoring to adopt a new and untried means of raising revenues based on the productive industry of the country and one that which will make even larger demands on our pecuniary resources. But we have abundant ability to meet these claims. A very small part of the profits of our industry will be sufficient to supply the public treasury with the means to prosecute the war and furnish a sound foundation for public credit."[14]

Connecticut was a manufacturing state whose profits would be taxed as would those of out-of-state stock and bond holders. Buckingham was an early supporter of the Lincoln administration and pledged whatever manpower or financial resources were required to severely punish the sinners whose crime was slavery and rebellion. In response to Lincoln's request for aid, on July 3, 1862, Connecticut's war governor, William A. Buckingham, sounded a clarion call to all citizens.

> In the name of our common country, I call upon you to enroll your names for the immediate formation of six or more regiments of infantry to be used in suppressing the Rebellion. Our troops may be held in check, and our sons die on the battlefield; but the cause of civil liberty must be advanced, the supremacy of the government must be maintained. Close your manufactories and workshops, turn aside from your farms and your business, leave for a while your families and your homes, and meet face to face the enemies of your liberties!

Buckingham's generosity to the state was matched by financial and social aid for soldiers and their families. Widows, stranded destitute wives, mothers, and wounded and sick soldiers received his attention and generosity even when legally not mandated. He gave heartfelt

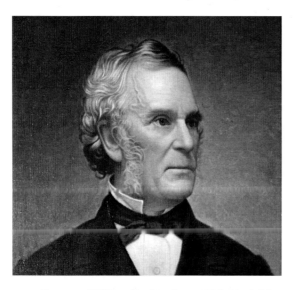

farewell and "Godspeed" to departing regiments and welcomed home the survivors. Having lost his only son, two-year-old Willie, gave him insight into the pain and sorrow of families of the fallen.

He received hundreds of letters from soldiers in the field and hospitals, wives, fathers and mothers and their surrogates pleading for transfer, furlough, discharge, or financial aid. Institutions we take for granted today did not exist. There was reliance on the "organized mercy" delivered by the Christian and Sanitary Commissions and the Ladies Aid Society, whose virtue included paying their own way. The United States Sanitary Commission was a private organization founded by prominent ministers, scientists, doctors, and high-society women. Its goal was to "find out what the

Governor William Buckingham, 1804–1875 (Museum of Connecticut History.)

government will do and can do and then help it by working with it and doing what it cannot," while supervising the general health, sanitation and welfare of the army. It provided for the medical, social, and personal needs of the soldier and was a precursor of future organizations. This included providing diverse goods for soldiers, improving sanitary conditions, and educating nurses and doctors. Specifically, the commission would "inspect recruits and sanitary conditions, train nurses, restore and preserve health, provide provisions for cooks, nurses, and hospitals, and prevent sickness."[15]

The commission provided myriad items ranging from fresh vegetables to bandages, socks, blankets, and reading and writing materials. Trains were converted to moving hospital cars with hanging litters. Waterborne hospitals were created by converting ships into operating rooms, dispensaries, and patient wards with all the necessary equipment and staff. Better stretchers, ambulances and transportation from the battlefield followed. The commission established hospital directories where friends and relatives of soldiers could obtain information without cost as to a soldier's place and condition for a year after becoming a hospital patient. By war's end their records held 900,000 names.

Lincoln called the Sanitary Commission his "fifth wheel" since it took up valuable space on his administration's carriage and because its critical nature made it an unwanted liability. The commission's work filled a need, and did so effectively with the encouragement and oversight of Congress. But a more systematic approach was needed to provide the best in medical care.

Buckingham's foresight extended to the consequences of war, both its length and ferocity. By May 1861 the governors of New York and Massachusetts had appointed agents in Washington to supervise the soldiers' general welfare and take care of the sick and wounded that might appear from their respective regiments. Buckingham's soldiers walked on hallowed ground. Not satisfied with reports from regular army channels, he sent his own agents to ascertain the health status of his soldiers. They were authorized to send home every sick or wounded Connecticut soldier well enough to travel and were instructed, "You will find many privations incident to the camp and a state of war which cannot be relieved. But when you discover grievances that can be redressed, you will give your efforts to accomplish that object through proper officials and benevolent associations which are organized for that purpose."

He dispatched retired Colonel J.H. Almy to live in New York City, covering expenses only, to deal with soldiers' needs and wants. Many soldiers received no pay for months and required medical care, shelter, food or a ticket home. Almy gave the governor a graphic picture of pain, suffering and loss that demanded a systematic approach for the coming thousands of stranded souls in March 1862. Families needed to know the status and whereabouts of loved ones:

> Yesterday morning I was notified that 42 wounded soldiers of the 10th Connecticut regiment had arrived at Jersey City. I immediately made arrangements for their removal to the Park Barracks where after giving them suitable refreshments I obtained orders form Col. Tompkins for their transportation to their homes. I regret to say that the New Haven Rail Road refused to transport the men upon the order of Col. Tompkins and I was obliged to pay their fair [*sic*] in full. The other routes accepted the orders without demurring. I had the wounds dressed and gave the men money for their immediate necessities, called in surgical aid and sent them off cheerful and in good spirits. Some of the men are badly wounded but the majority is doing well. About twelve are so feeble that they were unable to move without aid. These I had carefully placed in wagons and delivered at the various stations. The men expressed themselves grateful for the attention we showed them and [I] did not complete my labors until midnight.[16]

Colonel Almy next contacted Secretary of War Stanton about the need for immediate financial aid from the paymaster.

> Several hundred sick and wounded soldiers returned form [*sic*] Gen Burnsides division have not received any pay since they left Annapolis. They are furnished with transportation to New York but arrive here penniless and in urgent need of money. They bring with them the necessary certificates but on application to Major Leslie the paymaster I learn that he has not the requisite funds at his disposal to meet their wants. If you would please order funds to be forwarded to Major Leslie for that purpose you would perform a noble act of charity towards these brave men who have vindicated our country's flag with such honor during the past few weeks.[17]

The response was the immediate transfer of $10,000 with directions to pay the returning sick and wounded. This was mostly in response to the Lincoln administration's high regard for the governor. Stanton personally wrote Buckingham about other matters on April 16, 1862: "Accept my heart-felt thanks for your kind note. In the midst of toil and care that wearies my spirit and exhausts my strength such words of comfort renew and strengthen me greatly." And on March 21, 1863, he wrote, "If I can do anything to assist you in the coming election let me know and it will be done."[18]

Almy, for his part, corresponded with the *Hartford Courant* to give the public up-to-date information on loved ones and neighbors. April 11, 1862: "Three hundred sick and wounded soldiers from Gen. Burnside's division have arrived here since the battle of Roanoke. Sixty are from Connecticut regiments and have not been paid since the expedition left Annapolis. "To the editor he entreated, I write to ask of you the favor to state in your paper that all sick or wounded soldiers who will send me their description lists or if discharged their certificates of the same can obtain their pay without delay. These men seem especial objects of charity for they arrive here penniless and without any means or provision even to reach their homes."

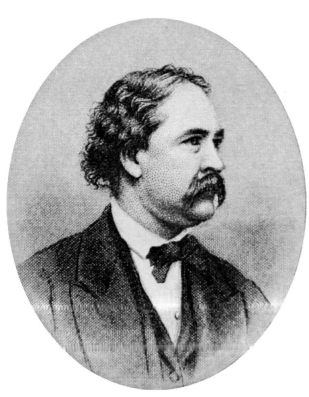

Both the living and the dead had to be dealt with, and the latter can't buy tickets home. Economy of effort and cash was essential. Almy proposed an inexpensive and novel way of transporting the deceased.

> I chose a plan by which the bodies of those who have been killed in battle at Roanoke as also those who have died from sickness can be returned to Connecticut at a trifling expense. Capt. Ferris of South Norwalk has lost a son in the 8th Regiment and is anxious to recover his body. He has been in the coasting trade and is familiar with the Hatteras coast. I can obtain a cargo for him to Hatteras, from Col. Tompkins and he will personally attend to the

Colonel J.H. Almy, Connecticut agent in New York City (Connecticut State Library).

return of the bodies, bringing them on his vessel. I submit the plan to your Excellency and ask for an early reply.[19]

By May 1862 arrivals from the South became overwhelming. There were soldiers with amputations and those "toning" up to have such surgery; those with infected wounds and other illnesses. They knew no holidays. The system was in overload and chaos.

In five days have received over 1800 sick and wounded mostly from Yorktown. 600 more expected tonight or tomorrow. The scenes I daily witness are heart rending and painful in the extreme. About 300 of those lately received were wounded severely in the battle of Williamsburg. 1000 sick of typhoid fever and the balance recovering from their wounds. Our hospitals are nearly full and I do not know how we are to provide for them properly. A large number are able to go to their homes a few days after their arrival and I have sent off over 1000 within the past 4 days. Thanks for your kind message about me to the legislature.[20]

From his office on Broadway Almy could see the "sharpers and runners" preying on the unsuspecting volunteers, charging $5 for a hack when 50 cents would do and stealing their bonus money. "I suggest that an order be issued to all of our regiments requiring them to report to me on their arrival in this city. I have made arrangements for punishing those who defraud our soldiers at no expense to the state of Connecticut." He was now boarding vessels to be the first contact for hometown boys.[21]

At the battle of Antietam the Sixteenth Regiment was decimated. Almy's report in the *Hartford Courant* claimed the death of Lt. Colonel Frank Cheney, whose actual wound was slight, although he mustered out just months later. His letter of apology followed. "Please bear in mind that this was the first authentic news received from our Connecticut regiments. I felt very badly that I had not telegraphed you more guardedly but my information seemed so inclusive and so direct that I could not question its correctness. My information was the 16th was all cut to pieces and they had lost nearly one-third of its numbers in killed and wounded."[22]

Directing a regiment to barracks for breakfast, providing steamship or train home, information about Connecticut soldiers' whereabouts and designation, recording details about the sick and wounded in New York hospitals, escorting a woman with her children to see her dying husband, providing back pay and newspapers while receiving and transporting the dead was the colonel's job.

Following the losses at the Battle of Fredericksburg, the State Legislature on December 16, 1862, authorized a committee of four to evaluate the military health care system concerning the seven Connecticut regiments who took part in that engagement and render whatever aid and assistance required. Drs. S.T. Salisbury and T.B. Townsend (the junior partner of the chief of the new army hospital in New Haven) were joined by legislators L.W. Coe and O.J. Hodge. They found that shelter tents seemed inadequate for the cold weather, rations and supplies uneven in quality and availability. The new emphasis on sending the severely injured directly to division hospitals, bypassing the regimental, seemed to be working. Teams of more experienced surgeons could evaluate and treat, getting additional consultations on the spot if necessary. The conditions and morals of the volunteers were found "better than anticipated." Lack of pay was the greatest complaint. The condition of the sick and wounded in hospitals in Washington and immediate vicinity was "very satisfactory and we are certain that a great majority are under better circumstances for speedy recovery than they would be at their own homes." They concluded that the state should appoint an agent whose duty should be to attend to the wants of soldiers in the field, reside in the city of Washington and be paid by the state.[23]

The governor took that mandate as authorization to send agents to any military hospital holding Connecticut soldiers. New York, Washington, Philadelphia, York, Jersey City, Newark, Baltimore, Annapolis, Memphis, Cairo, Chattanooga, Nashville, Lexington, Cumberland and Portsmouth Grove could expect regular visits by agents because the governor demanded frequent detailed reports. Patient's name, company, regiment, hometown, hospital, ward, bed number, diagnosis and prognosis for transfer home were to be reported. Hospital surgeons' names were useful as they allowed the governor to inquire directly about the status of individual Connecticut soldiers.

Agents' pay was $50 a month plus expenses. Dr. W. White from Fair Haven was somewhat "corpulent," according to Colonel Almy, and when in Washington stayed at the toniest place in town, the Willard Hotel where board for one week was $24, meals extra. (Privates were paid $13 a month.) The agent in Philadelphia was Robert Corson who submitted a three-month bill through December 31, 1864, for $350 "for the aid and comfort of Connecticut soldiers in hospitals in Philadelphia and elsewhere."[24] He billed for car tickets, postage stamps, stationery, tobacco, visiting hospitals, office expenses and cash for soldiers, and visiting paroled prisoners at Annapolis.

Agent C.B. Webster described his experience covering Tennessee and the environs in July 1864. The "principal wants" were tobacco, postage stamps and paper, often supplied by the Sanitary Commission which also provided vegetables and other stores for those "decidedly scorbutic." At the governor's request, Webster tried to have one Private Starkey transferred home. "He has lost his right arm but in other respects he appears in good condition and is worthy of the affection that his wife cherished for him." The surgeon did not have the authority to transfer men beyond his own department. That required an order from the secretary of war, who provided such orders for groups only and not individual cases. The agent denied a hometown newspaper account that "our men are suffering dreadfully." All patients received the same treatment; "it is absurd and untrue that Connecticut men do not receive the same care as do others. There are 20,000 patients in hospitals of Nashville and Louisville and many are suffering with amputations and infections. Some are constitutional grumblers, but the food is good and there [are] little to no complaints. The doctors are fine and they are building pavilions."

Agent W.A. Bennett noted that soldiers' clothing allowance was only $3.50 per month and that he had no clothing to give them. "We must have a fresh supply of underclothing for our soldiers. All should be furnished with warm flannels." He visited eighteen hospitals in the Washington area and 199 Connecticut soldiers, "quite a number of whom will never be able to return to duty and will probably be discharged when their condition permits them to leave the hospital."

By May 1863 the military hospital in New Haven could accommodate 550. Dr. Coggswell of Plainville and Dr. White were appointed by the state legislature to visit the sick and wounded soldiers in military hospitals and obtain discharge of those unqualified for service, while transferring those well enough to travel to the hospital in New Haven. "By an understanding with the surgeon general we hope to have as many sick and wounded of Connecticut soldiers transferred to this hospital as the buildings accommodate. Such transfers will be made with small companies as it will be impossible to give attention to individual cases."

They visited hospitals in Baltimore, Fredericksburg, Washington, Alexandria, Philadelphia, Providence, and smaller towns in New York and Pennsylvania, reporting on the quality of food, living quarters, grounds, clothing, heating capacity, sanitation, staff attitudes and professional skills.

We found many whose usefulness as soldiers was at an end. We noted immense pressure of business upon the surgeons in charge and some may have been overlooked or neglected and urge speedy transfer and elimination of *red tape.* Surgeons were employed who had never before seen a gun-shot wound or a case of camp fever. War upon a gigantic scale burst suddenly upon a country used only to peace wholly unprepared to meet the demands made upon it by the sudden gathering of such vast bodies of soldiers, casualties of battle and inevitable sickness. Surgeons have become thoroughly educated to the work at hand. The Sanitary Commission and various soldiers' aid societies have done much to alleviate the suffering of the inmates of the many hospitals.[25]

No detail was too small for the governor. Written reports were required twice monthly. Orders to investigate just one soldier's status were usual. Dr. White, stationed in Washington, was told to investigate a case in nearby Virginia: "The governor desires me to call your attention to the case of John Wellman of the 2nd Regiment who is sick in the hospital at Alexandria. His Excellency will be glad to have you afford any assistance which may in be in your power."

To Dr. White, July 9, 1863: "Charles R. Bagley of Co. E and Edwin H Eggleston of Co. B 20th Regiment Conn. Vol. are with five or six other sick and disabled soldiers at Fort Schuyler New York and desire to be transferred to the hospital at New Haven. If the way shall be open for such transfer and it can be received without injury to other good men I would like to have it made."

To Dr. Coggswell, July 7, 1863: "I learned from Dr. Jewett that a transport with sick and wounded soldiers recently arrived at New Haven and by some mistake left at the hospital forty five Massachusetts and other New England men who were designated to be ordered to Portsmouth Grove Hospital and sent sixty to that hospital who were to have been left at New Haven. You will have the goodness to go to Portsmouth Grove and see if the exchange cannot be made and give your efforts to secure that project."

To Dr. White, September 1863: "Advise me of your mission in Portsmouth and of the condition of the sick and whether you have secured the transfer of Connecticut men to New Haven. Upon your early convenience you will visit the sick in Philadelphia and while there learn as possible the condition of Peter Reed Co. H, 20th Reg. who is in West Philadelphia." (He was wounded and captured on May 3, 1863, at Chancellorsville, pardoned on May 15, 1863 and eventually discharged.)

To Dr. Coggswell in Washington, January 4, 1864: "There are reports in circulation unfavorable to the conditions of the men at the Hospital in Cumberland. You will proceed at once to that station and would enquire into the condition of the men at that place and report the results of the investigation to this office."[26]

Agent reports were not just lists of names but included graphic descriptions of desperate human conditions. Robert Corson in Philadelphia confides to the governor in February 1863, "This has been a very sad case. The man had applied for a discharge and had his application approved and the papers were in the process of being made out. Nevertheless under the present regulations these matters cannot be hurried and the unfortunate man had been disappointed once or twice in regard to the time of receiving his final papers. He had maintained a uniform cheerfulness in regard to it. Indeed there was no cause for the indulgence of any other feeling yet in the utter surprise no less than the horror of it all he was found dead, having hanged himself with a curtain cord in a retired closet. He must have labored under a temporary depression that amounted to insanity."

The spring offensive brought an onslaught of casualties reported by Agent Corson based on recent visits to six hospitals in Washington.

On my visit to Belle Plain and Fredericksburg I found long trains of ambulances awaiting their turn to have their occupants transferred to the steamers for Washington. Some of these wounded had been two nights on the passage over roads cut to pieces by supply trains and suffering from hunger and loss of blood; several died when taken out. On arrival they were furnished by the Sanitary and Christian Commission with tea, coffee, or stimulants and made comfortable as possible. I accompanied a boat load to Washington. The condition of the men at Fredericksburg I found bad although everything possible was being done by the government and commissioners owing to the pressing demand for supplies at the front. The men, many with amputated limbs were lying with nothing between them and the hard floors, even those who had blankets suffering for want of straw. Before I left supplies had begun to come in and roads were becoming better. Volunteer surgeons and nurses were arriving in large numbers and were of the greatest service. Many of those remaining were badly wounded and I fear will not recover. All the wounded that I have seen seemed cheerful even in death. There were no complaints and no regrets at having entered there [*sic*] service.[27]

As regiment after regiment marched south, Buckingham devoted time, energy and personal resources to maximize their equipment and comfort as a father would his departing son. He was present at each regiment's departure, traveling with his volunteers as far as Bridgeport and visiting them near the battlefields.

A witness recalls his accolade for his noble band of men: "Remember the government makes ample provisions for its defenders. Whatever the government provides your men are entitled to receive. See that they are thus provided. If through carelessness of officers on the higher staffs such provision is not made, do not hesitate to make your complaints until the grievance is remedied. If you cannot get redress otherwise then write me the facts fully and I will apply to the highest power in the land for you." During a visit to Washington, Buckingham told an agent, "You will see a good many battles and much suffering; don't let any Connecticut man suffer for want of anything that can be done for him; if it costs money, draw on me for it." After the battle of Gettysburg the same agent telegraphed the governor about the dead and wounded who responded "Take good care of the Connecticut men."[28]

In January 1863, the city of Philadelphia held 130 Connecticut soldiers in ten different hospitals. From October 1, 1864 for a period of six weeks, the list of Connecticut soldiers in hospitals in New York City alone came to 295 names. Governor Buckingham had promised that all Connecticut soldiers would be treated in New Haven where they would "receive the best treatment and we think no soldier can find any fault with the medical treatment which they may have received at the hands of the surgeons in this hospital."

No chief executive officer was more skilled, dedicated or effective than Governor Buckingham. He was instrumental in providing competent doctors, tending to and personally financing soldiers' needs, and providing a sanctuary in Connecticut for returning hometown troops. His efforts were duly noted on August 26, 1863, in the *New Haven Daily Palladium*.

Governor Buckingham has completed arrangements for the sick and wounded soldiers of Connecticut to be brought home and cared for instead of being left to the mercies of scattered hospitals in which they happen to fall. Officers in Connecticut regiments are to report to the Adjutant General the names and places of such soldiers in accordance with this plan.

Forty-two years later, Dr. John B. Lewis reminisced about his experiences with Governor Buckingham's effectiveness.

Prior to the war all medical supplies had been obtained through the Purveying Bureau of the army, but the rapid organization of a large volunteer force soon exhausted the purveyor's stores and in the emergency a regimental medical outfit had to be otherwise looked for. Once making the facts known to Governor Buckingham, he promptly authorized the surgeon to make liberal provision for the care of the sick and wounded of his regiment by direct purchase of articles needed before a government supply could be procured. Connecticut Volunteers were able to proceed to their destinations with adequate preparation for all exigencies. Soon the medical purvey was prepared to promptly fill all requisitions and throughout the whole war I found no difficulty in obtaining all medical supplies wanted for field or hospital use.[29]

Behind the scenes and on the front page of local newspapers, the governor was a guiding hand in dealing with the health and welfare of Connecticut's native sons. At this time, Lincoln struggled for reelection and won by a narrow margin. But as the war dragged on, Buckingham became more popular, in his election, eventually carrying every single county. In April 1865 he won by over 10,000 votes. In a rare display of humor, he attributed his victory to General Grant in a note to Jewett concerning hospital contracts: "It is reported that Grant has taken Richmond for the very purpose of influencing the Connecticut election. Should not the president propose a higher rank for him?"

If money was needed, the governor often used his own checkbook. In visits to the camps, soldiers complaining of back pay had their problem solved on the spot with his personal funds. He would even send money to family back home. Cold cash solves many problems as he wrote to hospital surgeon Bromley in Memphis, Tennessee. "I learn from Captain Galloupe who recently visited your hospital by my direction that there are now seven sick soldiers under your charges belong to the 21st Connecticut Regiment, that most of the sick will be able to leave for home and that a small allotment would be a great assistance in allowing them to obtain food suitable for their feeble condition. If they cannot be furnished enough travel rations, I take the liberty of asking you to approve for them transfer and if advisable will furnish them with a small amount say $5 each. And for each man I will enclose it by mail if you prefer to move them out."[30]

Covering so many general hospitals in so many states demanded a number of field agents, whose behavior would be carefully monitored. In July 1864, William Benedict, a new hire from Plainfield, got a specific and detailed job description with his orders.

> You are hired to act as an agent for Connecticut with power to do whatever you can for the comfort and efficiency of the troops in the service of the U.S. Your compensation will be $125 per month and necessary expenses. Proceed to Washington and make that city your headquarters. Lease a room, convenient for an office, get a secretary, and advertise. Visit sick and wounded, aid any that may properly need your assistance in obtaining furloughs, discharges or pay. Correspond with various ladies aid societies in Connecticut and distribute to Connecticut soldiers articles as may be furnished for their benefit. Keep record of your doings, make brief report of the service to this department on the 1st and 15th of each month. Keep a correct account of expenses and submit vouchers.[31]

The governor's puritanical wrath could be considerable, as a lazy and or incompetent agent would soon discover.

> It has been a month and there is no report. I hear nothing from you and know nothing of what you have been doing to secure transfers and to give information which is satisfactory either to their friends or me. You will give this subject your attention and advise me at once as to transfers which you have received within the past month. Look up the hospitals in New York, New Jersey, and Pennsylvania and keep me advised of your work as often as once in ten days. You will regard this as an essential point of your duty.[32]

Buckingham's frustration was mounting as hundreds of requests poured into his office. He advised an attorney representing the family of a hospitalized soldier far from home, "Write at once the surgeon in charge of the hospital and inquire whether he can consistently recommend his discharge. This is the only way to rescue him. I have not been able to get a man transferred to New Haven except in squads and then only when the War Department favors it important to make changes. They cannot do individual applications. It has been some time since I applied to the proper officers to have all the Connecticut sick in the Department of the South sent north and hope yet to secure their transfer." In another letter he protested, "I find it impossible to do justice to our sick and wounded soldiers."[33]

In 1864 Coggswell and White repeated their tour, which included hospitals in Florida. They noted much improvement, but perhaps through rose-tinted glasses.

> There were excellent conditions in which the General Hospitals were found as was the ability, skill and general kindness of the officials and cheerful endurance of the men themselves. No government on earth ever made as liberal provisions for its armies and especially for its sick and wounded as ours. In all wars there must be of necessity be much of unavoidable sufferings, but here as little exists as ever did in any war due to liberal provisions of the Government and the twin sisters of civilization and humanity — the Sanitary and Christian commissions — who robbed the war of half its horrors and the battle field the hospital and even the bed of dying soldiers is rendered comparatively comfortable and happy. No soldiers in the Union army are better cared for than ours and no other state has as great a proportion of their sick and wounded within their own borders for treatment and restoration to health as Connecticut.[34]

The governor was inundated with requests from job seekers, soldiers, their family and elected officials for transfer to the hospital in New Haven, medical furloughs or discharge, back pay, bounties, promotions, and relief from the charge of desertion. In 1864 he issued a detailed printed document listing duties assigned to others and not his jurisdiction. Paymaster General Fitch in New Haven handled all bounties. Promotions were decided by the officers of the regiment. Discharges and furloughs were the province of regimental colonels with approval of the general of the army corps. Medical discharge required approval by the regimental surgeon or the surgeon in charge of the hospital. The Medical Board appointed army surgeons.

> As I have no authority to discharge a soldier or to grant or extend a furlough and as my time will not allow an investigation of the many applications, I feel obliged to refer all persons interested to the officers above named. Drs. Jewett, Cogsell and White will enable transfer of many disabled Connecticut Volunteers to New Haven. That hospital will not accommodate all but I have reasons to believe that transfers can be made to an extent equal to its capacity. This subject that is of so much interest to the sick and their friends shall have my earnest attention, but the surgeon general cannot attend to individual cases or consent to a transfer except in squads from one hospital.[35]

This document to the contrary, Buckingham was directly involved in all aspects of the soldiers' welfare and especially the sick and wounded whose pleas flooded his office.

The past employer of Charles Brayton of the Eighteenth Regiment asked for his transfer from a hospital in Annapolis to New Haven, where his wife and child resided. He sustained a fractured femur from a Minié ball in June 1864 and was first treated by the rebels, leaving him with a leg two inches short that requiring crutches for him to ambulate. He was transferred to the Veterans Reserve Corps (VRC) in April 1865 and discharged disabled in December 1865.[36]

Henry Thompson of the Seventeenth Regiment sustained a gunshot wound of the right arm at Gettysburg and was in a hospital at Hilton Head for fifteen months. "My arm is not yet healed nor will it ever in this climate and the Doctors say that I never will have the use of it. Could I have a transfer to New Haven or a discharge?" He was transferred to the VRC.[37]

Chauncy Park of the Fourteenth Regiment was wounded in the shoulder by a Minié ball at Fredericksburg in December 1862 and was a patient at Knight hospital, where the ball was extracted. The wound healed and Park was discharged five months later. The agent hired to obtain bounties wrote the inquiry. "He needs the bounty due him $75, but the reason for disability was not stated. Jewett refused to sign letter about that. Will you governor? He is a laboring man and has a family to support." He was discharged disabled May 1863.[38]

William Strange of the Thirteenth Regiment wrote from the Chestnut Hill Hospital in Philadelphia. "I have two fingers amputated and have lost the use of two more in the right hand. I want transfer to New Haven. I have a wife and family near there I wish to hear from them soon. My hand is no good so I can go home as soon as you do this for me." He was transferred to the VRC three months later.[39]

Charles Crane of the Twelfth Regiment pleaded his situation from the same hospital a month later. "Will you please notice the request of a poor soldier? I have had my limb broken and now it is out of place and my health is very poor. My Doctor advised me to address you a few lines and ask you if you would please inform the Surgeon in charge here and have me transferred to Connecticut. I live near New Haven. It has been over two years since I was home. As it is it will be some time before I will be able for duty."[40] He got his wish and was discharged ten months later.

Harvey Hancock was in a hospital for several months in Virginia recovering from an "accidental" gunshot wound to the hand in February 1864 while in New Bern. He was discharged in June 1865. "I am in the hospital with nothing to do. I thought I would write to you and ask if I could not get transferred to the Invalid Corps at New Haven. The ball passed through my right hand and disformed my hand so that I can't shut it. I have had to lose one of my fingers from the wound and I have done no duty since. It is very lonesome here lying around with nothing to do to pass the time. I think I could do duty in the second bitallion [*sic*] invalid corps and it would not seem half as hard as laying around here doing nothing. If I was able to do duty here I should not ask this favor."[41]

Ben Brown of the Eleventh Regiment was wounded twice in a four-year tour of duty, the last time at the Battle of Petersburg. He made this plea three months later. He was transferred to the VRC and discharged in November 1865.

Dear friend. I set my self down to write you a few lynes to ask you if there hant some away that I can git to my own state hospital. I am in a hospital where there is all rebils prisoners and I am wounded in the head and have had ten pieses of scull taken out of my head and its is very bad yet and I would lyke to git two my one state if it's a possible thing and if you will teel me how ican git there I will thank you very much for your kindness to me and I have ben in the service three years and I have down my Duty and if you can do eny thing for me I wish that you wood. Will close for this time co good by.[42]

Wounds that would not heal or those with amputations meant walking with crutches if at all. "I am wounded in the right ankle so I am not able to walk without crutches." "I would like to be transferred home where I could be of use to whatever you see proper to put me at." "I have a gunshot wound through my left shoulder. Can you do anything for me, please let me know." Such were the pained and frightened voices of those who bore the brunt of war.

George Brigham of the Fourteenth Regiment was promoted from private to first lieutenant and wounded twice, and became a prisoner in between. In January 1865 his father wrote the governor, an old friend, about getting his son a job. Buckingham wrote Surgeon

General Barnes about the several battles in which he had participated: Antietam, Chancellorsville and Gettysburg. Accommodation was made and the favor granted. He was discharged disabled in December 1865.

> His wound, which he supposed by this time when he was with you last would be almost if not entirely well, had troubled him exceedingly this week and upon examination by a surgeon more pieces of bone were taken from it which prevents him from very active service. It is quite a trial for him as his heart was fixed to return and do all that was in his power to help finish up the evil which has brought to our beloved land so much sorrow and suffering. It is the opinion of his physician and friends at Rockville that he will never be free from trouble with the wound in his limb. There are positions in the army he could fill such as quartermaster so that he could ride and thus favor his limb. Anything you can do to aid him — we will consider it a great favor for any service you can render.[43]

Citizens from Buckingham's hometown got more than a passing notice. A letter from the governor in February 1863 sought a return home for Private George Huntington of the Fourteenth Regiment, a fellow resident of Norwich. "He is in the hospital under your charge and has been sick most of the time since he entered the service. May I ask you to examine into his condition and see whether this is a case in which the further interests will be promoted if you recommend a discharge." Surgeon Bauds responded,

> He has been an inmate of this hospital since August 1862 when he mustered in. There has not been much the matter with him during his stay here save an attack of the mumps. He is now about ready to return to duty. The only grounds on which he could be discharged would be *under age.* Unfortunately he is now under charge of desertion of his company commander having reported him to this hospital as a deserter asking that he be returned under guard. While this charge is against him he cannot be discharged nor receive pay. I will have to return him to duty that he may if possible clear himself of the accusation.[44]

Huntington was transferred to a reserve corps shortly thereafter and discharged with disability two months later.

Surgeon Vanderkluper, in charge at a hospital in Smoke Town, Maryland, was queried by the governor in March 1863 about two hometown constituents. Adams was from East Windsor and Chamberlain from Norwich. Both were discharged disabled in April 1863.

> Henry Adams and George Chamberlain of the 16th Regiment were wounded at Antietam rendering them unfit for duty and to be discharged from the service. The mothers of these soldiers have been attending them during their confinement in this hospital and holding themselves in readiness to go home. I request they be provided with transportation to their respective homes.

Surgeon Charles Carleton of the Eighteenth Regiment reported on two other Norwich sons while apologizing for not answering sooner due to his "poor health" (pulmonary tuberculosis) and "arduous duty" in March 1863.

> Private Thomas had typhoid fever and was in the hospital for six weeks. He had slight affliction with rheumatism, was free from pain but weak. I see no reason why he will not yet make a good soldier. Charles Lynch is in a hospital under another surgeon who thinks he will remain. If on his return to the regiment I think him unfit for military duty I shall discharge him.
>   Dr. Hough has resigned as I think you know and I am greatly in need of a 2nd assistant surgeon. I have not sufficient strength for the work I am obliged to do now. I have worked twelve hours today, Sunday. Some days, I have more to do than this. Here's hoping that you will remain "Our governor."

Thomas died in June 1863 and Lynch completed his tour of duty in June 1865.
Some soldiers were unable to send money home to their dependents. The governor

received numerous letters from dependent parents, wives, and children of volunteers. Mothers whose children served in out-of-state regiments were by law not eligible for state benefits; "There is no law in this state which extends aid to the *mothers* of soldiers,"[45] he wrote. That is not to say he did not provide for them regardless.

Mrs. C. M. Garrett made a case for transferring her son, wounded in September 1862, paroled as a prisoner and in an Annapolis hospital: "He needs to get home to his poor sick mother. He tried to get a furlough but all in vain. I am sick and need him and if you can do anything to relieve our necessities I do beg and pray that you will. He is my oldest son. His father died soon after he went in the army."[46] He was discharged in March 1863.

Mary Keith sought to have her son John transferred because of chronic diarrhea. "He is very feeble and unless something is done for him immediately I fear he will be past help. I can see him and give him those little attentions by way of nursing that would I trust soon restore him to health and active duty where as if left where he is will soon be past help and be sacrificed as to many of our noble young men are." He had enlisted in November 1861 and reenlisted December 1863. He was discharged in August 1865. No action was taken.

Mrs. H.M. Hopkins described her son suffering from "mumps, measles, and chronic diarrhea and the hardships of marching. His emaciated constitution has become so much shattered by sickness and hardships that he will never be able to endure service in the army. Can he receive discharge from where he is or if not be transferred to New Haven. It would be very gratifying to us to have him nearer home."[47]

The governor, responding to a mother's plea, wrote the hospital surgeon at Fort Monroe, Virginia, concerning Daniel Hayden of the First Connecticut Artillery. Three different hospitals reported and none had any evidence of his existence. He was later listed as a deserter.

> I am informed by the Surgeon of the 1st Connecticut Artillery that he is not fit to be a soldier on account of general debility. I ask you to examine and determine if his condition is such as to justify the opinion of Surgeon Skinner that you recommend his discharge. He is the son of a widower enlisted while under age without her consent.[48]

Mary Wilson felt her nursing care was the best medicine for her son George of the Eighteenth Regiment and offered to take him home if discharged. He had been captured at Winchester. He was pardoned a month later, in July 1863, and mustered out in May 1865.[49]

> My son is sick in the Hospital at New Haven and he has been treated by a band of Doctors and they say he is not able as he has got the chest dyseas and he has been sent from one hospital to another for the last years. He is my only. The Doctor think if I could get him home he would get better. I cudd take better care of him than they did there. There is no money and he is 18 years old and will have been in the army two years. He has had a low presence and found his health poor. I have cited that you cudd give him dysabilty and wished you wood do it as soon as possible.

A selectman described a soldier's "mother dying of cancer with two sons, one served 1 years in the other still in the field. Can the one in the army be sent home before she dies?"

Another selectman requests discharge for Charles Barley of the Fifth Regiment, who was on short furlough and then returned to duty. "The father is an old and almost helplessly decrepit man with a large family on his hands and is very poor. He has but one other son. He is also in the army and has been from the first. He assures me that he must have his son Henry here to lean upon for support or call upon the town." He served four years, mustering out in May 1865.

Charles H. Gary describes his son as a "consumptive" who "does not feel able to do military duty. I am an invalid, my wife and daughters are entirely dependent upon this young man. If he is drafted and forced to go we are completely broken and at the same time he will not be of any service to the government. He is totally unfit." He served out his nine-month tour without a hitch.[50]

Ellsworth Russell of the Second Regiment Heavy Artillery felt he was not doing well in a hospital in Philadelphia. "I have been pretty sick. The Doctor said that I had the consumption. I have spell of spitting blood. I spit 5 quarts in a week so the Doctor said that I would not live long but I hope that I shall. I cannot do any duty. If I do it will make me spit blood again the doctor said that I might outgrow it if I keep still. I should like to get to my own state whare I might be nearer home for I am home sick hear and I want to give most anything to get. I have got good many friends thare and my folks could come and see me often. If you would get me transfurd I be very much obliged." He had enlisted February 1864 and was discharged June 1865.

David Jennings of the Second Connecticut Heavy Artillery was sick in a hospital in Rhode Island with a broken and poor family to care for. "My wife died last May and left five small children and no one to see to them but one of the neighboring men and he wishes me to get a furlow to come home to see about getting them some places to live. I am a poor man without influence and the nabors can no longer offer their home and I apply to your honor to assist me to get a furlow to get home to see about providing a place for my five motherless children." He served out his tour, ending in August 1865.

Henry Dunbar of the Twenty-first Regiment was not entitled to discharge, according to his surgeon, because of a functional derangement of the heart due to tobacco and alcohol. His wife thought otherwise. "He is not well and has not been for some time. He has the heart disease and liver complaint besides he is ruptured badly. He also has two brothers in the service. He also has a widowed mother and two small children that need his help. I think this will suffice." He served out his three-year tour and was discharged disabled in May 1865.

Lydia Gatel of Lebanon lamented her fate. "I don't know if my husband is alive or dead and have not heard from him in a long time. I have no money and in no condition to get any. I would like some assistance if it can be had."[51] Another wife reported that her husband had reenlisted and then disappeared without a trace, leaving her family in desperation.

Soldiers wrote they were "sick with little improvement in health," or "ill," "unfit for duty and will be for some time," suffered with a "sick headache," "climate does not suit me," and requested transfer, furlough or discharge. Some complained that the hospital food was poor and the portions were too small! An anonymous soldier confided from a hospital in faraway Rhode Island, "We are not allowed to buy anything to eat for our own comfort and all that we get to eat is a little piece of salt beef and a half a slice of bread for breakfast and for dinner half a pint of soup and a small piece of bread and very poor at that and for supper two small potatoes a little salt beef and the same quantity of bread and half a pint of coffee. Other state soldiers get transferred out why does not little Connecticut do the same."[52]

The governor wrote the provost marshal of Hartford concerning Private John Kerr of the Veterans Reserve Corps. "He has been in a feeble condition for a long time. I would respectfully ask that he may be examined and as whether his physical condition is not such that the interests of the service would be promoted by his discharge." Major Jewett promptly examined him and recommended discharge in August 1864. He had been captured in June 1863, was paroled a month later and transferred to the VRC in March 1864.

A similar letter was penned to the surgeon of a large hospital in New York. "There are many Connecticut soldiers under your charge who were ordered to Connecticut but were detained in New York because the hospital in New Haven was full the time they arrived in New York. They were of course disappointed and if not inconsistent with the vested interests of the service I want to respectfully suggest that they receive a furlough with orders to report to the hospital in New Haven." The surgeon correctly replies, "I have no authority to furlough in the mode suggested but that the Connecticut patients will be transferred as rapidly as beds become vacant at New Haven. There are a large number of Connecticut patients to be transferred."[53]

The governor was also aware of the rules and regulations and often claimed having no authority in those cases he deemed nondeserving. Amongst the many pleas and requests was the all-too-common need to transfer the deceased home. The governor asked Stanton for such assistance concerning "a highly loyal citizen of Connecticut who lost her husband at Antietam and was desirous of the remains to be sent to the state to reside permanently."

A mourning father asked to retrieve his dead son buried at the Wilderness. "If you could just do what lay in your power for a broken hearted father, the Lord would then agree that I have given my sons to help to subdue the rebellion and I have lost two of them all good along with their father. One of my sons was killed at the battle of Rappahannock Station November 7, 1863. We got his body home and if only his brother could be buried at his side I could give them up and feel more content, but I cannot live long if I cannot get his body home." The War Department responded, "All the necessary permits will be granted upon personal application at this office, accompanied by proof of loyalty and identity. The orders of the Secretary of War however forbade passes to be issued to more than one person to procure the same body."[54]

A father tried to visit his wounded son in a Chattanooga hospital but "was not allowed to go any further. I would most earnestly with the feeling of a father like a pass to see my suffering son who has periled his life for our common country or if it not in your power to do so, invest yourself that I might get a pass."

The father of Lieutenant Jayson Snyder applied all the way to the secretary of war for a pass to see a badly wounded son with an amputated leg December 1862. "He desires a pass to see his son in Fredericksburg, to administer to his wants. Knowing he is a true and loyal man I am asking for a pass."[55]

Providing for so many in need through a new federal medical system demanded the best physicians available.

CHAPTER SIX

Regimental Surgeon

At the onset of war, 58 percent of the soldiers in the army of the Potomac had no preenlistment physical exam. Only 9 percent had a thorough inspection before, during, or after being mustered in. Fifty-three percent of those discharged with disability had the condition prior to enlistment. An 1861 Sanitary Commission report by A. J. Phelps declared that "feeble boys, toothless old men, consumptives, asthmatics, one-eyed, one-armed men, men with different leg lengths, club-footed and ruptured, and in short, men with a variety of disability, and whose systems were replete with the elements of disease were accepted as recruits and started to the field only to become a tax upon the government, and to encumber the movements of its armies."[1] In the last three months of 1961, there were 4,000 medical discharges of which 3,000 were for preexisting conditions.

In August 1861, the secretary of the Sanitary Commission, Frederick Law Olmstead, discussed the importance of pre-induction examinations with the governor. "We need perfectly sound, tough and strong men to endure the privation, fatigue and exposure. Inspection of recruits has been very inadequate. Men who cannot lose a meal or two without becoming ill and disheartened, and men who when slightly indisposed need domestic comforts and tender care are of no use as soldiers and but impede."[2]

Part of the problem was the inexperience and capability of army doctors. They served as gatekeepers, exercising critical judgment as to who was able and who was not. The Sanitary Commission's report on regimental surgeons early in the war indicated need for improvement. "The Surgeons of 176 out of 200 regiments were sufficiently well qualified; four were incompetent, and thirteen of doubtful competence. In seven regiments, no surgeon was present. One hundred twenty-nine Regimental Surgeons were not only competent but have discharged their duties with creditable energy and earnestness, twenty-five with tolerable attentiveness; ten have been negligent and inert. For twenty-seven surgeons no distinct opinion is expressed."[3]

There were regimental surgeons who had never seen an operation, much less held a scalpel. Some had never gone to medical school, much less graduated. Of the first six Connecticut regiments, one "surgeon" was actually a dentist and another an apothecary. They were appointed based on popularity and political connections rather than competence. In

May 1862 the newly appointed thirty-three-year-old Surgeon General William Hammond ordered preinduction testing for all doctors by a certified medical board appointed in each state. Army surgeons were the only officers required to prove competency by taking written and oral exams prior to induction. Politically appointed generals whose main virtue was family prominence and/or ability to get votes were allowed to lead thousands of men into battle with often disastrous consequences. The Connecticut legislature passed a resolution on May 22, 1861, seconded by the medical society, *one year* before Hammond's national decree.

> In compliance with request of the governor, the Connecticut Medical Society should designate a small number of the profession who should act as an advisory Board in future appointments of Surgeons and Assistant Surgeons to the Connecticut Volunteers. Whereas, the fact of an impending war exists which may be both prolonged and calamitous and whereas this convention regard the health, comfort and well-being of the force of this state to depend very largely upon the qualifications of its Medical Staff: and whereas none can so well ascertain from the very nature of the case the qualifications of those who apply for the position of Surgeons or assistant surgeons as their peers, the Physicians and Surgeons of the State represented in this Convention appoint a board of medical men so that none but the best and most competent will be able to secure the officers in question.[4]

The need for an effective medical hierarchy with a chief of staff was obvious. On May 6, 1861, Pliny Jewett applied to the governor for this position and without salary if need be. Like many others who volunteered to leave their homes and jobs, this doctor was willing to sacrifice his considerable private practice to serve.

> Since our conversation in Hartford as to organization of the Hospital staff of the different regiments; it would be well for you to appoint someone as surgeon in chief whose duty it should be to attend under your direction to the proper organization of the medical and hospital staffs. To see that they are properly supplied with instruments, medicines, etc. to assist the mustering officer in the inspection of recruits etc. If on reflection you should think it best to make an appointment of this sort, I wish to offer my services *gratuitously*. I am aware that it will occupy a great portion of my time; but still as I am so situated as not to be able to offer my services in another capacity, I am willing to make the sacrifice.[5]

A week later the dean of the medical school, Worthington Hooker, recommended another candidate, Jonathan Knight. He recognized the importance of teaching "medical and surgical care which is due to our solders in hospitals." A systematic approach by a man with experience "would be a great relief to you with all your other duties and would be effective in providing properly for the care of our soldiers." Two recent medical school graduates enlisted as common soldiers with the idea "that they might if necessity required, aid the surgeon in his duties." He recommended following the plan of New York where each regiment had 1,010 enlisted men and officers with one surgeon and two assistant surgeons. The governor realized this demanding job required stamina and perseverance better suited to a younger man rather than one older and more venerable.[6]

The fire of patriotism burned brightly amongst the medical society of Hartford County. All but one physician signed a petition offering assistance and several sent letters requesting medical service in the army. They would make the same sacrifices made by thousands of volunteers, leaving behind family, home, and profession along with welfare, safety and comfort.

A committee was formed of practicing physicians from each of the eight counties. The medical board's actual work was conducted by three doctors from Hartford, New Haven and New London seeking "none but the best and most competent." Competition from non-traditional health care providers had always been an issue and efforts were made to keep them out. As early as 1857, Jewett sponsored the following at the CMS proceedings: "It is resolved on motion of Dr. Jewett that William Sage of Unionville be expelled from this Society under the by-law which makes it the duty of the Medical Society to expel any member *notoriously* in the practice of homeopathy, hydropath, or any other form of quackery." The resolution was unanimously adopted and passed, expelling Sage from the society. A second motion by Dr. Jewett also passed: "that the several county meetings be requested to investigate the subject of members of this Society consulting with irregular practitioners, and enforce the by-law in such case made and provided." Doing commerce with the non-traditional health care providers would not be tolerated.[7]

Gurdon Russell was forty-six years old, a Hartford native, and a graduate of Trinity College (1834) and Yale Medical College (1837). He was a founder of Hartford Hospital and of the Hartford Medical Society, the president of the CMS, and the first medical director of the Aetna Insurance Company, a post he held for fifty years. He chaired the Committee on Delinquent Members and wrote, "If you don't pay dues, out!" When asked by Dr. Lindsley in 1865 to address Yale medical students at graduation, Russell asked that his name not be advertised, as he claimed not to have a lot to say: "I agree to address the graduating class but do *not* publish. I do not see that anything special would be gained by its publication."[8]

He had a distinguished appearance, with a gray beard and full head of hair, an intellect and temperament to match. He practiced into his seventies and died at age ninety-four. He was childless, and his life insurance listed the state medical society as beneficiary. He was an excellent judge of people with a rare ability to get them to work together and resolve issues, a talent which served him well on committees.[9] Descriptions of him noted that he was "interested in knowledge of men and affairs, possessed of unfailing tact, unselfish honesty, and fond of history."[10]

His quiet elegance was a counterpoint to Pliny Jewett, who was about the same age. Jewett was physically imposing, autocratic, positive in his opinions, forceful in their expression and vehement in their defense. In 1857 both Russell and Jewett were appointed to the committee to receive reports and examine biographical notices of deceased members for the past year and to the Standing Committee on Publication to which all communications would be referred from the several counties. They had worked well together before and performed most of the medical board's work.

The third judge was Dr. Ashbel Woodward, age fifty-seven, born in Willington,

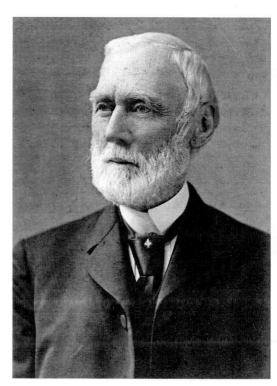

Gurdon Russell, M.D., 1815–1909, circa 1897 (Hartford Medical Society Historical Library, University of Connecticut Health Center, Farmington).

Connecticut. His ancestors had arrived in America in the seventeenth century. Woodward graduated from Bowdoin College Medical Department in May 1829 and later earned a second medical degree from Yale Medical School at the end of the Civil War. He was president of the Connecticut Medical Society from 1858 through 1861, a devout Christian and deacon, collected rare books, and wrote a two-volume biography on General Nathaniel Lyons that was published in 1862.[11]

In 1860, he addressed the Connecticut Medical Society's convention on medical ethics. He felt that the press and public unfairly censured and criticized doctors and that it was self-evident that a medical association should exclude those who openly violated its laws. He regretted there was no "coercive power" or "penal consequences" for breaking ethics statutes. His speech enumerated the difficulties of being a doctor. Even if one survived disease exposure, one might face the fevered wrath and impossible expectations of the public when things do not turn out well. Neverending work and thankless charity was the doctor's lot. Given one year prior to the onset of the Civil War, his address offers a prescient vision of what war would demand. Valor, self-sacrifice, exposure to life-threatening hardships, duty, honor, and nobility would be essential qualities for the military surgeon. "Instead of the tumultuous swell of music he hears the moans of the dying! Instead of gay pennons he sees the coffin and the crape: instead of the triumphal march, solitary hearses hurrying the dead to the grave."[12]

He advocated considering the whole patient, not merely focusing on an organ or disease, a potential problem with the new fields of specialization. In considering just the eyes or lungs, for example, one "misses the total picture."

At age fifty-seven, he volunteered as a regimental surgeon of the Twenty-sixth Connecticut Volunteers. He mustered in November 1862 and mustering out, along with the rest of the regiment, nine months later. Admiral Farragut seized Port Hudson, Louisiana, in May 1863 with this gray-headed surgeon at his side. Woodward was later promoted to medical director of the Gulf Department with the rank of major. Suffering a long and difficult bout with malaria, he returned home to recuperate that summer.

He wrote a dissertation while still on the field of battle that was published in the *Proceedings of the Connecticut Medical Society*, May 28, 1863. Entitled "Vindication of Army Surgeons," it describes the trials and tribulations of the army doctor and his role in society:

> The charges of incompetence brought against the medical officers connected with our Volunteer forces, have been reiterated loudly and often. A majority of the younger members of the profession have been educated in excellent schools, and enjoyed the advantages of observation and study in the best-appointed hospitals. Extensive acquaintance with the theory and practice of medicine is now required by our medical schools as an essential preliminary to graduation. The standard both of professional and general culture among the present physicians of the country is unquestionably high.[13]

He decried the lack of rigor in medical education just a few years earlier, along with deficiencies in ethical and moral training. He was a witness of these young men on the field of battle and could vouch for their hard, effective work and sacrifice.

> No small number of the most skillful and honored members of the profession have been constrained by motives of patriotism and humanity to leave the enjoyments and profits of domestic life to minister to our suffering soldiers in the field. Few men of wide experience with families to support can afford to exchange the lucrative practice of large cities for the comparatively small compensation paid to surgeons in the government service.

Overseeing the medical board was the fair-minded governor, whose goal was finding the best support for his state's soldiers. He was intimately involved with the creation of Connecticut's regiments and was personally connected and committed to officers, enlisted men and doctors alike. He wrote to the secretary of war during the peninsular campaign, "If during siege or anticipated battle of Yorktown or at any other point the army should require additional surgical aid, I will be pleased to send forward good experienced surgeons for temporary service on receiving notice by telegraph."

The first meeting of the medical board was held July 26, 1861, in the Allyn House in Hartford. In attendance were Jewett, Russell and Woodward to appoint two regimental surgeons. Initially only state residents could apply. A month later eleven candidates were interviewed and nine appointed. Subsequent meetings were held in New Haven at the Tontine Hotel and then at the army hospital as it became established. Flow charts outlined in red were made listing the surgeon, first assistant and second assistant, which by 1863 supplied eighteen regiments.[14] Written recommendations were forwarded to the governor, who had final say. He advised but never overruled.

In April 1862 Dr. Jewett wrote the governor, "I enclose a list of surgeons who have consented to act as volunteers in Virginia in case of necessity. They are all *good men* and *true*. I shall be glad to do anything in my power to assist in forming a corps of volunteer surgeons from this state. I have already tendered my own services and they have been conditionally accepted by the surgeon general. I am visiting Norwich on the 19th and would like to visit with you personally."[15] Buckingham did not attend the board's meetings but met often with Jewett and seemed to have a personal as well as professional relationship with him.[16]

What were the criteria for a successful army surgeon? Dr. Jonathan Knight had terminal rectal cancer and had but one year left when he penned his recommendation for a recent (1862) Yale medical graduate, J. W. Terry. Half a century of medical practice and illness had altered his once bold to now tremulous writing, but not his incisive intellect.

> He is a modest unassuming young man of gentlemanly habits and unblemished character as a student and diligent and successful and familiar with the principles of his profession. He has worked in a hospital in New Haven for months — faithful and skill full. The officers of the institution were confident in him when given care of patients. The experience which he acquired here in taking care of the sick and wounded soldiers prepared him to perform the duties of an army surgeon. I have no doubts of his fitness to perform the duties of a regimental surgeon.[17]

Henry Stearns of Hartford was another Yale graduate (1850s) who also studied in Paris, London and Edinburgh for two years. He was house physician for the Retreat of the Insane under the direction of Dr. John Butler, who described the character and requirements of an army surgeon. His analysis of job and candidate presaged a remarkable three years of duty for Stearns.

> He is a delightful fellow, well grounded, posted up on the advances, and fully competent. He is unassuming with sound judgment, calm, judicious, intelligent and resolute. More men are killed or disabled by the neglect of hygiene, bad or insufficient food, good food badly cooked, needless exposure, bad air, bad location or arrangement of camp or quarters and the fevers and disorders consequent upon this neglect than by the gun and sword. Not an old man, not a larger practical experience but old men even if they would take this position would be poorly fitted for the arduous duties of such a post. I am a warm friend of this young surgeon.[18]

Dr. Thomas Miner of Hartford recommended J.B. Lewis because he "understands his business and loves it." The candidate's credentials were excellent: he was a graduate of New

York University Medical School with eight years of practice under his belt. His mentor stressed the importance of sanitation and general medical knowledge.

> The surgeon will find much to do to keep him off the sick list and free from the complaints incident to an entire change of living and climate. He should be a man of large experience in medicine as well as surgery. It is the whole duty that does not consist just "cutting off legs and arms" but he should be also able to suggest those prophylactic means that are conducive to health.[19]

Descriptions of being "a thorough gentleman," "well read," an "efficient practitioner of guaranteed ability" or "accomplished professional and general scholar" did not automatically lead to approval. L.S. Pease made his case in an unorthodox manner to his hometown governor: "I have been fifteen years in a successful practice and can send recommendations. I will recall a circumstance of early practice which may illicit [*sic*] your interest. I had the satisfaction of adjusting the dislocated shoulder of your venerable father." He was appointed and later promoted. Dr. Curtis of Hartford described Pease as a "careful, correct and humane man."

Some claimed prior military experience in the Crimean War (1853), the Mexican War (1846) or the Seminole Indian War in Florida (1835). Their age and experience ranged from medical cadet to senior citizen. Jewett writes Russell in October 1861:

> I do not like the stand taken by the governor before the medical board saying positively that we should not appoint Dr. Leavenworth. I shall not consent to examine any more candidates for surgeon until the present list is used up. There is too much red tape in this to suit me. I consider the whole thing an insult to the profession and especially to the medical board.[20]

In April 1861, 65-year-old Dr. Leavenworth applied to become regimental surgeon of the Fourth Regiment of Volunteers. He felt "entitled" due to his age and experience. "I am senior to most of the gentleman constituting the medical board but I should rather solicit than avoid an examination." He acknowledged a "pecuniary" need to support his family, namely a sister and her offspring, but was rejected. Dr. Jewett pleaded on his behalf, advising the governor, "He has lost his property and is now poor, with a deceased brother, and family to support. He is well qualified to act as surgeon. His medical and surgical acquirements are good and in addition he has a large experience in the army having been in actual service for some ten or fifteen years in Florida and elsewhere." He was offered the lesser position of assistant surgeon of the Twelfth Regiment and was sent to Mississippi in the fall of 1861, stationed outside New Orleans. By November 1862 he was dead. Surgeon Brownell reported to the governor, "His health has been very feeble the whole summer and I could see that unless he returned home he could not long survive. His unit went on detail and he was to work at a hospital. He died very easily and of no particular disease working the day before he died. The cause of death was the "debility incident of his age."

Why expose a man this age to southern diseases to which younger men had succumbed, not to mention the general hardships of military life? Dr. Leavenworth graduated from Yale Medical School in 1817, having apprenticed under Eli Ives and Jonathan Knight of New Haven. A botanical garden was established at Yale in 1817. Dr. Leavenworth was sent forth to make a collection of indigenous plants for this garden, soon believed to be the best in country. Due to lack of funds it was abandoned, but not without gratitude for the effort. Leavenworth toured the South to study botany and entered the drug business in Georgia for four years. As an assistant surgeon in the U.S. Army, he was stationed in Florida for the next eleven years and was in government practice during the Seminole War. He returned to Waterbury, Connecticut, in 1842 to practice, "but he never seemed quite contented and seemed to long for the free social enjoyments and intercourse incident to camp life." He had "spotless integrity and purity of character" but never married. He supported his sister's children and orphans.[21] Dr. Jewett had tried to honor the wishes of a Dr. Knight apostle rather than appoint by intrinsic merits. Legacy issues and political correctness could not trump needs for the best interests of the service.

Frederick Dudley was an apothecary in New Haven for four years with just one term at Yale Medical College when he was successfully supported for assistant surgeon by Dr. T.B. Townsend and Pliny Jewett, who added "I cheerfully concur with Dr. Townsend. He has been a student in our office for a few months."

Other candidates claimed only brief experience as a hospital steward as justification to applying for position of surgeon. Andrew Gibson, a private, served in that capacity for the Fifth Connecticut Volunteers. Surgeon Brunette described him as "gentlemanly, temperate and kind to the sick. Of his ability as physician and surgeon I have no opportunity to judge." Gibson also claimed to have been steward of a hospital staff in Frederick, Maryland, and that the Medical Board had assured him of the position of assistant surgeon especially in view of "the sacrifice I made at the call of my country, services rendered, and privations endured. I am poor with a wife and two children and have not been paid for a year. To take exams cost two months' salary and the money was borrowed." He was not appointed.

The motives to apply for surgeon included need for a paying job, patriotism, desire for adventure, and perhaps an attempt to find meaning in life. The consideration "in these crises every man should so do something for his country" or "being a professional physician and surgeon with considerable experience" were valid but no guarantee for a job. Nor was "intimate acquaintance with all diseases of camp and their successful treatment" or "my reputation as a physician in this place for the last twelve years will perhaps entitle me to your Excellency's consideration at the earliest possible moment," or "I do not seek a place for compensation however much I may need it."

At first a flood of candidates appeared. Upon the advice of the adjutant general, the governor ordered public notice given as to when the medical board convened so all who desired could present their case. "You will consult with Dr. Russell and ascertain what time will be convenient for him to call a meeting of the medical board. You will then advertise the same giving notice three or four weeks before the time fixed up."[22] This increased the board's work, as on August 8, 1862, a dozen candidates appeared, only half of whom could be adequately examined. A second session was held a week later.

The governor was inundated with requests from elderly or infirm "doctors" along with recommendations from regimental commanders for their favorite candidates. The regimental commander of the Ninth Volunteers protested in September 1861, "I spoke to your Excellency with reference to the appointment of a surgeon and mentioned Dr. Gallagher of this city. I feel very anxious with sufferance to this matter and have induced the doctor to make an application for an examination. I can fully vouch for the doctor's *character* and *standing* in *every* sense as a gentleman and a citizen and he is quite ready to stand his examination. I am very far from being satisfied with either the moral character of or the medical ability of the man whom Dr. Jewett of this city has said we must have. I cannot understand why we must have him on any ground of benefit to the public service. I know about the man whom he has recommended. I do not want him on any time."

By advertising in the newspapers, the governor could now deflect all these appointment requests to the medical board, whose approval was mandatory. He might suggest a candidate or even discourage one from applying further, since the board's decision was final: "I would say however that there are many applications for the positions," or "I will advise you if I can fill the vacancy but it is doubtful," or "Contact the medical board which meets next month."

Some surgeons were dispatched south before there was a medical board and were ordered to take an exam back home or by the regular army board in Washington or Philadelphia. Some commanders sent telegrams indicating dire circumstances for regiments left with no medical coverage. The exam itself was anxiety-provoking for some, especially the more senior who had no book learning for years. Surgeon Samuel Skinner was forty-two and a Yale graduate who required prodding by his commanding officer Colonel Robert Tyler of the First Regiment C.V. Heavy Artillery. He passed, advancing from regimental to divisional headquarters as a colonel in a distinguished career. "Surgeon Skinner was somewhat reluctant to stand his examination as you requested but an intimation from me that he will otherwise be obliged to take an army board has I think decided him to try it at home. I would prefer that he would accept the army examination as the state board if it finds him deficient can do nothing while the army board can recommend that he be discharged. One would think that the inducements of pay and position held out by the service ought to receive a superior class of medical officers. I confess I have no desire to see any further appointments into the regiment unless practitioners can be found of education more liberal and experienced and more extended than those whom I find with the regiment."[23]

Colonel J. Hawley of the Seventh Regiment sent exasperated messages from Hilton Head, South Carolina, concerning Assistant Surgeon Hines' order to take medical board examination. "No request to attend sessions received here. We have as yet no surgeon. I cannot possibly spare either of the assistant surgeons. Ought his devotion to duty to stand in the way of his advancement? It is the sickly season with possible yellow fever cases so can't spare Hines to go north for an exam."

Even religion might play a role. Dr. Nathan Mayer was the son of a rabbi. This had no deleterious effect on his application or career. Dr. H.L. Hewitt of Bridgeport had prior experience as an army surgeon in the Mexican War and declared that "All of my ancestors have served the state. I volunteer and will take such position as my qualities may seem entitled to." A letter of recommendation was encouraging except for a notation in large black capitals and underlined indicating he was a *"member of Roman Catholic Church."*[24] He was rejected. Governor Buckingham was liberally minded. He advised adding Catholic chaplains to the army for the growing number of Catholic soldiers and authorized building a Catholic church near the rubber company he managed. Dr. Jewett's father was known as discouraging any "Romanizing influences," a sentiment common for the era.

Colonel Wright of the Fifteenth Regiment minced no words with the governor on his views for replacement of assistant surgeon in September 1862. Their surgeon, Dr. H.V. Holcombe, had several medical furloughs, granted by Dr. Jewett, and had been largely absent. His ailment was tuberculosis, from which he succumbed in 1872.

Doctor Barnes of Oxford Connecticut is to be appointed 2nd assistant surgeon of the 15th Regiment. Do not I beseech you visit that affliction upon this regiment. He is a fool and an ass and utterly incompetent to fill the place. The two companies from Meriden where he was once settled would not take his medicine for an ordinary colic and my other two surgeons than whom no better men can be found have expressed the preference to do all the work rather than be subjected to an association with him in the medical duties of the regiment.[25]

Some candidates seemed too frail for combat, but appearances can be deceiving. Dr. Jewett worried about Dr. Nathan Fisher of Norwalk; "I have some doubts about his qualities. He had been a dentist and had no practical experience. He was a feeble looking man."[26] They consented nonetheless to his appointment as assistant surgeon to the Thirteenth Regiment. He was offered promotion to regimental surgeon in October 1863 because of a job well done, but he declined reenlistment.

Dr. Jewett's views on most subjects were unvarnished and direct. In November 1861 he wrote Dr. Russell about various applicants.

> We shall have four candidates for examination; Dr. Ward, Dr. Backus, Dr. Holcombe, and Dr. Harrison. Dr. Harrison is mistaken in supposing that I am prejudiced against him. It is true that I do not like his treatment of the protrusion of the uterus nor do I like the mode he has adopted for securing wounded arteries.
>
> Dr. Lewis of the Fifth Regiment passed his exam for Brigade Surgeon and is waiting an appointment. An effort is being made to promote Dr. Bennett for surgeon of the regiment. It is my opinion he is too young. It would also be unfair to give him an appointment more fairly given to Doctors Warner and Holcombe.[27]

Dr. Jewett's views on quackery and homeopathy were no secret. An unsolicited letter to the board by Dr. A. Lewis of Litchfield in August 1862 may have sparked some interest. "Personally I have had contact with Dr. Vail and I think it right you should know that he has been in all kinds of quackery practicing (according to a reporter and I believe him) at one time as a 'German piss doctor,' dabbling in homeopathy and making rostrums. You can use this any way you please, but use it amongst your selves." Another local physician wrote, "I am told he has been selling pills the past three years to prevent conception" and notes the respectability of Dr. Lewis, author of the previous letter. The applicant, from Rochester, New York, was denied an examination.

Dr. Baker of Middletown notified the board that a Dr. A. Pratt of Chester had twelve years earlier been expelled from the local medical society for quackery as well as selling nostrums and potions: "He is a notorious quack. He advertises claiming to cure all diseases with a new science, which he termed 'magnopathy.' He claims to know vastly more than others. He later became a hydropath physician with a 'master cure.'"

Dr. Woodward wrote about a "witless" candidate. "A physician told me that Dr. Minor said that a candidate was rejected because he did not know how to make beef tea! I fear all his talk about the phalanx is humbug and am annoyed by his pertinacity. I suggest we do not examine him."

Surgeon Sabin Stocking of the Seventeenth Regiment was stationed in St. Augustine, Florida, and requested a discharge or transfer because it was too hot! "In accordance with the opinion of the medical faculty here I have offered my resignation. Immediately after coming into this department I found that the climate did not agree with me. My health has gradually declined and I now find myself unfit for the duties of a Surgeon in this climate. In more northern latitude perhaps my health will be better. Should there be an opening in the state for a medical officer I think my health may be so far recovered as to allow me to serve my country still longer." His request was denied and he was mustered out in July 1865.

Surgeon Ira Winsor of the Ninth Regiment submitted his resignation. The governor responded, "I would be happy to comply with your request but there is not now a medical man in the state who I can legally appoint as assistant surgeon who is willing to accept. The Medical Board will meet again soon and if there are men who meet with the proper qualifications they will advise and I can fill in vacancy." He served a total of six months.

Dr. Charles Hart wrote to Dr. Russell complaining about his lack of promotion. He was a native of Hartford who at twenty-four years of age graduated from the College of Physicians and Surgeons of Columbia College in New York after two years of study. This was followed by a three-year apprenticeship and then two years in practice. He was appointed second assistant surgeon in December 1861, and then first assistant surgeon of the Tenth Connecticut Volunteers in August 1862. He protested, "I am thoroughly sick of the position of assistant surgeon and seek promotion. I hardly think it necessary to trouble you with my reasons which could only be appreciated by one who has seen active service in the field (twenty-one months)." Dr. Russell responded that there were more senior and experienced candidates deserving promotion. Hart replied that he was "still alive" and "all alone," reminding his superiors that he was the only physician for his unit. His proclamation "being out in the field" was meant as a demeaning reference to physicians in the North who did not suffer the same danger of exposure to the Confederate army and southern diseases, either of which could be fatal. In the minutes of the Hartford Medical Society for April 1862 Dr. Russell describes his visit to army hospitals in Washington, D.C., where neatness, ventilation, and good management were stressed. He saw the residuals of battle as well as cases of measles, pneumonia, and groin abscess from typhoid fever.

Hart was present at and survived the battles of New Bern, Fort Wagner, Petersburg, and Appomattox Court House. He was also stationed in Kinston, North Carolina, Charleston, South Carolina, Saint Augustine, Florida, and the Bermuda Hundred in Virginia.[28] His was a varied career lasting four long years, and he had undoubtedly earned promotion. Evidently squeaky wheels do get oiled, for Hart was promoted to regimental surgeon in November 1864.

The mother of Dr. Hart asked the governor for approval to send "my son the doctor" a replacement horse. The delivery service would be Private A.F. Adams, wounded at Petersburg, recuperating at Knight U.S. Army General Hospital and soon returning to her son's Tenth Regiment. The governor was advised of her plan in September 1864, and apparently acquiesced, like Dr. Russell not wishing to trifle with the Harts.

> My son the doctor has had the misfortune to lose his horse and wants another, saying he has more uses for one now than for some time previous. He is in charge of the whole regiment and is at present working as chief medical officer of that division.[29]

In January 1863 Levi Jewett was the only doctor for the Fourteenth Connecticut Volunteers. He felt this entitled him to promotion to surgeon, even if that meant transfer to another regiment. His father agreed, writing the governor that his twenty-nine-year-old son's wife and child were living with him and describing the young doctor as "a hard working religious man who should be promoted." At Ream's Station, Virginia, in August 1864, he suffered serious fractures of the face and skull from a shell explosion. He was discharged disabled in January 1865.[30]

Applications for surgeon or assistant surgeon were often filed with accompanying letters of recommendation. Surgeon J. Hamilton of the Twenty-first Regiment helped his assistant William Soule, a graduate of the Medical Department of Yale in 1851: "He should be promoted as he is cheerful, assiduous and skillful while working on the sanitation of the men. As a surgical operator he has proved himself equal to any in the division."

A successful quest for advancement was achieved by Samuel McClellan of the Sixth Regiment, who noted that "several officers in habit of drinking" had their names submitted by the colonel but his had not: "Since last summer he noticed a decided change for the better in this matter. I do not deny that I unconsciously fell in the habit from it during service, unfortunately the prevailing custom in the army but that I ever drank to intoxication or was ever unfit for duty I deny."[31]

Pliny Jewett, himself not bashful about the grape, found drinking to excess a hopeless trait as indicated in this assessment to the governor about the proposed replacement for the deceased Leavenworth. "Dr. Fletcher was very intemperate before he joined the army. He may have reformed. If so it will be a rare instance under Army influence."

Requests for promotion were based on higher pay, prestige, a desire to be placed in a hospital setting for career advancement, and a need for change of scenery for personal issues. To forestall morale and administrative headaches, Dr. Russell proposed a system to deal with the issue of promotion in March 1863. "As the difficulty of procuring medical men for the army increases, we shall be obliged as the post of Surgeon becomes vacant to promote those now in the service and to rely upon the younger men of the profession for recruits." Six months later in a letter to the governor he revisited the issue of medical manpower as they were running out of volunteers. "So many have entered it that the services of those who remain are in constant demand and for the most part those who offer themselves hereafter will be young men, just entering upon the profession. Of these are well educated, active and the good of the service will not suffer."[32]

Several of the state's surgeons were performing detached service in hospitals or clerical duties on general staffs, leaving the assistant surgeons to provide care for the regiments. "This becomes more questionable when so many surgeons and assistant surgeons of the volunteers are appointed by the General Government for the performance of these very duties." In a parochial sense, Connecticut doctors should take care of Connecticut soldiers. "The state should retain the services of her officers and the national government should provide them for general purposes. In the mean time we propose to write to prominent medical men in all parts of the state, desiring them to inquire if there are any in the profession who are able and willing and who can be spared from their private practice to enter the army. We think this appeal to professional pride and to honor a public necessity will be sufficient."[33]

Requests for assistant surgeons became more frequent at the regimental level. The governor responded to Colonel Abbott of the First Connecticut Artillery, who suggested hiring J.S. Delavan, a contract surgeon from New York whose father was a doctor. "It is however very difficult now to find men who are willing to go and who are competent for the position. I have been disappointed in some who have been approved. I will not forget the importance of the subject and then do the best I can for your regiment."

In June 1864, Dugold Campbell was a private in the Second Connecticut Heavy Artillery seeking discharge because of "severe indisposition by rheumatism." "By profession I am a surgeon with a diploma from Edinburg Scotland in 1861. I would like to apply as assistant surgeon or contract assistant surgeon and am willing to undergo examination by your boards." The governor referred the case to Jewett, who offered an exam if a diploma was produced. It was not.[34]

The requirement for a surgeon to be resident of the state was cancelled. Russell asserted that acceptable candidates must be "capable, of good character and professional standing, and a graduate of some regularly established and constituted medical college." George A. Hurlbut was born in Glastonbury, studied at medical college in New York City and later practiced there. A legislator described him as "fully competent not only as a surgeon but as a man whose influence and character would eminently fit him for the place," noting he was a nonresident of the state. He was declared eligible, served in eighty-eight engagements, and was present at Lee's surrender to Grant and the Grand March in Washington at the war's end.

Some candidates were rejected with or without being interviewed. Two out-of-state candidates requested reimbursement for applying, including travel expenses. Dr. Grant (rejected) asked for a list of those candidates (ten) who had not been passed by the medical board and of those not allowed a formal exam. Dr. Russell cautioned, "I trust that Dr. Grant will not make any unnecessary public use of the same as we have been desirous of treating kindly all that may have been rejected by the board."

The governor investigated charges made against doctors, especially when death intervened. Lieutenant Samuel H. Thompson of the Sixteenth Regiment mustered in August 1862, survived the battle of Antietam and just weeks later was admitted to the regimental hospital with a sore throat and fever. Assistant Surgeon Nehemiah Nickerson consulted with Nathan Mayer, who felt he had "sub-acute inflammation of the tonsils" and recommended tonic and stimulant. After a couple of weeks of treatment in the field he was allowed to return to Connecticut, where he died in October. Charges of negligence were filed by friends and family asking for the governor's investigation. The area medical director described Nickerson as "upright, conscientious, energetic, patient and a skillful surgeon." William Thompson, a minister, noted that his son was coughing up blood, had chest pain and was exhausted upon arrival home. He claimed the doctor feared being the "laughing stock of the regiment for allowing absence to a man just because he has a sore throat" while calling it a "trivial disease" and the patient "very fretful and childish." The personality change was from the fatal disease and failure to allow earlier medical furlough was from officer meddling. Still the minister "prayed that in this day of trouble and rebuke the governor of Connecticut and all in authority may be divinely guided." The governor's investigation required responses from both Nickerson and Mayer. Most of the blame fell on the junior surgeon, portrayed as "rough and uncaring." Mayer's defense noted that the patient was seen several times daily, consultation was held with senior surgeons, and an apparent clinical improvement had not delayed any furlough. Despite being saddened and shocked by the officer's death, Mayer vouched for his colleague and explained the plight of all army surgeons.

> Charmed as I was by the good nature, brilliancy and attractive appearance of Lieutenant Thompson, I regarded him in the light of a dear friend and shocked at the news of his death. The difficult position of surgeon is little known. A new regiment subjected to great fatigues has caught its members somewhat indisposed in a very short time. All demand excuses from duty. Were he to do their will but the skeletons of companies would remain and the hospital would soon be the barracks of all. Yet these men are a little sick and bestow all their hatred upon the surgeons because he orders them on duty where they soon learn to bear fatigue and become inured to a soldiers' life. When a man has to treat a hundred patients in three hours, he needs all his time in reflection on the disease and has none to spare for flattering their weaknesses.
>   Believe me, sir, you're [*sic*] Excellency.[35]

Nickerson survived a bout with typhoid fever in 1863 that required prolonged convalescence in New Haven. He was captured at Plymouth, North Carolina, on April 20, 1864, and confined in Savannah. His wife pleaded for his release with Major General Foster on September 1, 1864. "Can you not do something to affect [*sic*] his release? I have just received a letter from the surgeon of the 104th Pennsylvania Volunteers dated August 20 saying that he had just been released from the prison at Savannah. He says 'it was by a special demand from Maj. Gen. Foster that he was released.' Now I do not wish to trouble you but my husband is sick and if he is not soon released he will never come home. He was well when he entered the service but since a severe illness in Washington eighteen month since he has never been well. Now I pray that what you can do you will do quickly as he may be dying of this. Do all you can to affect [*sic*] his release and my blessing shall be yours."

He was paroled on September 23, 1864. He was promoted to surgeon of the Twenty-first Regiment and mustered out on June 16, 1865. He began receiving pension benefits in 1881 for "typhoid fever and as a sequel phlebitis of the left leg causing swelling and pain on using the limb." Supporting reports came from Dr. Jewett, who treated him at the hospital, and Dr. Bissell, a fellow regimental surgeon. He received $20 monthly benefits for varicose veins for the remainder of his life, thirty-eight years.

Many doctors serving in Connecticut regiments were either approved by Dr. Jewett through the medical board, were taught by him, or were patients given medical furloughs and respite from the battlefield. Two physicians benefited greatly from his generosity and kindness. One, Nathan Mayer, arrived in America in 1850, emigrating from a German town with thick accent, all five feet of him. He was known as the "leetle doctor." Dr. Mayer

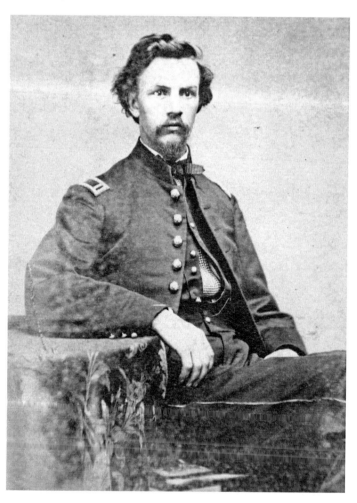

was appointed assistant surgeon in 1862 for the Sixteenth Connecticut Volunteers of Hartford County, and was promoted to regimental surgeon in 1863. Mayer's father was the first rabbi to practice in Hartford, ministering at Beth Israel Synagogue. He sent a note of sincere gratitude to the medial board for his son's appointment.

Where else but America could a newly arrived immigrant achieve such a prominent, sought-after position? Certainly not in his country of origin or anywhere else in Europe, where a rigid class structure existed and upward mobility was strictly limited by birth. Mayer survived being a prisoner of war and a yellow fever epidemic in New Bern, North Carolina, before returning home at the end of his three-year tour of duty.[36] Mayer obtained an extension of his furlough, generously issued by the surgeon in charge at Knight U.S. Army General Hospital, August 1863: "He

Nehemiah Nickerson. Assistant Surgeon, Sixteenth Connecticut Volunteers (Connecticut State Library).

is suffering from illness and is unable to travel. Extend twenty days, leave of absence. P.A. Jewett."

Doctors captured as prisoners of war were exchanged as a matter of course as a result of a gentleman's agreement agreed to early in the war following a battle in Winchester, Virginia. In a Hartford newspaper article of May 19, 1864, ran this notice:

> Nathan Mayer visited a few friends in the city recently. His regiment was captured at Plymouth North Carolina. He was taken with Colonel Beach to Richmond but both were exchanged after remaining there only four days. The Surgeon has leave of absence of twenty days.

The absence was authorized by Major Jewett, a compassionate colleague indeed for a young doctor in need. May 1864: "He is now suffering from illness and is unable to return to duty. Given fifteen days off duty. P. A. Jewett."[37]

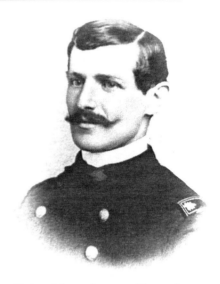

Nathan Mayer, Surgeon, Sixteenth Connecticut Volunteers (Connecticut State Library).

That came to five weeks home, a paid vacation away from the stifling, fever-ridden South, approved and blessed by good old Pliny. For an authoritarian with a temper and tough exterior, at least concerning fellow physicians, he could be a soft touch indeed. Connecticut doctors could count on a medical furlough from a sympathetic surgeon in New Haven.

Hubert Vincent Holcombe was regimental surgeon for the Fifteenth Connecticut Volunteers of New Haven, Connecticut. He studied medicine at both Yale and Castleton Medical Schools. He was the son of a doctor for West Granville, Massachusetts. Holcombe's family arrived from England in the seventeenth century and fought in the American Revolution. He had been in practice in Branford, Connecticut, his wife's hometown, since 1854 and had served as assistant surgeon for the Eighth Connecticut Volunteers in New Bern, North Carolina. He replaced another Yale medical school graduate, Dewitt Clinton Lathrop, who died of "fever" after six months active duty in New Bern.[38]

At six feet four inches tall, Holcombe's nickname was the "long, tall doctor." He too was a prisoner of war and survived the same yellow fever epidemic as Mayer. While Mayer had a long postwar medical career and died in his eighties, Holcombe succumbed to tuberculosis at the age of forty-five, just a few years after the war was over. He developed symptoms of the disease while in the service, his ill health being first noted by Dr. Jewett, who wrote furlough extensions for him as well.[39]

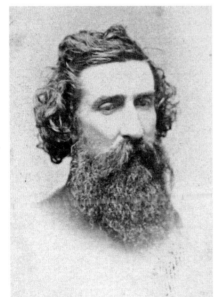

Hubert Vincent Holcombe, Surgeon, Fifteenth Connecticut Volunteers (Connecticut State Library).

August 13, 1863
He is suffering from scorbutic disease and chronic diarrhea and is unable to travel for twenty more days.
   P. Jewett

September 16, 1863
He is now suffering from illness and is unable to travel.
   P. Jewett

October 6, 1863
Extended twenty days. He is now suffering from chronic diarrhea and inflammation of the liver and is unable to travel.
   P. Jewett

December 16, 1864
He is suffering from inflammation of the liver and is unable to travel. He has suffered from the disease since September 1864. Twenty more days.
   P. Jewett

This last note refers to the yellow fever epidemic which began at the end of August and ended with the first frost in November. Being appointed regimental surgeon was a heady accomplishment for any young doctor. Drs. Russell and Jewett must have appreciated this remarkable circumstance, having reviewed numerous applicants for the job. One was a blue-blooded scion of a well-established American family, the other a recent immigrant and a non–Christian. America was strengthened by millions of these newcomers, benefiting from their hard work, skills, drive to succeed and sometimes genius.

Thirty-one sessions of the medical board were recorded, with applicants coming from several states, including New York, Vermont, and Massachusetts. Twenty-three percent of the applicants failed, the percentage being higher earlier in the war. Graduates of known medical schools were by definition already vetted and outliers were not. Each board member was paid $200 at war's end for the four years of work, which amounted to $6.40 a session.

Evelyn Bissell was a twenty-three-year-old graduate of Yale Medical School when he volunteered for the Fifth Connecticut. He described his oral and written examination for assistant regimental surgeon: "After an ordeal of four hours, I successfully passed." This "ordeal" would be a mere tune-up, for he was twice taken prisoner of war. After he was released by Stonewall Jackson at Winchester as the first designated "noncombatant" prisoner, he was recaptured, reparoled, and served three more years. The examining board did him and the soldiers he would treat a major service. Table 2 summarizes Drs. Russell, Jewett and Woodward's efforts.[40]

TABLE 2. RESULTS OF EXAMINATIONS FOR SURGEON BY THE MEDICAL BOARD

Year	Sessions	Candidates	Pass Assist. Surg.	Pass Surgeon	% Pass
1861–62	12	57	25	14	68
1862–63	8	49	32	9	83
1863–64	7	18	17	0	94
1864–65	4	11	8	0	73
Totals	31	135	82	23	77

Dr. Jewett and others made great financial sacrifices that went unrecognized and unappreciated. Promotion was a limited and unlikely benefit, as the highest rank for most doctors was major, which few attained. The entire medical department had one brigadier general, two colonels, and sixteen lieutenant colonels. This was a point of contention in the medical community as it limited their members' income and authority. Dr. Frank Hamilton, professor of surgery from Buffalo, addressed the issues of rank and medical authority:

> In this voluntary service they are the only class of officers who by education have been previously prepared to learn their duties in the field. With few exceptions they have been men of education and in many cases of large experience. They have been as a class superior to the field officers of the Regiments in which they have served, and at first sight nothing appears more immeasurable than that men of education superior to that of the Regimental officers, with a knowledge of their own duties far more complete than that of the latter class of theirs, should in any respect be subject to these officers in their own sphere. It cannot be denied that the medical officers are entitled to the questions of rank precisely as other officers are, and that they have been badly treated by Congress in its legislation on the subject. They should be on the same footing that the other staff officers are.[41]

Dr. Woodward defended the surgeon's role in battlefield treatment, relating the difficulties not seen back home. Civilian doctors did not see hundreds of patients at a time and in a hostile environment.

> Sick soldiers receive as good treatment in our general and regimental hospitals at the seat of war, as they would at their own homes. The soldiers are well prescribed for and carefully nursed. Hygienic conditions are as fully observed, as the exigencies of the service will permit. Many imagine that he is chiefly occupied in amputating limbs, probing gunshot wounds, extracting bullets, sewing up saber cuts and dressing bruises. Operative surgery furnishes but a small proportion of the cases, which he is called upon to treat. The time and energies of the medical department are mainly devoted to the treatment of diseases.[42]

Dealing with mass casualties is always a difficult and complex matter. Triage separates the treatable from the hopeless. Transporting soldiers with long bone fractures was a particular logistical nightmare in pain, suffering, and secondary infections. Few splints were available and traction a new procedure. It was easier and less painful to transport patients with the injured part removed. It was safer to remove an extremity within forty-eight hours of injury than when infected, when loss of life became probable. If there was absent circulation or nerve function, or poor soft tissue coverage, then amputation was essential. Teams of surgeons developed expertise in deciding when to operate and what type of surgery offered the best chance of success.

Silas Weir Mitchell reminisced fifty years after the war, soberly and without twentieth-century prejudice. He congratulated the difficult and largely thankless work done by Civil War doctors: 2,100 regimental surgeons, 3,650 assistant surgeons, and 5,500 acting assistant surgeons. He noted that 28 percent of amputation patients and 61 percent of skull trephine patients died. "These surgeons appeal to me as unrecorded heroes, I have known of men who dressed wounds and did the gravest operations until they fainted beside the operating table or fell asleep to find in an hour of slumber strength to go on with their work." Fifty-one doctors were killed outright or were mortally wounded. Four died in prison. Two hundred eighty-one died of disease incident to active service.[43]

Dr. Ashbel Woodward defended the medical system and the trials and tribulations of the army surgeon.

> In passing judgment, the conscientious surgeon must stand faithful to the government on the one hand and do impartial justice to the applicants for relief on the other. If a doubt exists as to the fitness of the person he allows him the benefit of the doubt. In this way all injustice is avoided. The dishonest and lazy soldier is sent to his appointed tasks. He seeks revenge in

denouncing the officer in letters and in conversation and communications to the press; he gives ventilation to his rage. The surgeon is denounced as a tyrant and an imbecile, and in the minds of the thoughtless, prurient sympathy is excited for the victim of his imaginary cruelty. There are cowards and shirks. Draftees fall to a lower plane of morality and aspiration. Some never rise to the level of true manliness. They are fertile in low expedient, ingenious in fabrications, dead to pride and seek only of securing safety and ease. They have little respect for justice, are supremely selfish and hopelessly debased. They condemn and abuse officers who compel them to discharge their duties. There are able-bodied soldiers applying to the surgeon for discharge. If you say no, the surgeon's reputation suffers due to misstatements of soldiers and their friends and relatives. The army is the best school for the improvement of surgery that the profession has had in any age or country.[44]

The army surgeon's primary responsibility is to keep the soldier healthy and on the battlefield. The civilian doctor has as his primary goal the welfare of his patient rather than the government. This might include keeping him from harm's way and thus off the field of battle.

Families write letters to elected officials, newspapers, and commanding officers applying pressure on the honest military doctor who then faces a moral dilemma. The surgeon who excuses one soldier from his duty, by necessity orders someone else's son to take his place. Separating the sick from the not-so-sick, the injured from the pretenders, the totally incapacitated from those partially able requires wisdom and experience. To be an effective army surgeon required being fair and even-handed as well.

Walt Whitman, America's resident poet, spent long hours on hospital wards comforting and encouraging wounded and sick veterans, including his brother. He wrote from the heart and his own experiences about the army doctors' performance:

I must bear most emphatic testimony to the zeal, manliness and professional spirit and capacity prevailing among surgeons, many of them young men in hospitals and the army. I never ceased to find the best young men and the hardest, most disinterested workers among these surgeons in the hospitals. They are full of genius too, and this is my testimony.[45]

In *Life on the Mississippi*, Mark Twain wrote that "war talk by men who have been in war is always interesting, whereas moon talk by a poet who has not been on the moon is likely to be dull." The romance and majesty of war can be seen only from a distance and mostly by those who have not endured the searing experience. Close up, war is cruel, indiscriminate, unforgiving and deadly.

CHAPTER SEVEN

The Elm City

The New Haven Colony was founded in 1638 by a band of merchant pilgrims from England headed by the Reverend John Davenport. The Quinnipiac Indians fished and hunted there while fighting the incursions of the Pequot and Mohawk tribes with little success. They were glad to cede this parcel of land thought not worth its troubles. It was located at the confluence of two meandering rivers and one moderate-sized river; the West, Mill and Quinnipiac. They emptied into a harbor protected by natural land outcroppings later called Long Wharf and Steam Landing. The land was flat and sandy and not much above sea level, offering easy access by shipping.

By the 1860s the center of town was the railroad depot, with its northern entrance off Chapel Street. It was notable for its large tower with clock and bell reminding passengers of the many arrivals and departures. Locomotives announced themselves by belching smoke and fire. The New York and New Haven railroad arrived daily, 5:30 A.M. till 11:20 P.M., ten trains arriving and ten departing daily. Some continued on to Meriden, Hartford, Springfield and Boston. The trains were rarely late and usually within a few minutes of schedule. From the west came the Derby Railroad. A line extending east was the Shore Line Railroad to New London and then Boston, six trains leaving and six arriving daily. The large Merchant Hotel was adjacent to the depot and hacks were available at fifty cents a passenger and thirty-five for two including trunks. A horse railroad was established for local transport at just six cents per customer.

In the nineteenth century, transportation was by water or rail, both of which prominently featured in New Haven, a growing manufacturing town which by 1860 numbered 35,535. Four steamboats a day ran between New York and New Haven. River, ocean and rail transportation allowed unimpeded delivery of immense amounts of goods and, if necessary, sick and wounded soldiers. This, combined with the availability of fresh water (New Haven Water Department), gas outlets for lighting (New Haven Gas Company), and terrain suitable for septic systems, made it an ideal location for a large army hospital.[1]

The broad main streets of Temple and Chapel were lined with 150-year-old elm trees. Columns of hardwood trees reached three stories high, draping their branches and lacy leaves like soaring gothic arches over adjacent brick and wooden buildings. They provided quiet, deep shade for the summer and elegance the year round. The elm trees withstood salt air and the fire and smoke of locomotives but not a disease inadvertently imported from France by a bark beetle, a condition ultimately uncompromising and devastating, much like the war.

In the center of town was an emerald jewel, the public square or town green, a stage for parades, political discourse, picnics, and military processions. It was silhouetted by statuesque trees, carpeted with green lawn, framed with an iron fence and serenaded by migrating birds and loquacious, opinionated residents. In its center was the Liberty Pole, from which hung the national flag when an appropriate occasion arose. Nearby was one solitary gas lamp and in the southeast corner the town pump, supplying cool water in the warm months. Just down the block was the massive statehouse, made of brick and mortar with marble steps and immense columns. On Temple Street stood Trinity Church, Centre Church and the North Church. For amusement one could rent velocipedes at Hoadley's restaurant. The restaurant also included a bookstore for college students. A. J. Beers on State Street was a wholesale fruit store renowned for ice cream and strawberries as well as nuts of all kinds, oranges, raisins, bananas, jellies, sardines, pickles and candies. Nearby, Hyde and Hibbart sold the best fresh fish, lobsters, and clams.[2]

The shopping center was Chapel Street. Ladies' silks, linens, laces and thread could be found here. On the corner C.A. Bradley offered silk hats, soft hats, cloth caps and furs. Benjamin and Ford, also on a handsome street corner, sold watches, fine jewelry, silverware and rings for all occasion. There were haberdashers and tailors for every price range: Atwater's Parlors, Bliss, Fitch, Merchant, Manchester, Mason and Son, and Kingsley and Sons. Shoes, carpets, dry goods, hardware, saddle and harness, stoves, furnaces, tin flooring, steam piping, furniture, groceries, and newspapers aplenty were available for purchase. Moses Thomas sold coffee, tea and spices, O'Neill repaired and sold watches, Baumgarten sold organs and Steinhart specialized in sheet music and pianos. Weed offered the latest in sewing machines, including Singer, Florence and Osborne. Wilcox and Hall had the best in silks, linens and wools, and the Cutler establishment sold paintings and engraved art.[3]

Also on Chapel Street was Minor and Company, an import-export company. One Minor graduated from Yale Medical School in 1863 and became an army doctor. The store sold crockery, glass, and kerosene oil. Henry A. Peck was a photographer, two of whose relatives were Union soldiers who died in the war. He sold stereoscopic views, frames, oil paintings, and offered "old pictures of deceased persons enlarged and finished in the finest style, carte de visite and everything pertaining to the arts." He was co-owner of "The Cheapest Book Store," Peck and Coan, which was convenient to the college and sold schoolbooks and notebooks as well.

The government post office was on Church Street with its wide granite steps and two thousand private boxes for the public. Near it and the depot were four banks, Western Union Telegraph and printing offices of three local newspapers. Also available were papers from New York, Richmond, Boston and London. The Connecticut Mutual Insurance Company was one of the local insurance companies, competing with Boston and New York firm's branch offices.

Just outside New Haven were the coal- and iron-casting works of Fitch, employing 125 men. The Rogers & Smith Company, a silver plating outfit, employed a like number. The Steam Saw Mill Company made logs into lumber, and the Phelps brewery made beer. The largest carriage makers in America were located in New Haven; their operation was later converted to war products. Casting factories, machinery for iron wares, clock and lock works, fish hooks and machinery, and shirt manufacturers flourished.

Benham's New Haven Directory of 1863-64 listed thirty-two places of worship: three Catholic churches, two Baptist, ten Congregationalist, seven Episcopal, eight Methodist, and two synagogues. There were five hotels — the New Haven, Tontine, Tremont, Madison and the Union — three tobacco shops, four dentists, forty-two physicians, and fifty-six lawyers. No fewer than eight photograph and ambrotype shops and four picture frame manufacturers are listed. Photographs in the form of cartes de visite were popular with the troops and their families, at a cost of a dollar apiece or less.

A year's subscription to the *New Haven Daily Palladium* newspaper was $6.50. The city's total yearly expenditure was $61,500. The annual salary for the superintendent of schools was $1,200 and for the governor $1,100. The chief of surgery at the medical school earned $4,000, Dr. Jewett, chief of staff at the army hospital, $1,920, and his former junior partner billed $5,400 plus an additional $1,200 as a contract surgeon.[4]

In 1861, there were 1,149 births, 392 marriages, and 851 deaths. Of 7,525 children, only one-third went to public school. One out of four children died before the age of five. In New Haven in 1862, of 935 deaths, 473 were children under the age of six. (See Table 3.) Half the deaths were children less than six years of age.[5] These were the stark, immutable facts of life facing the young men who were willing to accept the challenge of being a doctor in the mid-nineteenth century.

TABLE 3. DEATHS IN NEW HAVEN, CONNECTICUT IN 1862

Male	484	30–40	66
Female	451	40–50	42
Younger than 1	189	50–60	56
1–5 years of age	284	60–70	34
5–10	72	70–80	44
10–20	56	80–90	16
20–30	83	90–100	3

The town's main attraction was then and remains Yale College. It was a five-minute walk from the depot; 519 students from places as diverse as California, India and China came to study for four years with a faculty of sixty white Christian men. Open to the public were the daily student morning prayers, 7 A.M. to 8 A.M. These were held in the Chapel and lasted ten minutes so the students could rush off to recitations and other classes. On York Street was the medical school with its own tower, bell and clock, a convenient three blocks from the State Hospital.

A booklet encouraging tourism described New Haven as having "few domestic infelicities" and noted that there were "many men of virtuous and substantial character." The police blotter suggested other possibilities more consistent with human nature. A glimpse of the cantankerous side of this society can be seen in the police blotter. Of 1,497 total arrests, 783 were for intoxication, and 110 were for intoxication and disorderly conduct. The other causes for arrest in 1863 were assault and battery (195), desertion (139), theft (134), prostitution (72), keeping a house of ill fame (24), breaking windows (18), malicious mischief (5), adultery (10), peddling without a license (5), and manslaughter (2).[6]

Connecticut regiments whose ranks were filled with citizens of New Haven County and environs had their farewell hurrah at the town green. Surrounded and cheered by loved ones, local citizens, and dignitaries, regiments marched proudly to the center green. Flags flew, bands played patriotic tunes, ladies waved encouragement, and politicians speechified. The *Palladium* described one such farewell for the Fifteenth Connecticut Regiment Volunteers, New Haven's own, on August 28, 1862.

> They marched up State Street, then on to Chapel Street, then on to Church, then Crown and York streets, then on to the town green and state house. There they were regaled by one of Major Mansfield's splendid collations. The Fifteenth left New Haven this afternoon at 12:30 on a train of thirty cars drawn by two locomotives. An immense crowd was on hand to witness the departure. The Fifteenth struck their tents like the Arabs and went away amid sunshine, tears and hearty good-byes; some to victory, some perhaps to die for their country! How shall we rejoice if some time in the not distant future we may welcome them back — their banners bright with victory to a state grateful to them for noble deeds? The Fifteenth has gone. Our hearts, hopes, and prayers go with them.

The advantage of having soldiers as customers and part of the consuming public was not lost on the local merchants. If onlookers were bored with the festivities, a number of shops had items that might appeal to them. "Steel" armored vests, for example, were sold at Bliss's shop at 336 Chapel Street. Deluxe models were advertised in the *Palladium* as follows:

> The Brave are fallen!
> Many of them might have been saved by using
> Atwater's Adjustable Armor
> This fact has been demonstrated beyond a doubt.

> The following extract from a private's letter says Colonel Briggs of the Massachusetts 10th was hit in the region of his heart with a Minié ball but having on one of Atwater's Patent Armors his life was preserved. Every test that has been made proves the Armor an absolute protection against saber and bayonet thrusts and pistol balls at any range and from rifle balls at the ordinary range. The armor covers every vital part except the head and is so adjusted to the presence as to have free use of all parts of the body. It is made in sections and is easily detached and packed in a big knapsack. The material is the best of steel, made expressly for armor purposes.

Those who bought these iron life preservers first swore at them as they fell apart and did not fit, and then threw them away as worse than useless cardboard. The most effective means of protection from saber and bayonet thrusts was to avoid the intoxicated and criminal element. During the entire war only 960 cases of knife wounds were reported and most of these were from felonious assault or accidents, often relating to drunken behavior. Very few were battle-related.

Hospital patients were ready customers whose interests and needs were not always satisfied by government sources. Many items for sale could be found on the last page of the *Knight Hospital Record*, where a variety of ads were directed at the enlisted soldier. Pricing was important, as a thirteen-dollar monthly paycheck determined types and frequency of purchases. Items for sale included inexpensive coats, pants, boots, and shoes made expressly for soldiers' wear. Tailoring could be provided for any military uniform. Also promoted were photographs tinted or not, photograph albums, books, magazines, and newspapers including all the daily New York papers. Advertisements for clothing included "cheap" shirts, collars, military hats, caps, gloves, trunks with traveling bags, woolen shirts, and the best socks in town. Cotton and woolen socks sold for thirty cents a dozen, while knitted gloves and cloth gloves were fifty cents a pair. Buck gloves and mittens were $1.50 a pair, linen and silk handkerchiefs fifty cents a dozen. All these great prices were available because, the seller claimed, "most [were] bought very cheap." There were ads for an auction house, picture frames, sewing machines, and military goods of every description. The notary public handled bounty, pensions, and any legal problems, including back pay. One could buy hardware and mechanical tools, sheet music, musical books and instruments, snuff, cigars, cigar holders, tobacco and plain and meerschaum pipes.

Having a healthy set of teeth was most important for one's health. Dentists did a brisk business in New Haven. Hartford's late Horace Wells, the discoverer of nitrous oxide as general anesthetic, would have been pleased to read about the enterprising Dr. Strong in the *Palladium* ad of April 1863:

> Laughing Gas
> Aching Teeth
> Extracted
> Without the slightest pain! With the
> Nitrous Oxide or laughing gas made
> Perfectly pure and fresh every day

Also on Chapel Street next to the depot was a drugstore whose proprietor Whittlesey was "as good a doctor around was he to choose to practice." He owned another establishment specializing in chandeliers, lamps, china, crockery, cutlery and silver plated wares. In case of an accident or need of a doctor, further up Chapel Street was "Apothecaries Hall," and separate drugstores run by Noyes, Leavenworth, Beers, Dickerman and Dow. Below the depot was Daggett's drug store; the Daggett family included doctors and an assortment of elected officials. Dr. Daggett had his office on Wall Street; Dr. Pierpont on York, Dr. Townshend was on the Tontine block, Dr. Ives on Elm. Nearby were Drs. Tyler, Park, Whitmore, Hubbard, and from the medical department of Yale, Drs. Sanford and Bacon.

By 1862, the city of New Haven had forty-two physicians, six homeopaths, one hydropath, two Indian medicine practitioners, one psychological specialist, and four female medical caregivers as listed in the town directory. By 1866 the number of doctors in the city limits climbed to forty-five and by 1871 to fifty. Forty of the latter group graduated from Yale Medical School.

Downtown New Haven offered a smorgasbord of products and services geared to the departing soldier, some destined to return sick, wounded or not at all. Aid and comfort from disease or injury included armored vests, knives, flannel abdominal supporters, water filters, Dr. True's Liniment and folding cups.

CHAPTER EIGHT

Building a Hospital

One of twelve patients died of wounds, a rate of 13.8 percent. Scaled to today's population, a proportionate number of war's dead would be over six million. The scope of the medical care required was staggering. After each major battle a cascade of names covered the front page of newspapers and overflowed onto the next, names painfully familiar to the hometown residents. Ships docking in northern cities began unloading hundreds of desperately ill and wounded with no hospitals or facilities to receive them.

The first army hospital was erected in Washington in May 1861. At first public buildings, school houses, churches, hotels, warehouses, factories and private dwellings were used. A vast system of hospitals would of necessity be created under the command of medical and not line officers despite the fact that volunteer surgeons "knew nothing of military hospitals small or large."[1]

It was argued that hometown air, food, and loving care would speedily return each state's soldiers to health so that they could return to the battlefield and bring victory. Lincoln described an army like a sieve and said that keeping soldiers in the field was "like shoveling fleas." At Antietam 170,000 soldiers were paid but only 83,000 were accounted for. Authorized and unauthorized discharges, furloughs, and desertions accounted for major discrepancies in troop strength. If soldiers were allowed to recuperate at home, they would stay there and never return to the battlefield. State hospitals would serve as a haven for malingerers, deserters, malcontents, draft-dodgers, and bounty-jumpers — in short those looking to profit and escape the war. Lincoln's administration at first favored building hospitals near the battlefield, but convalescent facilities within cannon range was at best imprudent.

The army's medical hierarchy incorrectly believed that exposed Union soldiers became immune to local diseases in a process called acclimatization. Reinfection with malaria was common. Colonel Hawley of the Seventh Regiment reflected medical opinion about South Carolina in October 1862. "The troops who have been in this department a year ought to have a change of climate. The entire force has its vital powers greatly lessened by the continuous absorption of malarious poison, and cannot endure severe fatigue and long marching half so well as when it happens down here." Transfer to a seaport free of mosquitoes or to the disease-free North was required to break the cycle of persistent ague or fevers that plagued both armies. The morbidity and mortality of the febrile illnesses contracted in the South could not be overestimated. A nationwide hospital system would better serve the nation's needs for these reasons and more.

As the war ground on, it became clear that Lincoln's reelection would be difficult and uncertain at best. Showing the voters that everything possible was being done for their sons, husbands and fathers could pay dividends at the ballot box. An investment in hospitals might translate into votes. Having a brand-new hospital would muffle critics in the press and elsewhere on the subject of medical care. It would also facilitate transfer of soldiers home where they would likely vote for the Republican administration. There were 2.2 million Union soldiers.

The decision to build convalescent hospitals in each state left the question as to where and how. Proximity to transportation by rail or water, availability of clean water and other sanitary features were crucial. Lighting would be candlepower or gas, the latter four times more expensive. The effects on local business would be enormous. The need for food, building materials, clothing, drugs, hospital equipment, and soldier-related paraphernalia would create a financial boom for many providers.

G.B. Hawley solicited the governor on July 3, 1862. He was a property owner, physician, and original incorporator and officer of the newly founded Hartford Hospital (1855) in central Connecticut.

> We expect soon 300 wounded and sick. There is a need to build barracks and bunks for wounded with the appropriations made by the Legislature. The surgeon general has communicated with Dr. Jewett that the first hospital in the country shall be at Hartford. We need to make immediate preparations. Please inform us whether we shall immediately commence our barracks and bunks the expense of which to be paid from the fund appropriated for that purpose.[2]

A great white edifice had already been built in New Haven. In 1826 a committee of six, which included Drs. Jonathan Knight and Timothy Beers, founded the General Hospital of Connecticut, a charitable institution. In 1832 the citizens of New Haven complained about the "cruelty of doctors" in their apparent refusal to treat impoverished cholera patients. Private families and keepers of public houses were reluctant to assume fiscal responsibility for charity cases. The hospital served as a "refuge and asylum of sick and distressed," for the poor and the destitute sojourner needing "medical advice or skillful surgery."[3] It sat on twelve acres of land rising from the shoreline and overlooking New Haven Harbor and Long Island Sound.

An application to Congress for $25,000 was denied, leaving just the state for funding. No expense was spared. A three-story stone building was erected, 100 long and 50 feet deep with a Grecian portico, at a cost of $12,500. The walls were of Chatham red stone with three-and-a-half-foot-thick basement walls and two-foot-thick upper walls. All the rooms had fireplaces decorated with oak and chestnut. The attic was made of spruce and the cornices of white pine. The windows on the first floor were ten by fifteen feet, and the other windows eight by ten. The inside doors were two inches thick with the best English mortise locks available. There were seventy windows, mahogany sills, a piazza in the center of the building, a copper boiler, two ovens, and an operating room with circular seats with backs. The gutters were of copper, with two lightning rods. A brick cistern was of "twenty hogs head" capacity.[4]

By the 1850s, the hospital's average daily patient census had risen from two to fifteen. The board opposed having "indigent females" stay on hospital grounds or allowing homeopaths to admit patients. The latter group requested an equal number of beds but was denied. An offer to build them their own hospital contingent on their raising an equal amount of money was declined as they could not raise the $10,000.[5]

In 1860 the General Hospital Society had 198 patients, 111 of whom were from 33 different towns, and was aided by appropriation of $1,779 from the state. Average cost of each patient to the state was $2 per week while expense to the hospital was $3 per week. The average hospital stay was less than eight weeks. "Most if not all the attendance and valuable services of surgeons and physicians has been gratuitously rendered." Hartford Hospital was not yet opened for reception patients. That building was erected at cost of $50,000, of which $40,000 was paid by citizens of Hartford and the rest by the state. A grant for $40,000 from David Watkinson paid for the poor and sick of Hartford, but no provision was made for the admission of indigent patients from other parts of the state.[6]

Dr. Jewett had four weeks earlier applied to be chief of health care, but by June costs of medical board meetings and actual care of soldiers needed reevaluation with the governor. He wrote: "I enclose bill of General Hospital Society of Connecticut for board medical attendance and care of sick soldiers with a bill for medicines furnished by direction of the surgeons. I am not certain whether the bill should be sent to you or to Washington. The bill was contracted after the troops were mustered into service. If I have done wrong in sending it to you please return it and don't be obliged."[7]

Others were lining up at the governor's trough with products and services to sell, sometimes useful and even necessary, such as ambulances, boots or hospital beds.

Alex, Strong, Hayward & Co., Dealers in Boots, Shoes, Hides and Leather in Boston were ready to protect the soldiers' feet with "all kinds of boots and shoes and could get up the required goods as low as any manufactures in our state. We have formerly manufactured shoes for the U.S. government and have therefore the requisite experience."

In August 1861 Dr. J. Darrach, the superintendent of New York Hospital, offered his institution "for the relief of the sick or wounded soldiers of the state over which you preside as may at any time be in this city needing Hospital relief." The fee for privates was $4 per week and for officers $7. The offer was made because of "numerous applications for relief made at this hospital and there being no provision for it in the city."[8]

In November 1861, M. Armstrong & Co. offered discount ambulances at $120 that had just been sold to the federal government for $143 and transportation carts at $98 previously sold for $118.

Dr. Jewett sat on the state's Committee on Human Institutions, the Medical Board for appointing army surgeons, and the General Hospital Society of Connecticut, all of which planned the new facility in New Haven for returning sick and wounded. The governor's ability to attend their meetings was always featured in Jewett's letters: "It would give me great pleasure to see you at the same time. I will send my carriage for you." "If convenient I would prefer to have the meeting in New Haven." "The directors of the General Hospital Society of Connecticut request you to call a meeting on the special appropriation for hospital purposes at the hospital in New Haven at your early convenience. Please inform me of the time of the meeting."[9]

He quickly and affirmatively responded to requests from the governor, as in this note penned from the state hospital on July 30, 1862, "I shall be most happy to comply with your request with reference to Dr. Carleton. The only objection we had to him was his age. I shall hold myself ready to perform any duty under my command you may think best to assign me; and shall be most happy to assist in the organization of the medical staff of the regiments in any way in my power." Carleton was from Norwich and a graduate of Harvard Medical School whose career as surgeon of the Eighteenth Regiment ran the full nine months and was described in glowing terms despite his "weakness of the lungs [tuberculosis]," from which he died in 1866.

Jewett was to be chief of staff of the new hospital. He recommended that the directors of the General Hospital Society approve a contract with Surgeon General Hammond on May 14, 1862. The federal government would pay $3.50 per week for each soldier admitted to the hospital for all expenses. In Philadelphia and New York the rates were $4, assuming higher overhead in the large cities. The more hospital patients, the more beds full, the more money the federal government would pay. Because many of the overhead costs were fixed, keeping the beds full was an economic priority.

On May 17, 1862, a committee was appointed to solicit subscriptions in the city and adjoining towns for additional funds for managers of the hospital to provide for sick and wounded soldiers. The members of that committee were Drs. Knight, Jewett, Hubbard, and Daggett. Two ministers from each denomination in the city were chosen as hospital chaplains. The New Haven Water Company provided water at no charge for the temporary buildings. Another local company piped in natural gas. Provisional seed money came from the state legislature as well as private citizens of New Haven and other parts of Connecticut.

The original stone building, though colossal and extravagant, was unventilated and thus unsuitable for the care of the wounded. From a practical point, just one foul-smelling gangrenous extremity would make air quality in a closed building unbearable. The state hospital would be used for administrative purposes rather than patient rooms. Soldiers were thought to do better in terms of wound infection, diarrhea, and other medical conditions in open-air facilities.

Early in the war, the United States Sanitary Commission reported to the government on the general subject of military hospitals.

> No fact in sanitary science is better established that old buildings from want of systematic ventilation and other reasons are most unfit to be used as hospitals on any large scale and that even in inclement weather, tents or the rudest shanties are preferable. In winter months when doors and windows are sure to be kept closed, it certainly shows itself in the form of hospital fever, erysipelas and other formidable diseases and in the general depression and tedious convalescence.[10]

Surgeon General Hammond offered firm guidelines on the construction and staffing of these hospitals in his text on military hygiene, detailing building designs and operating specifications.

> The maximum air space allowance may not prevent hospital gangrene, pyemia and erysipelas. The 1,800 cubic feet of air allowed a patient may be foul air, and hurtful simply because it is stagnant. Sufficient space between the beds and a constant renewal of the air are more important elements than the number of cubic feet per bed. It is very difficult, in ordinary buildings used as hospitals, to secure ventilation without exposing the inmates to injurious draughts of air. This difficulty is avoided in the building now being constructed in accordance with the orders of Surgeon Letterman by means of "ridge ventilation" which keeps the air constantly pure without exposing anyone to unpleasant or dangerous drafts.[11]

This led to the construction of various vents that were retractable depending on weather conditions. In the winter ice and snow often froze the vents shut. The attempt to remedy this with floor vents seemed more helpful in allowing invading rodents and other vermin

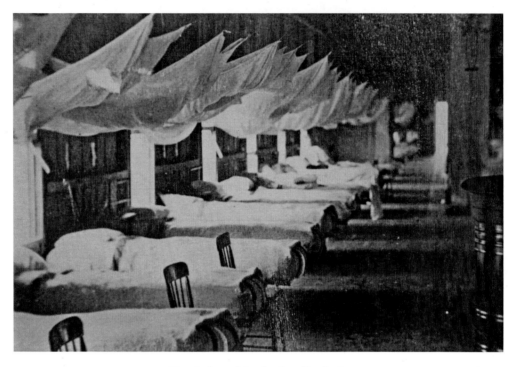

Hospital ward (author's collection).

than patient comfort or air flow. In Washington, air-cooling with hand-driven fans worked the best.

The legislature raised $15,000 to provide five new buildings for 500 patients. Temporary tents were later replaced by single-story wooden pavilion-like structures coated with white wash. The floor was eighteen inches from the soil, with fourteen feet from floor to eaves. The outer dimensions were to be 187 by 24 feet, with ample windows, allowing for adequate light and air circulation among the rows of 100 patients per building. The beds were in parallel rows, a bed stand between them for medicines, books and personal items. At the foot of each bed was a chair. A card on each table listed the patient's name, number, date of admission and disease. Each ward was supplied with gas, water, and toilets at each end. Each building was under the charge of a ward master and several assistants who were responsible for its cleanliness, appearance, and avenues of health care delivery.

Water closets were a topic of dispute, particularly over how to avoid pungent odors. Most effective was placing a small room at the end of the building completely separated from roof to floor, capable of cross-ventilation. Emphasis was placed on the proper removal of waste material. An adequate water supply driven by gravity enabled the flushing of waste in in-house toilets. In the absence of a water supply, privies separate from the wards were required with daily emptying and removal of waste from watertight boxes. Piped evacuating systems were the most sanitary and clean-smelling. Depending on the location, vaults, sinks, privy boxes, and slit latrines all had a place. At this New Haven hospital, frequent changes of trenches and the heavy use of peat moss as cover was effective maintenance of its septic system.

Secretary of War Stanton issued a directive in 1864 enforcing medical input on sanitation: "Buildings will not be taken or occupied for hospital purposes until after full exam-

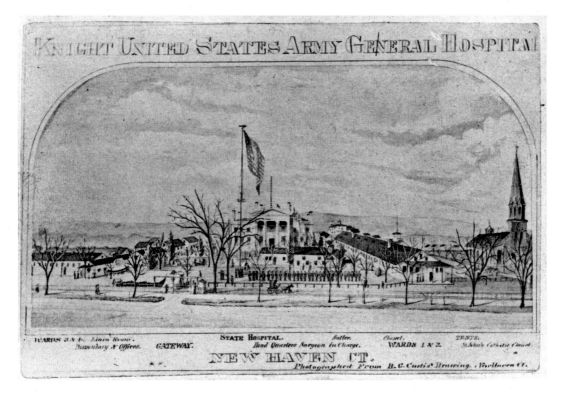

Sketch of Knight Hospital (New Haven Museum and Historical Society).

ination and approval by a medical inspector or other officer of the medical corps detailed for this purpose—all alterations will be made in accordance with plans submitted by him and approved by the surgeon general." The hospital location required well-drained soil remote from marshes or "malarious" sources and a plentiful source of water. The delivery of water required either a well or steam engine power. Hot water could be provided through iron pipes, as in Philadelphia's Satterlee Hospital which had sewage pipes connected to a distant sink. The economic status of the community determined the complexity of the facility. The wards could be arranged in echelon or V, circle, ellipse or rounded oblong with the administration building at its apex. Thirty feet separated each ward, and there were connecting covered walkways without sides.

The medical staff would consist of regular army doctors and contract or acting assistant surgeons from the local community, including medical school professors and students. Also required were clerks, cooks, carpenters, bakers, policemen, firemen, chaplains, administrators, printers, postal clerks, housekeepers, launderers, undertakers, hospital stewards, orderlies, nurses, and a host of other ancillary people to provide health care for thousands of returning soldiers. For every soldier fighting in the field, nine people were needed for support.

A city within a city developed, replete with its own police and fire department. At the ends of wards, one-inch rubber hoses were kept attached to water closets along with buckets and axes. Laundries with washing machines, wringers, and drying rooms were set up. At its peak the Knight hospital bakery made 30,000 loaves of bread per month. There were kitchens, cafeterias, food service for the nonambulatory, chapels, printing rooms, a butcher shop, a carpenter shop, a guard house, a pharmacy, the quartermaster's storehouse, administrative offices, a post office, and a library. Officers had their own separate eating and sleeping quarters, as did the female nurses and medical cadets. A knapsack room was lined with two-by-two foot pigeonholes for the patients' personal effects. These served as sad reminders of the deceased, for final dispensation required shipping possessions to their families.

The operating room consisted of two rooms each fifteen feet square with skylights. The first room, used primarily for surgery, was fitted with cupboards containing instruments, sponges and a microscope. The last feature required application to the Medical Purveyor Bureau providing "satisfactory [evidence] that the officer will use the instrument for the benefit of science and will report the results of his observations to the surgeon general."

The second room was used for the medical discharge board. Immediately next door but away from the wards was a "dead-house," also lit by skylight. It was fifteen by forty feet with a vault eight by four feet complete, with windlass and dumbwaiter ready to prepare bodies for burial.

On June 9, 1862, the New Haven hospital accepted its first patients, 260 casualties from the Battle of Fair Oaks, Virginia. Doctors Daggett, Wilcoxson, Lindsley, and Hubbard were there to greet them. Dr. Jewett assumed overall command with Dr. Knight as an active consultant. The rolling thunder of successive battles produced waves of hospital newcomers who were thankful and fortunate to be home and alive.

Getting a national hospital network up and running during a bloody civil war was a monumental undertaking. Dr. Jewett revealed the growing pains in a letter to Surgeon General William Hammond who, despite his youth, was already an accomplished professor and researcher with eleven years' experience as an army surgeon. He had published numerous academic medical papers, including an award-winner at a recent AMA convention, and was a university professor in Philadelphia and Baltimore. Descended from the founders of Maryland, he got the surgeon general's job with the backing of the U.S. Sanitary Commission, the New York medical establishment with whom he had his early training and the McClellan family of Philadelphia. His candidacy was initiated and advanced by the family of General George McClellan, the man Lincoln fired because of his "slows," and who became the Democratic Party presidential candidate in 1864. The candidate's father, George McClellan senior, was born in Woodstock, Connecticut, and graduated from Yale College in 1816 and later from Yale medical school. He also attended medical school at the University of Pennsylvania and subsequently founded two of his own, Jefferson Medical College in Philadelphia and the short-lived Medical College of Pennsylvania at Gettysburg. The senior McClellan was described as having the "heart of a lion, and the eye of an eagle," a description perhaps lacking in accuracy as he died suddenly at a young age in 1847. His brother Sam and other son John were also doctors. Medicine was the family business with diversions in politics, a prominent sideline.

Hammond stood over six feet, weighed 220 pounds and had an autocratic personality. He assumed office in April of 1862 and began the necessary radical changes of an antiquated medical department. Many regular army surgeons would relish his downfall as seniority no longer ruled. The Lincoln administration preferred a westerner like their favorite generals (Grant, Sherman, and Sheridan) but bowed to congressional pressure and accepted Hammond's appointment.[12]

Administrative problems left unresolved included who paid the bills and who was in charge. The original hospital charter stated "no physician or surgeon shall receive any compensation for his services," not an encouraging situation for those expected to spend long hours delivering wartime health care. This Christian community believed in the Talmudic teaching that "a doctor who charges nothing is worth nothing," or that "a doctor who charges half a kopek is worth half a kopek."

The state hospital was now a hybrid. On June 14, 1862, Dr. Jewett wrote from what he calls the "State Hospital" to ask Surgeon General Hammond to define the change in status.

> To prevent mistakes and to let our Directors understand just what the position of this Hospital is with the Medical Department; and also that I may be able to define my own position; will you do me the favor to send me my appointment in due form, with instructions. It would be well for our directors to understand that the institution is now under the care of the War Department so far as the sick and wounded soldiers are concerned.[13]

In September 1862, the governor's agent in Washington, J.E. English, reported his conversation with the surgeon general. "Hammond said if you have buildings and beds we should occupy them. The government will refund the amount. The Connecticut Hospital would receive sick and wounded soldiers with the promise of quarters, food, medicine and medical and surgical care for the considerations of $3.50 each per week. He proposed to agree to all or part of the agreement to the government for one year to be renewed not exceeding ten years."[14]

Of the first 555 hospital patients, 29 died, 110 returned to duty, and 89 men from Connecticut were discharged. Three hundred twenty-seven inpatients were left mostly living in tents. The bed crunch became severe, leaving Jewett to seek out the unfailing support of the governor December 27, 1862.

> I have never felt any hesitation in calling upon you for your influence in connection with the sick and wounded soldiers; and as you have never said <u>no</u>. The surgeon general has ordered through the honorable Mr. English <u>one hundred and fifty</u> Connecticut wounded to be sent to this Hospital. I have now in the Hospital over <u>one hundred</u> Connecticut men who have reported to me from time to time as their furloughs have expired. I shall have over <u>two hundred and fifty</u> Connecticut men in the Hospital when the new detachment arrives. I can just make more room for these by using a building that has been pronounced unfit for Hospital purposes by the Medical Inspector Dr. Lymans and by resorting to tents. My Plans and estimates for new buildings are now in the hands of the Quarter Master General for his approval. They have the endorsement of the surgeon general. Will you send a letter to General Meigs stating the absolute necessity for new buildings with the reasons therefore? You might mention the fact that we have but three military hospitals in New England, at Portsmouth Grove, Boston and New Haven. Please make the letter as urgent as you can.[15]

In October 1862, Jewett requested a consultation with Hammond. He had no experience concerning military rules and regulations, much less the financial intricacies of running a large hospital. The medical staff, composed of private practice physicians and university professors, was becoming increasingly reluctant to participate without compensation. In May of 1862 Jewett was appointed as contract surgeon, at a salary of $110 a month, having forfeited his private practice whose income was four times greater.

In November 1862 Jewett's special orders came through. He was now a major and surgeon of volunteers officially appointed by the secretary of war. The hospital's change of status became clearer. The surgeon general canceled the contract with the state hospital society, and on behalf of the federal government rented the grounds for $1,000 per year (though the asking price was $1,500). This placed the hospital under the control of the federal government and Chief of Staff Pliny Jewett. This was a federal institution, answerable primarily to Washington. Local interests would continue to influence events and require dutiful consideration, but the state charter still applied. Five more months of contract changes and bureaucratic consultations were required before reaching a final agreement.

Dr. Jewett continued to appeal to Dr. Hammond for support concerning the medical staff, the exact requirements of filling out reports, and understanding concerning his bare-bones support structure. He was a federal employee; the other staff members were not. He wrote on New Year's Day in 1863:

> You will see by my official communication and from the explanations of the Honorable J. E. English, that my position with reference to weekly reports is a very unpleasant one for me. The fact is, my dear sir, I found it impossible to make the attending surgeons of the State Hospital perform any extra duty, for the reason that under the charter they can receive no pay from the hospital Society. They have given their services freely so far as the attendance on patients and under the circumstances I have not felt like calling on my venerated friend Dr. Knight and others to make out the morning reports. I beg also that you may understand that we were all somewhat *green* in the management of a Military Hospital. I can assure you that you will have no further cause of complaint as to the reports. We are now in good working order. I trust ere long, you will see fit to put us on a purely military basis. We are neither one thing nor the other now. Trusting that you will excuse me for the trouble this may give you I remain.[16]

A second letter was fired off to Hammond on the same New Year's Day explaining why forms were not filled out, deadlines not met, and military rules and regulations violated:

> This Hospital is still under contract with the surgeon general, and has been so since the 9th day of June last. The medical officers, medical cadets, hospital stewards, and female nurses are all furnished by the General Hospital Society of Connecticut under the same contract. The same may be said of the male nurses and cooks. Until the 7th day of last November, I was acting assistant Surgeon under contract with the surgeon general. The attending surgeons of the Hospital have been on duty since the 9th of June last, under the charter of the Hospital Society and can receive no pay for their services. My time has been so fully occupied as the General Superintendent of the Hospital; and until I received my appointment as Surgeon of Volunteers, my pay was so small that I could not hire a clerk, to assist me even, in making my monthly and quarterly reports. If it is absolutely necessary I will have the weekly reports made up in the best manner possible and will forward them to you as soon as I can prepare them. In consequence of my being the only officer of the government at this Hospital, I have found full occupation from 8 o'clock in the morning until 11 or 12 o'clock at night. And even after devoting this amount of time in the care of the Hospital I know that I have "left undone many things that ought to have been done." I trust it will not be found that I have "done many things that I ought not to have done." I did not know that weekly reports were required of me until I received the letter from Surgeon McLaren, Medical Director of New England Department, under the date of Dec. 26th 1862.[17]

On March 4, 1863, Dr. White an agent for the governor, arrived with thirty-eight Connecticut patients from Fredericksburg. The hospital census was 355. Jewett was getting medical supplies from the federal medical purveyor and would soon have buildings completed despite the wintry weather. This would allow 200 more beds for returnees, taking into account the expected discharges.

By April 1863 the military hospital was given an existence independent of Yale College and the state medical and political bureaucracies. The grounds, buildings and employees were no longer under contract to the General Hospital Society of Connecticut. The medical director and quartermaster of the department sealed the event with a personal visit. This was a federal institution, financed and regulated by rules divined in Washington. The state could and would contribute but did not control the purse strings or the hospital's administration. Administrative workers and civilian patients belonging to the state hospital were moved to another building on Whalley Avenue. The original stone hospital building was now occupied by Jewett and officers on duty.

With the establishment of federal authority, doctors were paid as contract surgeons at $110 each month while maintaining their private practice of medicine. This luxury did not extend to Dr. Jewett. He was listed as a major of less than ten years' experience, and received $162 a month as full-time army surgeon. For field officers extra money was available for horses, servants (two), and meals. In comparison, a veterinary surgeon was paid $75 a month, a hospital steward $30, a private $13, and a nurse $12 a month. Doctors were still at a distinct disadvantage, for they were outranked by all other branches, and lacked control of supplies and ambulances, which were under the quartermaster department.

Ward masters, clerks, nurses, stewards, and others had to be hired, trained, and supervised. Daily, weekly, monthly, and quarterly statistics had to be filed accordingly while ships and trains were unloading on their doorstep sick and wounded men who desperately needed medical care. By April 1863 administrative control was centralized, and during the terminal illness of Yale's chief of surgery, the growing hospital known as U.S. General Hospital was renamed Knight U.S. Army General Hospital. Jewett described these events in a history of the hospital written eight years later:

> On 1 April 1863, the institution was placed on a strictly military basis and by permission of the surgeon general was called Knight Hospital in honor of Dr. Jonathan Knight who as President of the State Society and consulting surgeon had been foremost in the good work of establishing and sustaining the hospital. Since then, we have been moving forward on the full tide of a successful experiment.[18]

This experiment came with no guarantee. Jewett blamed his changing status for another administrative snafu in a letter to the medical director of the Eastern Department in New York in April 1863.

> I would respectfully report that there was no Hospital fund at this Hospital for the months of February and March, as I was there under contract with the Hospital Society. The Contract was closed on the 7th last. Hereafter I shall comply promptly with the regulations with reference to the Hospital Fund.[19]

Hospital funds, a requirement under the federal system, were simply credit on the books of the subsistence department for the rations that sick men did not consume. This was used to buy delicacies for extra diet or special foods in the kitchen. Convalescents caught fish and raised vegetables as a supplement. When a holiday occurred, special meals could be paid for with this fund, as could new equipment, decorations for the wards, or recreational materials. Such a source could pay for lighting the hospital with gas, which cost $225 per month compared to candles at $59.[20]

Since the fund was a credit, money could not be transferred or disappear into a dark drawer or someone's pocket. Keeping accurate records was essential to avoid inquiries about fiduciary responsibility. Jewett pointed out that he was under state, not federal regulations at the time of the alleged infraction, at which time the regulation did not apply.

Another such "piggy bank" was the slush fund, which was created by taxing the sutlers and by selling bones, fat, stale bread, slops, straw, manure, waste paper, old newspapers, and flour barrels. Some hospitals earned $200 to $400 a month this way. The head surgeon could use this fund to purchase books for the library, daily newspapers, chapel melodeon or musical instruments, a printing press, or to fund other entertainment for the patients. Photographers could be hired to document surgical cases, specimens taken, and the likeness of men discharged on surgeon's certificate of disability as a guard against fraud. If the hospital fund ran dry, this was a backup. Army regulations required accurate accounts of both funds and documentation of regular oversight. Failure to do so invited unsympathetic inquiries and could lead to administrative or judicial action against innocent or guilty parties.[21]

The state legislature's Joint Committee on Humane Institutions was financial overseer for the state hospital. On June 12, 1863, Chairman John S. Rice of the House and several other members of the legislature left Hartford at noon for New Haven, where they spent three hours touring the Knight U.S. Army General Hospital. The visit was conducted by Jewett and his assistants. He was described as being a unique surgeon for an army hospital because he treated soldiers with such kindness and knowing compassion: "Doctor Jewett is duty bound to preserve good order and discipline and yet he does not lose sight of the fact that the unfortunate soldier is a Man." His assistants Doctors Wilcoxson, Hubbard, Daggett, Lindsley, Hooker, Townsend and Bishop were "skilled in their profession all well known as kind hearted men and faithful in their duties." They visited the 513 mostly convalescent patients housed in three barrack buildings and tents grouped in a circle around the state hospital. Guard duty was performed by an invalid detachment. Eight medical cadets attended wounds and saw that the medicines ordered by the surgeons were properly compounded and distributed. The state civilian hospital was staffed by six doctors who spent two months each supervising with Mr. Lake as the hospital steward. There were twenty-five seamen patients who were paid for by the federal government. State patients were paid for by the state and private patients were paid for by their friends.[22]

Those soldiers who were able lined up for a dress parade and listened to the chairman speak about the interest and pride the legislature felt for these brave sons. This was "a perfect system and neatness is apparent on every hand." Jewett ordered three rousing cheers and the impressed and satisfied visitors arrived back in Hartford by 7 P.M. One week later the hospital received 140 soldiers from the battle of Chancellorsville.[23]

On July 9, 1863, Major Jewett marched along with hospital soldiers, guards, militia, Masons, pallbearers, the Drum Corps, and the New Haven Band for the funeral of Lieutenant Colonel Henry Merwin of the Second Regiment. He had mustered in August 1861, was captured at Chancellorsville in May 1863 and pardoned just weeks later, in time to participate at Gettysburg, where he died from a chest wound on July 2, 1863. New Haven was garnished in flowers and crepe as the Reverend Eustis proclaimed, "What honor would be too large for one who might sacrifice everything for the protection and defense of his country and his land?"[24] This was not the first nor last such procession for the surgeon.

The consequences of trench warfare were more sick and wounded. By July 29, 1864, the Knight U.S. Army General Hospital was full, with 1,000 beds occupied. Jewett proposed filling hospital beds with Connecticut patients, a theme previously stressed by the governor: "I have in the hospital a large number of New York, Maine, New Hampshire and Massachusetts men. Would not this be a good time to make application for their transfer to their own states? Please make no direct use of this letter with the department."[25]

The chairman of Townsend Saving Bank, Charles Townsend, reported to the governor in August 1864 that substitutes were now getting $1,000 bounty and added "the greatest number of patients in our hospitals is from other states while our brave boys are suffering in the hospitals of other states."[26]

The governor expressed these notions to the new Surgeon General Barnes on August 2,

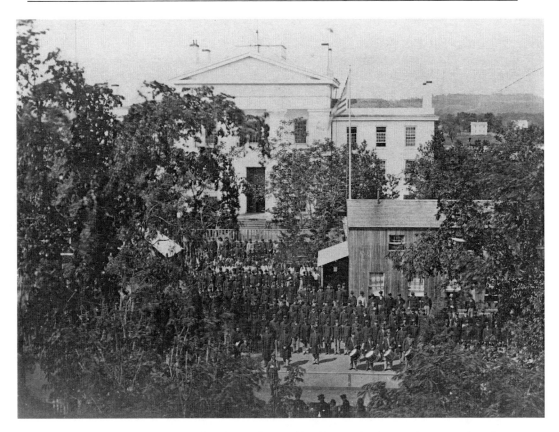

Knight U.S. Army General Hospital with state hospital building in background, surrounding fences and military guards (The New Haven Museum & Historical Society).

1864. "I would respectfully represent that the buildings of the U.S. Knight Hospital at New Haven was erected by the state for the purpose of receiving sick and wounded Connecticut soldiers and that if those now in the hospital who belong to New York, Maine and New Hampshire can be removed to their own states and other sick and wounded Connecticut men be transferred to take their places it would gratify our citizens and give strength to the union cause here." The first response came on August 12: "These transfers will be made as rapidly as possible. Due to the great crush of patients all the hospitals have been filled. Any rules to send them to their own states could not be wholly carried out with a due regard to their immediate comfort. They will be transferred as soon as there are vacant beds in the hospitals intended for them." By September 150 Connecticut patients were transferred to New Haven, with 150 more to follow. The same request to the previous surgeon general was denied. Such was the growing political power of the governor.

By December 1864, negotiations with the surgeon general for a new hospital lease were underway. The directors of the General Hospital Society of Connecticut voted to rent the hospital buildings and grounds to the government, which "will give us abundant room for additional buildings." William W. Boardman had financially supported the creation of New Haven's Fifteenth Regiment in 1862 and was president of the society. He was also a registered Democrat, state legislator, commissioner of Hartford County, editorialist and a successful businessman in real estate, wholesale coffee and spice. He suggested the governor offer less expensive and less desirable land to the federal government which could then be sold as a whole unit, assuming approval of the state legislature, which had refused to fund any new buildings: "One of the obstacles is the difficulty of procuring another location for the hospital and another is the reception such a procuring would meet in public estimation, thus giving up a good location without having first secured a substitute. We can find a place somewhere but then answer is to be given the U.S. at once and we can probably do better if we had more time."[27] There would be no new real estate deals. In Washington, Connecticut's Senator Foster and other state emissaries met the surgeon general on February 3, 1865. "The General would recommend to the Secretary of War that the U.S. government lease the state hospital and grounds connected therewith in New Haven as they add so much to which is now known as the 'Knight Hospital.'"

Governor Buckingham noted in his address to the legislature of May 1864 that enlarging the hospital was a priority: "The sick and wounded desired to be transferred to the U.S. Hospital in New Haven, and it was impossible to meet their wish for want of room." The hospital would be enlarged that winter with the construction of five new pavilions. On December 8 he replied to Jewett's proposal by asking for details as to "full and complete description of the materials to finish, an estimate of the cost of each building and what are the specifics."[28] No detail escaped the perusal of this experienced financier, manufacturer and businessman. "I care not how soon they complete the work or their calls for the money but hope two or three of the buildings will be ready to receive patients very early in February. Have the directors send me a list of those who proposed to build the pavilions and the sum for which they offered to do the work."[29]

The contractor Larkins and Pinney proposed to Dr. Jewett on January 9, 1865, "We will agree to build the five pavilions according to plans and specifications for $10,500. We will agree to complete them in forty fair working days. We could do them sooner we think if there were any objections. We understand that the state pays in cash."[30]

Jewett advised the governor that by early February all will be set as the builders seemed "*live men*." Just two weeks later he reported to Buckingham, "I shall have 100 beds ready for patients in the new wards in ten days. This will give me 115 vacant beds. Notwithstanding the bad weather three of the buildings are nearly completed. They will all be ready for patients the first week in February." Ahead of schedule and on budget, he reported on February 6 1865:

> The new wards are completed with the exception of the removal of the old buildings. The delay in removing the buildings is in consequence of my not having heard from Washington with reference to the lease of the old hospital building. The surgeon general has given his approval. The delay is with the Secretary of War. I suggest that you pay the contractors $10,000 and let the balance remain until the contract is completed. The balance of $500 will more than cover the cost of removal of old buildings.[31]

The legislature had not provided funding. As a consequence, the governor appealed to a "number of highly responsible and influential citizens" of Connecticut to finance the project. It should not be forgotten that fortunes were made because of this war. There were reasons other than patriotic ones for donations by beneficiary contractors and manufacturers.

The governor backed up his promises with two personal checks enclosed in a letter to Jewett Feb 7, 1865.

> As no provision has been made to pay from the state treasury for the five pavilions which have just been erected for the use of sick Connecticut soldiers, I have provided money from another

source which may or may not be returned and enclose a check on the Webster Bank of Boston for $8000 and one on the Ninth National Bank of New Haven for $2000 which you will hand over to Larkins and Pinney and make a receipt on the contract with the duplicate as paid by me. The balance I will pay whenever the work is completed. Say to the contractors that I am grateful with the promptness with which they have done their work.[32]

One week later the *Hartford Courant* reported the governor's achievement and generosity:

When additional room was wanted to accommodate the sick and wounded soldiers of Connecticut at the Knight hospital Governor Buckingham gave assurance that expenses for the necessary enlargement would be met. No provision had been made by the state for the improvement and now that the work is nearly complete and five new buildings each 25 by 100 feet nearly ready for occupancy. Governor Buckingham has sent his private check for $10,000 to cover the contractor's bills. The soldiers will never have to wait for the slow work of legislators as long as our present chief magistrate can look out for their welfare.

A week even before the additional buildings were open, the governor advised Dr. Jewett that efforts were being made to ensure the new beds would be filled by Connecticut soldiers. He had given marching orders to his agents in Washington, Drs. Coggswell and White. "The state has made provision for accommodating more of her sick and wounded soldiers on her shores. The hospital has room for 500 more. You will make the facts known to acting Surgeon General Barnes and respectfully request him to write orders to transfer Connecticut soldiers as fast as may be practical. I would especially like to have transferred men from Annapolis and Baltimore Maryland, Portsmouth Grove Rhode Island, New York, and Pennsylvania. If you can be of service in accelerating the soldier's [*sic*] home you will do so."[33]

He left nothing to chance, writing personal letters to the secretary of war, surgeon general, provost marshals, surgeons in charge of hospitals, and all his state agents in which he emphasized the need to keep the new beds full with Connecticut soldiers. Any limitation on that ability had his "earnest attention." Jewett never lost sight of the federal mandate, $3.50 a week per bed filled. Little fighting took place that winter and occupancy was down. He reported to the governor on April 12, 1865:

Vermont men are passing through this city almost daily from the recent battles. Why cannot the same promptness be used with reference to Connecticut men? I have nearly 400 vacant beds but have received none of the men from the recent battles. Vermont has but *one* agent. We have three.[34]

Keeping soldiers occupied can be a full-time job. Idle hands, unfocused minds, and unremitting boredom led to fights, desertion, and poor morale. Some passed their time using the universal Yankee jackknife to make intricate trinkets and ornaments from pieces of waste wood, bone, and whatever else was available. Baskets, fans, and picture frames were just some of the items offered for sale to the public.

There was musical entertainment, and patients could spend time at the library, stocked with newspapers, pamphlets, and magazines. The Castleton Medical School library in Vermont held 3,000 volumes, Yale's medical library held 1,200, and the McClellan hospital library in Philadelphia had 2,500. The Knight U.S. Army General Hospital had 800 books consisting of religious and scientific subjects, novels, adventure and travel stories as well as magazines and newspapers of all varieties. The more popular books were read so often that they wore out, requiring a steady inflow of new material.

The hospital library was open daily, except Sunday, from 1 P.M. to 3 P.M. The reading room was open from 9 A.M. to noon and from 2 P.M. to 6 P.M. The chaplain supervised the library, cemetery, and postal service. He kept addresses of the nearest relatives and, along with others, wrote letters for the illiterate or physically disabled. Initially only 20 percent of these newly formed hospitals had libraries, which were composed primarily of religious books generally donated by chaplains. There was an intense demand for other books and periodicals, generally of the lighter variety. An appeal for all kinds of reading matter was met by a generous public. An article appeared in the *New Haven Daily Palladium* requesting donations:

> Anyone who can furnish one; two, three or an even half dozen new books would make a large and beautiful library that would be fully appreciated by the soldiers and those inmates who follow. Give to the librarian or Mr. Wilson who is in charge. We request religious works, novels and tales as the most interesting for the soldiers.

A follow-up note appeared from Chaplain J.B. Cram in November 1864: "I have the pleasure of acknowledging on behalf of soldiers of this hospital a very liberal donation of books to their library from Mrs. Caroline E. Couch of the city. Old books are read so often, some now are unfit to read," he declared to the *Record*.

The Knight U.S. Army General Hospital offered every conceivable service that a small town could provide, including its own newspaper, which became the most desired reading material.[35] The *Knight Hospital Record* began publication on October 5, 1864 and ran weekly through July 12, 1865. The subscription price was $1.50 a year. Its contents were encyclopedic, and while the main audience was hospital patients, there was something in it for everybody. Soldiers liked stories ranging from the romantic to the adventurous, jokes, poems, national and local news, gossip, hospital goings-on, upcoming entertainment events, editorials and letters to the editor. Long-lost love, marital bliss in their future, aspirations for the girl back home, and future romantic rewards for the brave and patriotic were dominant themes. Copies were distributed throughout Connecticut and often mailed to soldiers stationed in the South. The workings of the hospital are described, including construction of the thousand-bed facility, and the details on how, when, and why patients were treated and transported from the battlefield. The numbers of hospital admissions, discharges, returns to duty, desertions, deaths, and transfers are dutifully recorded each month and often listed by the soldiers' names and regiments. The circumstances of dead and wounded members of Connecticut units still in the battlefield were listed in whatever detail was available.

Articles of interest were reprinted from other northern and southern newspapers, as well as the foreign press, especially England. Each four-page issue starts with a short story ranging from a couple of paragraphs to a full page. The American Revolution is a reference point, a symbol of all that was noble about America. The theme of bravery is extolled in the "Battle of Ticonderoga," a tale about Ethan Allen and the Green Mountain Boys in which courage and boldness ensure that Americans prevail. In another Revolutionary tale, a British spy swallows a silver ball containing secret information. His deception is proven by clever Americans who make him throw up the evidence and sentence him to hanging as a traitor.

In another story, an American seized by a British ship receives poor rations and rough treatment. He escapes and later captures the same ship in the War of 1812. The American has great charm and wit, and puts down the British officer's military ability by saying, "When a Yankee guesses anything, it's sure to happen." In case the point was still not made, a notation in the *Record* suggested a natural superiority: "Federal soldiers are two inches higher and weigh eighteen pounds more than British soldiers." The Union soldier is the defender of freedom: brave, courageous, resourceful, humble, and superior both morally and physically.

Another story concerns an avalanche in which all survive due to some heroic efforts and self-sacrificing teamwork. Individualism is extolled in a story about a six-foot-four-inch Texas Ranger who eludes capture by 100 Comanche Indians as he gallops through them to a forest sanctuary and its welcoming protective darkness. He demonstrates incomparable skill and bravery against an enemy superior in numbers but not in wit or daring.

But there is more to life than violent conflict; there is romance. One tale concerns a Revolutionary War soldier who confronts savage Indians to save another soldier's fiancée. In a similar setting, a woman disguises herself as a man so as to be near her loved one, much to his surprise and benefit. A few years later he becomes aware of the heroism and sacrifice made by his true love, and they live happily ever after. In an Indian story, a captured brave is about to be executed, but the chief's daughter sheds a tear, miraculously saving his life. The story's message is underscored by its closing stanza:

> Tis ever thus; when in life's storm,
> Hope, a star to man grows dim
> An angel kneels in woman's form,
> And breathes a prayer for him.

Prayer and the love of a woman can provide rescue and salvation even in the most hopeless of cases. A young girl living out west receives a letter each week from her loving soldier, but she is too poor to buy paper and writing materials and so cannot respond in kind. She uses her money for food and clothing so that she and her family can survive. Love finds a way and they later reunite.

In a story called "Love and Malignity," a soldier, deceived by another, believes that his fiancée fails to write to him because she is unfaithful. Wounded at Gettysburg, he suffers the amputation of his arm and subsequent debilitating fevers as his life ebbs away slowly but inevitably. He goes home to die, encounters the young lady again and discovers that in reality she was faithful. He becomes determined to survive and form a perfect union with her. "The old physician was more than surprised upon his next visit to find the patient whom he supposed past all recovery, sitting in an easy chair while beside him sat a woman who through adversity remained his promised wife." Hope springs eternal and once again the love of a good woman provides the strength to overcome the hopeless and seemingly incurable.

The soldier has hopes, desires, and needs. A warm touch from a loving hand or the laying on of hands by the doctor can soothe a painful wound or psyche. Such caresses can be hard to come by and by necessity may remain wished for rather than realized. Young men think about food, sex, and romance most of the time, and not necessarily in that order. Older men reminisce, if they can remember at all.

> I've ladies met, extremely fair,
> With soft blue eyes and golden hair,
> And those with orbs like raven's wing,
> That kept my poor heart fluttering;
> I've met girls with such charming ways
> They claimed my thoughts, for days and days;
> Yet none of them can cope with her —
> The dark-eyed girl of Dorchester.

But let the buyer beware, as this news story illustrates: "A pretty woman in Jackson Michigan has been recruiting in a novel manner. She married a man on condition that he gave her his bounty. She being pretty the man consents. After he goes off to war, she marries another and repeats this plot with four such marriages." Only with the last conjugation was she detected. Bounties of hundreds of dollars attracted gold diggers to the unwary and unsophisticated. Another story depicts an innocent young soldier proposing to a scheming adventuress while exposing his financial cache. She quickly arranges a consultation with her alleged father in order to discuss matrimony. They are soon married both legally and financially bound with the likely outcome left to the reader's imagination and experience.

Social gatherings where the two sexes could mingle were popular, allowing eligible young men to meet eligible women. Dances were a common social gathering, as the poem "Home from the Hop" portrays:

> Did you mind love When Gerald Lane
> Spoke this eve with you
> On the viranda [*sic*], in the air,
> How strangely white he grew?
> Was he ill, dear? For you know
> He's just fresh from the wards,
> And that horrible sabre-thrust
> May have given him cause
>
> Sleepy love? Well seek your pillow-
> What going and not kiss?
> Perhaps the Captain's —, Well, good-night,
> We should not part like this.
> I'll join you presently my dear —
> No? Well, once more good-night;
> You're strangely out of sort, it seems:
> I'll smoke awhile; good night.

The search for a soul mate brings up the age-old question as to what kind of gal would be best for you. Is it the gal who married dear old dad or just the opposite? Do the "orbs of Dorchester" match the importance of a kind soul and gentle touch? In the poem "I'm Not Particular," ground rules on the subject are defined. The young man's wish list includes "winning grace, pretty face, rosy health, untold wealth, that she be fair and young, and give hearty kisses." On the negative side are several cautions: "that she not scolds or is grave and not 'too good,' or dreadful bashful, and certainly not rude."

> Don't think I'm particular
> I love the ones that you can kiss and squeeze
> Now, don't think I'm particular
> I'm far from being that,
> Yet best I love the petite ones,
> And not the ladies fat.
> I am not fond of stately ones,
> For once I got so bothered;
> One kissed me in a drawing room,
> Until I nearly smothered.
> Yes, bless me, but I really thought
> That I was being smothered!

"The Sensitive Man" is a poem about the shy, perhaps timid, dreamy, self-effacing type and his struggle for recognition and achievement. He admires from a distance those who seem happily married and yearns for the same state.

> I envy you, you mated men,
> For all your wedded bliss,
> Your slippers, babies, cradles, and
> Your wives to love and kiss;
> Your shirts with every button on.
> Clear-starched and white as snow;
> Yet these, all these I might have had,
> but, feared a lady's no!
>
> I have not force of mind enough,
> In fact, I am not used
> To making love to ladies,
> For I dread to be refused!
> So to my grave I fear that I
> A bachelor must go,
> Unless some lady hints that she
> Is sure she'd not say-no!

For this readership, the details of how one courts and overcomes shyness are of no small concern. Clichés, gossip, and idle chatter do not constitute a workable manual for marital success. There is the hard reality of unyielding economic and socially unpleasant facts of life faced by many veterans damaged physically, mentally, or both. In the short story "Short and Sweet," we learn of the experiences of a recent widower and his search for a replacement companion.

> "When a man came a courting me, said Mrs. Dobson I hadn't the least thought of what he was after, not I."
> Jobie came to our house one night after dark and I sez, Come in and take a chance,
> "No Lizzie, I've come on an errant, and I always do my errants fust."
> "What is your errant?"
> "Courtin business. My wife's been dead three weeks and everything's going to rack and ruin. Now Lizzie if you've a mind to hev me and take care of my home and children I'll come in an takie a cheer. If not I'll get someone else tu."
> "If you come on this courting business come in I mus think of it a little."
> "No I can't til my errants done."
> "I should like to think about it a day or two."
> "You needn't Lizzie."
> "Well Jobie, if I must I must so here's to you then."
> So he came in. Then we was married right off. I tell you what it is, these long courtins don't amount to nothin at all. Just as well do it in a hurry.

The southern belle was just as refined and practical as her New England sister. Most cursed "those damn Yankees" with enthusiasm. However, flag waving and empty speeches do not put food on the table or clothes on one's back. Nor will it keep one's feet warm come winter. Consider this letter from a Nashville Confederate woman to her brother that was published in the *Record* in January of 1865. Tennessee was in firm Union hands and money scarce.

> Dear brother Tom,
> Things about here are getting worse daily. You will be astonished to hear that your friends of

the female denomination are dropping off every day. Yes dropping as willing victims into the arms of the ruthless invader. You had better come home immediately and look to your interest in that quarter as perhaps it may not be too late yet to produce a favorable change in your favor. Tell the boys down in Dixie; if they do not return soon they will not find a single girl or widow below conscript age in these parts as the watchword now seem to be "marry who can." My principles are unchanged and I am as true to the south as ever. We have a captain boarding with us merely by way of protection who appears to be a rather clever fellow for a Federal. He takes a sly glance at me at the table sometimes but of course, I do not return it. You know me too well for that.

    Your loving sister, Marie

    P.S. I. Do you think it would be a violation of my southern principles to take an occasional ride for my health with the Captain? He has such a nice horse and buggy. You know there can be no possible harm in that.

    P.S. II. That impudent fellow squeezed my hand as he helped me out of the buggy this evening. We had such a delightful ride.

    P.S. III. If ever I should marry a Yankee I would do it merely as the humble instrument to avenge the wrongs of my poor oppressed country. Little peace should he find by day or night, thorns should be planted in his couch.

    P.S. IV. Come home and take the amnesty oath for two months or so. On due consideration I have come to the determination to make a martyr of myself! Yes Brother Tom, I am going to marry on patriotic principles.

In spite of the best of intentions, unpredictable events, the relentless passage of time, and a host of other factors sometimes conspire to leave even a well-feathered nest inhabited by just one bird. Some remain mateless without hope of ever finding marital bliss. For others, this is not necessarily a bad thing. What follows are two laments, one from each sex, accompanied with advice for the lonely-hearted. Age does bring experience, which can be defined as the opportunity to make the same mistake more than once. The more mature applicants seem the most grateful, and likely to require a much lower level of maintenance. The old bachelor and old maid have the same fear, that of loneliness, both seeking the brass ring of happiness in the form of that someone special with whom to spend their lives.

The Old Bachelor's Lament
By Benedict
I sit in my dreary attic,
And ponder the long ago
What time with youthful ardor
I sought to be a beau;
My attempts were always bootless,
Tho' I made it the study of life;
Oh, why are women so foolish?
None ever would be my wife!

My age, I will not deny,
Is a trifle over two score,
But my looks are excessively youthful,
Tho' I'll never be handsome more!
What a shame that girls should marry
A man that's more of a boy!
Why don't they wed? Well they shouldn't
Matured men's hopes destroy

Now listen; my heart beats warmly
With all the impulse of youth;

I can swear that I'll love dearly,
And what more can I do for soothe?
Should any young lady desire
To change her name for mine,
Just let me know by over-land-route,
For "now" the accepted time.

The Old Maid's Lament
I sit in my lonely chamber,
And think of the days long ago,
Of days when I struggled and labored:
So hard to catch me a beau.
But my efforts were all unavailing,
I am doomed to live a lone life;
Oh! Why were the men all so foolish?
As not one to want me for wife?

I've been forty for twelve years,
And not a day older I'll be,
What fools men are to wed young girls;
When old ones are steady and staid.
Oh dear, if I only was younger
I would not now be an old maid.

The predicaments of those already married with children waiting at home were more complex. Some strayed from their vows while others remained steady and just yearned to be home. Furloughs were infrequent, especially for the enlisted man, for whom returning home was beyond reach. Letters became the only source of communication unless the wife traveled a long, hazardous distance at great expense for a reunion. Most could not afford the loss of both from the home. The thoughts of a family man are considered in the poem "Just before the Battle":

No, I'll not forget you darling
But oh, the time has been so long
Since the morning that you left me
To defend the right from wrong,
Till now I feel my sad heart sinking,
While I think you may not come,
When this raging strife is ended
And your comrades reach their home
No, I'll not forget.

In addition to reading, recreation for patients included arts, crafts, card playing (some times with gambling), as well as baseball and football. Daily hospital routine often consisted of just passing time rather than preparing for the future, a conundrum for the sick and wounded. Meetings and educational discussion groups were provided on a variety of subjects, including books, mountain climbing, religion, botany, geology, and general health care.

The importance of getting mail cannot be overemphasized. For the soldier it can be the most important event of the week. Good news or bad can determine subsequent behavior, for the good or not. A newborn baby, reminiscences of family or friends, an unfaithful sweetheart, an ill or departed loved one, or failing business interests back home are items communicated in letters that can alter soldier morale. A poignant article on this subject appears in the *Record* in 1865:

The Mail

How often I would sit on the bank of the beautiful Potomac, and watch the coming of the mail boat that daily plied between Washington and our little encampment near the bank of that grand old river. We all watched to see if there was a large mail, if there was, what a feeling of joy would creep through our heart, for then we could hope for a letter. If it were a small one, we would turn sadly away and think of home and the loved ones there. But they know not how eagerly he watches for that little epistle of love and hope that comes from home. He is alone, surrounded by temptations and in the midst of evil companions. He hastens to the company and waits for his name. There is one for him. He looks at the postmark. It is from home. His heart beats with gladness for he knows he is not forgotten if he is far away. He sister sends words of love and hope and the many little things she is getting ready to send to him. No one knows that amount of good a letter does to the soldier. It buoys up his spirits when he feels lonely, and keeps him from temptation and sin.

"Write me" is included in most soldiers' letters of this or any war. Health is discussed, as are current events, the quality and quantity of food, and inquiries about goings-on back home. But always there is the plea "Write me," do not forget me, and remind others to do the same. In just the first week of December 1864, the Knight hospital processed 1,000 letters. This number does not include packages containing foodstuffs, clothing, books, and newspapers. A complete hospital post office dealt with this torrent of communication.

Technology seems to be the main aspect of society that improves with time. Politics, morality, religion, philosophy, and economics may seem inscrutable and inflexible, stuck in the morass and certainty of human frailties. At this time, the telegraph was becoming prevalent in both military and civilian worlds. Faster than mail or even the Pony Express and much cheaper, it offered speed and efficiency. As described in the *Record*, it amazed an elderly lady who received a yellow envelope with response to her message in just a few hours. She proclaimed, "All the way from Wheeling and the waifer's still wet. That's an awkward looking box but it can travel like pisen."

What was life like on the wards of Knight U.S. Army General Hospital? The *Knight Hospital Record* provides us a picture window. The ward master ensured discipline, sanitation, and appearance of staff and patients. Decorations of the wards by soldiers and their families were encouraged. This article appeared just after the presidential election in November of 1864:

There are probably people in this community as in every other who suppose that a Hospital must of necessity be a gloomy, forbidding looking place, where nothing pleasant or cheerful is to be seen, and where everything only serves to remind the observer of wounds and sickness and sorrow. Such persons would be agreeably disappointed and surprised by a visit to Wards No. 3 and 4 of Knight General Hospital in this city. Upon entering either of these, they would see wreaths and festoons of evergreens suspended from the ceiling; and in the latter they would further observe banners and portraits wreathed with evergreens and gaily decorated with ribbons. In Ward 4, as you enter, you perceive in the center, a fine portrait of Washington. On the right of this is a motto "In God we Trust," and on the left is another motto, "My Country, 'tis of thee, of thee I sing." In back of this is a banner bearing the names of Lincoln and Johnson, with the picture of Uncle Abe, on the right and Andy Johnson on the left. Two patriotic young ladies, Mrs. Samuel Dunn, presented the mottoes and banners in Ward 4 and Mrs. Royce, both soldiers' wives. The husbands of these ladies have fought bravely for the glorious old flag. Sergeant Dunn died in battle. Lt. Royce still is in the field. On the Third Ward are pictures of Washington, Grant, and Lincoln that are appropriately embellished.

Our readers will see from the foregoing that Hospitals are not entirely gloomy institutions devoted to suffering and sorrow but that they are often made pleasant and cheerful asylums, where the brave soldiers may renew their health and vigor and usefulness. And the ladies will also see how they may contribute with a small outlay of time and labor to this desirable end. Why not all the wards should be made to present this lively and pleasant aspect!

Nearly everyone is briskly employed all day; everything goes on systematically and like clock-work and that everything possible is done to make the brave boys who have lost health or limbs or been wounded in the Country' services, as comfortable as possible. This military hospital is a creation of this terrible War. We have enlisted and secured the services of some of the best professional talent in the country.

Hospital plans and construction were detailed. The pavilion buildings were described as to appearance and function. The mess hall or dining room was just over half a football field in length, and on each end was a kitchen. One served a special diet for those who could not come to the dinner table. The apothecary, or dispensary shop, made up another building. It was described as less fashionable than a city drugstore, but showing a "neat, and orderly, and well stocked shelf rather than just soaps and perfumery. Uncle Samuel is mindful of the health of his brave boys, and furnishes without stint everything necessary for them in this line." Another department was the commissary, in which sat a multitude of barrels, boxes, and packages of sugar, coffee, tea, crackers, and flour. The quartermaster building contained shirts, pants, shoes, belts, socks, underwear, linens, and a host of other soldier materials. There were two washhouses where a warm or cold bath was possible. In the main room was a row of basins whose faucets and chains were kept bright and shining through the diligent efforts of recuperating soldiers.

The gloom of that winter was dissipated by spanking new quarters. Suffering from chronic diseases and pain from battle wounds can sometimes be tempered with humor. The *Record* published various stories, puns, jokes, and satire not as predictably funny for future generations but successful in tickling the fancy of its readers. Many involve the Irish, slaves, free blacks, army officers, southerners and romance.

The *Record* also covered a wide variety of medical subjects pertinent to soldier life both in the field and as inpatients. How are field hospitals organized and intended to function? How does one build and run a 1,000-bed hospital basically from scratch? How many loaves of bread must a bakery produce daily to feed this new city? Who was admitted, who was transferred, who returned to duty, and who died? What can a soldier do for himself to maintain his health? What should a soldier do to prepare for civilian life?

In the field, sick call was held at least once and often twice daily depending on demand. The first sergeant for each company handed the surgeon a listing of those seeking attention. The surgeon recorded who returned to duty or quarters as convalescent; what duties the convalescent was capable of and who was transferred to the hospital.

The route of evacuation for the wounded soldier is described over several issues. The confusion and disorientation of battle sometimes influenced the treatment and planned evacuation of large number of casualties. Eventually plans for an orderly and effective ambulance department were realized and staffed by dedicated and well-trained doctors and assistants who converted the chaos of mass casualties into a workable system.

The field hospital was the first line of defense. The assistant surgeon rendered initial treatment at the battle site. Each regiment had several ambulances by war's end and one or two large hospital tents set up nearby but out of range of shot and shell. Heat for the winter, appropriate ventilation, water sources, fresh diet, and a fully stocked dispensary are just a few things to be provided for total patient care.

Explanations of the duties of department medical director as well as brigade, regimental, and assistant surgeons are clearly outlined. The scope of the Medical Department's involvement in the health and well-being of the soldier from latrines to kitchen hygiene is defined. Aside from knowing the art and science of their complex business, sacrifices are shared by all. "The medical officers have shown as much skill, courage and endurance to say nothing of patriotism as any other class of officers. More casualties, deaths, wounds or captures have been sustained by medical officers than any other class of staff officer in the army in proportion to numbers of each."[36]

Soldiers found themselves surrounded on the battlefield with those suffering from painful open wounds draped with blood-soaked bandages. They inhaled the stifling, pungent odor of old standing blood mixed with infection. A cynical newspaper described hospital surgery; "The most attractive feature is the amputation table where the surgeons cut off limbs with as much composure as a butcher would saw a leg of mutton for your dinner table; where legs and arms, feet and hands, toes and fingers are heaped together in one conglomerated mess."[37]

The extraordinary hardships of getting wounded soldiers home are portrayed to a knowing reader. Patients with open wounds or broken bones despite the gentlest handling of surgeons traveled rough and unforgiving roads in ambulances that lacked shock absorbers. The shrieks and groans from uncontrollable movements of an unstable extremity spoke of more pain and bleeding. The washboard-like road caused jolts of pain "like the incision of many separate knives. With each revolution of the wheel is the eerie cry of pain, frequent through solitary roadside burials on the way. This is the worst if one judges by cries."

They were transported to a convalescent or general hospital, where regular hot meals and clean beds might be available. The final leg of transportation by rail or boat also had its hazards. Despite the yeoman work of the Sanitary Commission and army medical officers, death and disease continued to take its toll. Stretchers for some and straw for others provided bedding for the casualties, sometimes in groups of hundreds. It was a struggle to survive on dimly lit ships perfumed by the stench of infection and gangrene. Nurses and doctors did what they could for the agonized sufferers. Ships arrived at the docksides of many a bustling city where "soldiers like Rip Van Winkle awakened from slumber." The hospital was their new home until the wounds healed and they became well. If they did not heal, it would serve as a way station on their final journey. One-third returned to duty, some were medically discharged from the service, and some succumbed. "Many have already received final discharge and await reward of heroism and sacrifices in another world; may it be ample."

A common theme in the *Record* was the relationship of mother and son. This poignant and often heart-rending subject is the subject of poems, songs, and short stories. But while degrees of sacrifice vary, virtually all of society shared the experience of loss. Everyone knew young men who did not return and others who survived only to return deformed or chronically ill.

In a story called "Roll Call," a severely wounded soldier lies in a large city hospital, resolutely courageous and hopeful: "I am better off than many others; I came out to endure the hardships of a soldier's life, and I shall not complain." As the hot days of July wear on, he is afflicted with fevers and his wounds refuse to heal: "I want to talk to you about my mother. I dreamt about her last night and it frightened me that I could not sleep again." His father died when he was quite young and his brother from a battle just past. He had enlisted to avenge his brother's death, on behalf of the surviving family including mother and sister. With the progression of disease comes delirium. He has dark dreams about loved ones he can't reach but must answer the call to duty. Delirium ensues and he dies the next morning.

> Tell mom and sister to have my room ready for when I get home. Do you hear that roll call? They are coming. Do you see the captain of that company? That is my brother Charles. They told me he was dead. Now I see he commands that company, and I shall take him home to mother, what a joyful meeting that will be. I must go to my brother, good-by my friends good-by.
>
> Look no more for thy boy, fond mother. In a land of strangers he has found a Soldier's grave. Look with eye of faith to home beyond the grave and there amid that shining throng, that has fought, bled and died for country. See your boys, they beckon you. This way mother, although the throng is great, fear not; there's surely room for mothers who have given their sons to fight in such a cause and may you meet them there never more to be separated from them.

In a story called "Mother and son, the last word from his lips," a bright-eyed young lad of sixteen is wounded at Fredericksburg. He dies in the halo of nostalgia and motherly love.

> He appeared more affectionate and tender than his comrades. He longed for the arrival of his mother who was expected for she knew his wound was mortal and that he was failing fast. He thought she had come, for a kind lady visitor was wiping the death sweat from his brow as his sight was failing. He rallied a little and whispered "Is that mother," in moans that drew tears from every eye. Then drawing her toward him with all his feeble power, he nestled his head in her arms like a sleeping infant, and died with the sweet word "Mother" on his quivering lips.

"Kiss Me, Mother, Once Again" is a poetic tribute to a wounded New England soldier at Gettysburg. Comrades find him the morning after, lying among the dead and dying, stiff bodies layered in scattered piles like a forest carpeted with broken trees after an ice storm. He was still alone, "this bleeding hero, in an infant's quiet sleep, with a smile of angelic beauty, and a peaceful end unafraid to meet his maker." The scene is set before his last breath:

> On a field of bloody carnage
> Where the gory wavelets swell,
> Over wan and ghastly warriors
> Who have nobly fought and fell
> Lay a young and daring soldier,
> Weary, wounded, bleeding and fair!
> But a smile overspread his features,
> Such as angels only wear
> Smiles of sweet, angelic Beauty
> O'er his placid features spread,
> And his eyelids slowly opened,
> Gently, softly Willie said,
> Comrades! Tell my darling mother
> I am freed from earthly pain,
> But I longed once more to see her —
> Kiss me, mother, once again!

The difficulties of the sick and wounded especially in hospitals were confronted by chaplains and ministers alike. Surrounded by strangers, there is longing for a mother's love that can soothe and heal. The biblical notion of what it means to be a sojourner in a foreign or hostile land and how a righteous person should interact with them is a common theme.

This is not home! Perhaps a Hospital is to be thy last stopping place, and strangers to do thy last offices for thee; if kissed at all, by unknown lips. A man from Maine, a stout and manly youth living in New Orleans for but a short time was attacked with Yellow fever and soon died with no mother or relative to soothe or sympathize. He died among strangers and buried by them. When they were about to close coffin an old lady said "Let me kiss him for his mother"! May her sons, when they die, not lack a mother's sympathy or at the least find one who will kiss them for their mother![38]

The thoughts of a dying man are likely to be focused on the source of dependable love and comfort. As a boy, whom did he run to when he scraped his knee and was afraid? What better companion than the person you can unconditionally count on? In the poem "Thy Mother prays for thee," the gold standard of comfort is hauntingly portrayed.

> Such thoughts as these passed through my mind
> And as I lie thus musing
> And had a vision bright.
> A loved one's form before me stood,
> With voice both clear and free;
> And whispered, Fear not!
> For at home Thy mother prays for thee.

In the following two stories also from the *Record*, getting to heaven requires suffering and faith, as peace and glory conflicts a fevered and painful brow. Patients with penetrating chest wounds, infected stumps, or life-threatening diseases do not make speeches glorifying war, politics, or religion. It may be difficult enough just to breathe besides suffering the spasms of excruciating pain, without searching for additional strength to wave a flag, tell a clever joke, or quote prophecies from the Bible. It is also true that no mortal pilgrim having entered the hereafter has ever returned to advise us as to what it is like.

A Touching Scene
A minister describes an event in City Point Hospital noted by the chaplain of Christian Commission. He was moving through a long line of suffering soldiers while administering the consolation of the gospel when he approaches a gallant fellow who was severely wounded. His earthly march was nearly ended but when asked if he was prepared to die motioned for pencil and paper and wrote with tremulous hand "I am prepared to go to heaven; my trust in Jesus Christ is perfect and under these words assured victory over the grave: Come, rally round the flag, boys." The chaplain took the paper, and standing up read it with a loud voice. Just as he concluded, a soldier who had recently lost a hand sprang from his bed, and waving the mutilated stump in the air burst forth with the glorious song his dying comrade had suggested. The effect was electric. A thousand voices took up the chorus, and the place of suffering was made to fairly rock with thunders of melody. As that vast soldier choir ceased singing, the chaplain turned to look upon the dying brave. He was just in time to catch the last faint smile that flickered across the sun burnt face, as the soul wafted on the strains of that Union music to the throne of Liberty.

The second segment, *Touching Scenes in Military Hospitals,* tells of a Quaker lady who felt the war was justified and that the power of Christian faith eased both suffering and dying. She recites hymns to dying soldiers who think she is their mother.

> "Jesus can make a dying bed
> Feel soft as downy pillows are,
> While on his breast I lay my head,
> And breathe my life out sweetly there"

A soldier exclaims, "Mother, I knew you would come. Mother I am going to Jesus" and then succumbs. A little drummer boy, also near death, is whispered to by the same Quaker lady: "Rock of ages, cleft for me, Let me hide myself in thee." The boy recites the stanza as his mother had taught him, and he too passes.

The Angel of Death facilitates the soldier's passage to the beyond, representing mother, faith or spiritual strengths from within. "Be not afraid for I am with you" offers guidance derived from biblical lore. Returning to the comfort of home and mother is a recurrent theme. The sanctuary is home, being surrounded by loved ones, and being aided by a strong belief in salvation and the hereafter. In the following poems, it is opined that God wears Union blue. The heavenly shield is extended to the loyal defenders of the Constitution and Union.

> Washed in the blood of the braver and blooming,
> Prophets of Baal,
> Justice, mercy,
> God bless the flag and its loyal defenders.

The shield of faith serves to protect the traveler from the fiercest storm, the most terrifying experience, and from the fear of death itself. A soldier writes his wife in "The Night before the Battle." He is alone in the thick dew of morning, as "the cannon's rage will stun the ear and fill the soul with fear." He continues, "Blood may flow and I give myself to God's sweet care. And murmur soft my boyhood's prayer Dear Savior, guard me in my sleep. All danger in the distance keeps!"

Another poem written for a soldier who died of disease in North Carolina confirms the same sentiment: "Trust in God, to land free from sorrow and pain, believe in heaven, from this world to another, and trust in God, trust in God." Understanding the twists and turns of life may in the end be impossible for mortals. There may be no logic or fairness in the experience of war, and that for some is its ultimate horror. For no obvious reason a limb becomes useless or absent and a life is ended. Faith in a higher being that knows all and comprehends a universe that man cannot, serves for many as a passport through bitter, frightening, and life-threatening experiences. If man did understand the why of early death, would that make the loss of a loved one any less painful? According to John 11:25, "I am the resurrection and the life: he that believeth in me, though he was dead, yet shall he live." This requires an unshakeable religious faith, spirituality that helps confront the grim business of the battlefield. Some soldiers believed in this covenant, but some could not and did not. For them, once fallen, there would be no resurrection.

On a more practical earthbound footing is the notion that if your time has not come, even the doctor will not succeed in killing you. Although everyone claims to know that they are going to die, few actually believe it, especially the young. Supreme Court Justice Oliver Wendell Holmes, Jr., wrote about his personal experience as a soldier wounded in the neck at Antietam, tempered by years of judicial reflection: "Faith is true and admirable which leads a soldier to throw away his life in obedience to a blindly accepted faith, in a cause which he little understands, in a plan of campaign in which he has little notion, under tactics of which he does not see the use."[39] He added later with great pride that the "wounds they bore would be the medals they would show their children and grandchildren by and by. Who would not rather wear his decorations beneath his uniform than on it?"

Some soldiers dreamed of death, whether from the cacophony of battle or from the insidious cough of consumption. Poems invoke the earth of a battlefield soaked in blood, while grieving parents sob in the background surrounded by the solemn sounds of a church choir. A calm and peaceful aura envelops the stricken soldier who is then joined by other veterans, all very still with cold marble faces and sunken unblinking eyes. Courage in battle was defined as a duel with death: "Upon the first fire I immediately look upon myself as a dead man. I then fight the remainder of the day, regardless of danger, as a dead man should be. All my limbs which I carried out to the field I regard as so much gained, or so much saved out of the fire."

Death was the commonest theme for poems. The authors were soldiers, wives, journalists, literary figures, and the anonymous. The titles included the words "after battle, coming home, going to grave, grave site, death, dying, fallen, fatal, missing, returning, unreturning, and unknown." The sadness is gut-wrenching and unchanged from generation to generation. Birds fly freely in the bright blue sky as the damp and the cool earth serves as resting place for the once warm living body. For the survivors, the newly childless mother and father, there remains perpetual heartache in solitude.

A lifeless boy soldier lies in a field amongst other dead soldiers, yet he is quite alone. Another fallen is both father and husband and will return home in spirit only. Willie is a mother's beloved son, angelic and forever still. A bloody photograph of a beautiful fiancée is found on a deceased beau, a lost dream of happiness. The plea "Will you visit me in my grave?" repeats the fear of being lost and alone. What shall we do with all these unknown soldiers: faceless and nameless, their marker gravestones identical like a forest of white picket fences? How will their mothers visit and mourn them? How awful and horrific is the battle carnage resulting from shot and shell that has become so efficient in its work. "Tell mother and sister not to weep, but remember me, if you will." And finally "they are coming," the soldiers are coming home but not her dad; not today or even tomorrow and certainly not in this life.

The notion of mortality was a distant galaxy for those under twenty-six years, which was the average soldier's age. They ordinarily did not give it much thought except when in the natural course of events it occurred to others. The notion of immortality is appealing for those without a blemish or an ache, a full head of hair, unlimited stamina, and bottomless urges to prove one's manhood and bravery.

Missing-Dead
Undaunted by the battle shock —
Shrouded in the cannon smoke,
They still pressed on for woe or weal.
Right up to the cannon's breath,
Right up into the jaws of death,
They hewed their way with steel and lead
Till when the tide of battle turned,
And up the east the round moon burned
To look upon a sea of dead.

A Grave Site
A Union Soldier Mustered Out
Mustered out from din of Battle,
Clouds of smoke and wreaths of flame,
From the muskets' ceaseless rattle,
Scattering showers of fiery rain;
From the booming cannons' roar
Mingled with the groans of dying,

Passing to the farther shore.
Think of that great BOUNTY given
Where our soldiers MUSTERED IN!
Think of changing Earth for Heaven,
Throwing off the yoke of sin!
Leaving mortal for immortal,
Grieves below for joys above,
Entering the heavenly portal,
Happy in a Savior's love.

The Unknown Dead
By Fred Willoughby
Mayhap, a mother's loving eyes
Looked down on them from paradise,
And smiled, and beckoned them to come,
And share with her that happy home;
But some there were whose faces bore
The look that martyrs often wore,
And these unknown soldiers!

Just After the Battle
David Pratt, Company I, Eighth Connecticut Volunteers
Still upon the field of battle,
I am lying, mother dear,
With my wounded comrades waiting
For the morning to appear.
Many sleep to waken never
In this world of strife and death,
And many more are faintly calling,
With their feeble, dying breath.

Oh, the first great charge was fearful
And a thousand brave men fell,
Still, amid the dreadful carnage,
I was safe from shot and shell,
So amid the fatal shower,
I had nearly passed the day,
When then the howling shell struck me,
And I sunk amid the fray.

Oh, the glorious cheer of triumph,
When the foeman turned and fled,
Leaving us the field of battle,
Strown with dying and with dead.
Oh, the torture and the anguish,
That I could not follow on,
But here amid my fallen comrades,
I must wait till morning's dawn,

Death of the Soldier
By Hattie Bell
Tell my fond and gentle mother
Not to weep when I am gone
Tell my loving little sister
We shall meet on earth no more

Comrades see my breath grows fainter
And I scarce can see you now.
Tell my loved ones to forget not
Him who in life's morning died.

Captain Joseph Toy from the Twelfth Connecticut Volunteers, a father of three, died of typhoid fever while stationed in New Orleans. His sermon was delivered by the Reverend Ichabod Simmons in Simsbury July 12, 1862. This soldier's time had come, his lips frozen still and his tongue now silent. The tears on his cold frozen face were not his own but from his family. The minister discusses "our sons' blood flowing in the destruction of war," patriotism, duty, justice, and Christian faith.

> While the war rages, amid roaring broadsides, delirious screams of charging brigades and shrieks of brave patriots dying in the ranks, we ignore roll calls and inspect no company to see who have fallen. It is when night shuts down on the battle field and weary warriors lay him down to dream of wife and child, when the smoke rolls away — only then do we scan the lists of killed and wounded. When the soldier returns to his home, not as he went in joyful prophecies of happy victories but enshrined in the uniform of the dead and weeping ones gather to tender him their last offering of love. It is then that war's history is dreadful and our own attention is arrested by painful truths. Earth has no sorrows that heaven cannot heal.[40]

At the Knight U.S. Army General Hospital, wounds were healing and for most life got better. Every day except Sunday, the drum corps sounded reveille, or morning call, at 5 A.M. in the summer and 6 A.M. in the winter. Patients well enough to make their beds washed and fell in at roll call. Breakfast was prepared, the flag run up, and wards and offices swept clean. At 7 A.M., the drum again sounded and ward masters formed columns of men who were then marched to the mess hall for morning meal. Meals were delivered to the beds of those unable to walk.

The Veteran Relief Corps then performed "Guard Mounting." The grounds were policed and cleaned of the previous day's debris. At 9 A.M. came the surgeons' call. Assistant surgeons then saw each patient and prescribed medicine and diet. All was inscribed in a register brought to the dispensary where the prescriptions were filled and then brought back to the wards.

Afterwards patients might exercise, read, play cards or other games, visit the chapel or library, go downtown and shop, or visit friends. At noon the dinner call was sounded, and the same ritual repeated as for breakfast. At 5 P.M. a second surgeons' call was sounded and rounds were repeated where necessary. At sundown the drum corps played "the retreat," and the flag was lowered with a salute from drums and fifes followed by supper call. In summer, men sat under the skies in open tents and swapped stories about their past exploits for the amusement and edification of any who wished to listen. After final roll call, the drum corps played tattoo. A half-hour later, three taps on the bass drum meant lights out except for officers and the very sick. Chapel services were on Sunday, and the weekly inspection by the surgeon in charge took place each Saturday morning.

The requirements of furnishings, food, and equipment were staggering. A three-month return policy was instituted to protect the hospital from shoddy goods. Nationwide, soldiers were issued boots, coats, and blankets that fell apart weeks after receiving them. Drugs diluted with filler and containers fraudulently packed with stone instead of product plagued distribution centers. The Medical Department in Washington attempted to avoid price gouging and poor quality by building army laboratories for in-house drug manufacture. Some of the technicians were German druggists or chemists, some of whom became hospital stewards. Government laboratories in Philadelphia, New York, and Memphis turned out whiskey, sherry, quinine, calomel, mercurial ointment, and chloroform. Fortunes were made in the drug industry as some of America's largest companies got their start here. At war's end, the richest man in America owned the drug company that held the license to import the malarial drug cinchona bark, and synthetically manufactured quinine. Below are some of the needs listed in the *Knight Hospital Record* for its burgeoning institution.

OUTFIT OF A GENERAL HOSPITAL OF 1000 BEDS

Iron bedsteads	1,000	Socks	2,000
Hair Mattresses	100	Dressing gowns	1,000
Straw	1,000	Caps	1,000
Linen sheets	4,000	Knives and forks	600
Linen pillow cases	2,000	Mugs	600
Mosquito bars (if needed)	1,000	Plates	600
Shirts	1,480	Table spoons	600
Blankets	2,000	Teaspoons	600
Drawers	2,000	Bedside tables	500
Slippers	1,000	Towels	840

ARTICLES CONSUMED IN A HOSPITAL IN THE
SIX-MONTH PERIOD ENDING OCTOBER 1864

Fresh beef	116,000 lbs.	Tea	831 lbs.
Ham	8,832 lbs.	Sugar	12,480 lbs.
Fresh fish	23,112 lbs.	Soap	908 lbs.
Chickens	4,351 lbs.	Potatoes	72,998 lbs.
Beans	5,170 lbs.	Milk	48,637 qts.
Rice	1,461 lbs.	Butter	11,839 lbs.
Cornmeal	1,025 lbs.	Eggs	5,893 dozen
Coffee	2,282 lbs.	Soda crackers	1,782 lbs.

The diet in Connecticut was complete and nutritious, for fresh fish, meat, and vegetables and fruit were readily available. In the field, it was another story. The listings of materials, from bedding to butter, illustrates the need for local support and the difficulty in supplying a large army in enemy territory. Honest manufacturers and brokers did exist, but vigilance and oversight were essential on the part of the hospital's administration. Overpriced, shoddy goods were readily available for the unwary or the bribed. This was a large operation started from scratch and run by people who were mostly on-the-job trainees. How does one buy, on the average, 390 eggs a day? Multiple sources of supply were needed, including wholesalers and farmers alike who required cash, not IOUs. There is the question of price, quality of goods, availability, and the effects of the free and black markets.

By September 1864 there were 202 general hospitals and 136,894 beds in the Union army. Maintaining these hospitals with appropriate medications, bedding, furniture and food was a major undertaking. Below is a listing of a few items and quantities purchased by the Medical Department of the Union army during the war.[41]

Medications

Spiritus frumenti (whiskey)	1,907,145 (32-ounce bottles)
Spiritus vini gallici (wine)	582,187 (32-ounce bottles)
Vinum album (sherry)	736,459 (32-ounce bottles)
Chloroform	1,146,982 ounces
Ether	1,002,045 half-pound tins
Extract cinchona	518,957 ounces
Opii pulvis	552,196 ounces
Opii tinctura camphorata	993,311 ounces
Pilule opii	813,156 ounces

Bedding

Blankets	1,165,000
Sheets, linen	1,638,000
Mosquito bars	221,058
Pillowcases	1,050,166

Furniture and Appliances

Basins	92,000
Bedpans	38,000
Bedsteads, iron	274,000
Lanterns	39,000
Medicine panniers	5,830
Spittoons	89,000
Cooking stoves with fixtures complete	1,800

It appears that there was a spittoon for almost every soldier in every hospital. Huge quantities of spirits (three million 32-ounce bottles) were consumed for so-called medicinal reasons. Opium mixed with camphor was a common cold remedy, and in the plain form a painkiller.

And so the ship called Knight U.S. Army General Hospital was created, an ark in a turbulent sea. It provided health care, order and tranquility in a time of political conflict and unremitting violence. It gave shelter to fallen soldiers along with the stiff-necked and incessant grumblers. Father Abraham was the righteous and unwavering patriarch striving mightily to steer this vessel to a safe haven, where the false God of slavery would exist no more. His progeny would be like the stars in the firmament, saving the innocent and punishing the wicked, a blessing for all the states and the nations of the world. A critical part of the ship's crew for this noble undertaking was the men of the caduceus, the medical staff with the faith, humanity and skill necessary to allow entrance into the Promised Land.

For some states there was no haven, no ark, and no state hospital for sick and wounded returning soldiers. As late as August 1863, the governor of Wisconsin pleaded his case with Secretary Stanton: "While men from other states who have done better by their service to their country are constantly being sent to their own states, where their friends can reach them, and where they can become invigorated by breathing home atmosphere, no such right or privilege is given ours. Privileges are constantly being obtained for soldiers of other states, while we cannot obtain them for our soldiers. There is no hospital in Wisconsin."[42]

He noted that the surgeon general issued orders concerning Illinois soldiers that permitted transfer home furloughs when medical opinion considered that necessary for recovery.

Connecticut's military hospital maintained patients' belongings and sent home pay to support their families. Soldiers not able to plant, tend, or harvest had to rely on others, as explained to Major Jewett.

> Dear Sir,
>   I have just learnt that wife's pay has not bin sent to her yet and the reason no not and you would oblige me if you could see to it as I cannot git there.[43]
>   Yours respectfully,
>   H. V. Sims
>   7th Connecticut Regiment

While many prisoners of war died in captivity or shortly thereafter, others suffered the consequences of this experience for a lifetime. Pain, suffering and personal indignation can follow. H.V. Sims was 24 years old, 5 feet 9 inches tall, a blue-eyed Englishman who was a teamster when he enlisted in the Seventh Connecticut Regiment in September 1861. He sustained a gunshot wound on June 16, 1862, to the left side of his head, incurring a skull fracture with subsequent abscess and loss of vision in the left eye. He was furloughed home in the fall but failed to contact his wife. His father-in-law notified the provost marshal who then listed him as a deserter, not knowing he was a patient at Knight U.S. Army General Hospital. He advised Major Jewett about the financial difficulties in May 1863. He was returned to the battlefield as a cook with the Nineteenth Regiment and was captured at Drewrys Bluff, Virginia, on May 16, 1864. He was sent to Andersonville Prison and paroled on February 24, 1865, mustering out in May 1865. He was variously described as either missing in action or as a deserter. The head injury originally described as "not serious" clearly was, as subsequent hospital records indicated.

In 1868 he was divorced by his wife of eleven years for "committing adultery with diverse lewd persons" and being a steady drinker. His second marriage, in 1870, was also unsuccessful, although his second wife enjoyed for many decades disability benefits for a blind and brain-traumatized veteran.

CHAPTER NINE

Medical Staff of
Knight U.S. Army General Hospital

Getting doctors to work together has been compared to herding cats. They are individualistic, authoritarian and highly skilled, and do not like being told what to do, how, where or when. The chief of staff had the task to appease, encourage, regulate, and enforce. We can gain insight into Major Jewett's capability and likely responses to his job from the work of his eldest son, Thomas Backus Jewett, who was twelve years old when he began accompanying his father on Saturday medical grand rounds at the new military hospital. The young "doctor," like all visiting children on hospital wards, was a welcome sight to the staff and convalescing patients, bringing cheer and hope.

Thomas Backus Jewett graduated from Yale Medical School in 1879, simultaneously becoming a fellow of the Connecticut Medical Society (CMS). His graduating term paper "Temperaments" describes the five types of human behavior first discussed by Hippocrates and then Galen. The first is "sanguine," characterized by people who are "energetic, lively, sparkling, chest full and broad, action of heart quick and strong, impressions easily made and changed, judgment not as sound as imagination, of acute sensibility, great irritability, and a spirit of go ahead."[1]

The second type is the "bilious" or "choleric and ambitious." They have a "love of authority, haughtiness, and passions lively and strong." He further describes them as "inflexible, irascible, matter of fact men, often non-humorous." They are concerned with the "destiny of nations," and exhibit "undaunted courage, great endurance, audacity, and combine that with virtuous or infamous qualities." They are firm, decisive and determined and may become eminent due to this virtue or infamous on the same account.

The two temperaments can coexist and perhaps did in his father, autocratic but willing to sacrifice for the greater good. Patriotism meant making real sacrifices, financial, social, professional, and physical. The surgeon in charge was "entrusted with full and complete military command over the persons and property connected with the hospital." Pliny Adams Jewett was born for this job.

Next in command was the executive officer, Dr. L. C. Wilcoxson. He joined the Connecticut State Medical Society (CSMS) in 1842 and lived in the South until 1861 when he returned to New Haven. In December 1862, he was appointed acting assistant surgeon in the role of chief executive officer, maintaining his office on the first floor of the old state hospital next to Jewett. He was responsible for the day-to-day administration of the hospital and in the city directory of 1863 listed his home address as Knight U.S. Army General Hospital. He had charge of office and records, clerks and orderlies, supervised preparation of all reports, promulgated all orders and conducted general correspondence, and made appropriate distribution of patients received for admission. The department medical director required written reports daily, weekly, monthly, and quarterly; the surgeon general and adjutant general required them monthly; the adjutant general and paymaster required bimonthly muster and payrolls; the surgeon general required quarterly reports of property purchased with hospital funds and annual returns of medicines and hospital stores; and finally the quartermaster general required returns of camp and garrison equipment. All reports were required in triplicate. Books were kept on records of admission, a hospital register of sick and wounded, and an alphabetical register of casualties, deaths, discharges, and transfers. He was also responsible for order books, accounts of hospital and slush funds, and the maintenance of hospital property.

He ran the examining board for mustering out and medically discharging patients. This procedure required five detailed, handwritten copies per soldier, on a schedule that rarely missed a day, excluding Sundays. Those approved were assigned certificates of disability and were awarded a pension commensurate with their rating. After the hospital closed he was sent to a post hospital in Macon, Georgia. He returned to New Haven after the war and resumed activities at the state hospital and continued private practice for a number of years.

For those who were unfamiliar with army culture and thought these reports unnecessary, edicts were issued, like this one from September 1863, by Dr. C. F. Campbell, the medical director of Fort Monroe, Virginia.

> The want of printed blanks is no valid excuse for reports and requests required by regulations. Requests for supplies are to be ordered by the quarter. If you run out you will be held strictly accountable. All letters must be folded in three equal folds, parallel with writing and endorsed in the fold. No patient shall be sent to the general hospital if he can be treated at the regimental hospital. Medical officers are too apt to send cases, which are a little troublesome to the General Hospital. This practice must cease. All subjects fit for the Invalid Corps or discharged from the service are to be sent to the General Hospital.[2]

Keeping patients at the regimental level meant keeping them near the battlefield, which lessened their chance of disappearing in the chronic care facilities or being prematurely discharged from the service. Failure of the regimental surgeons to send their sick to general hospitals when patients were "past cure" was thought critical. The sicker patients were the ones transferred and would thus have a higher mortality rate. Transfer to the rear was desirable for the unscheduled patients who often arrived grateful for a regular hot meal and glad to wait for official administrative or medical dispensation, in biblical years if possible to avoid returning to the battlefield. If the general hospital was full and especially if legitimate documents were not available, patients might be turned away despite a long and tedious journey. The Sanitary Commission described some of the problems:

> Mortality in general hospitals are [*sic*] thought to be accounted for by this alleged fact. Some men spend the night in an ambulance at the hospital door. There is little room for doubt that many lives have already been lost from mere technical and formal obstacles to their preservation.

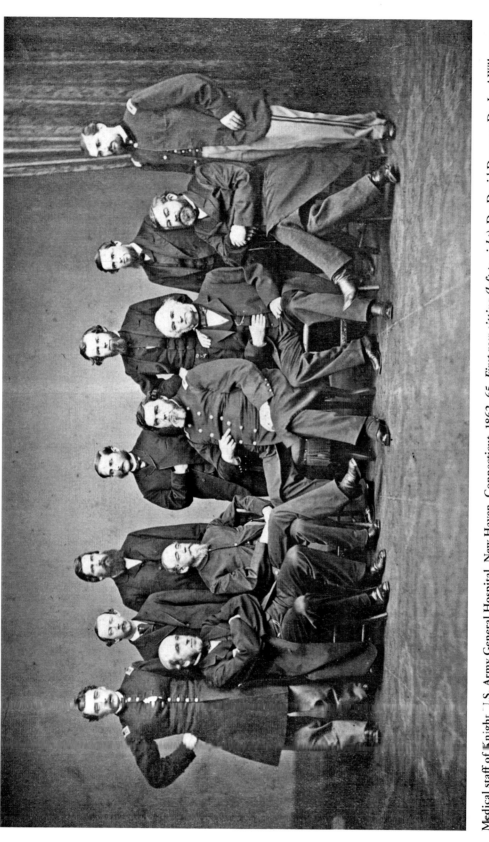

Medical staff of Knight U.S. Army General Hospital, New Haven, Connecticut, 1862–65. *First row sitting (left to right):* Dr. David Daggett, Dr. Levi Wilcoxson, Dr. P.A. Jewett, Dr. Worthington Hooker, Dr. W.B. Casey. *Second row standing:* unidentified army surgeon, Dr. T.H. Bishop, Dr. H.S. Pierpont, Dr. T.B. Townsend, Dr. Charles Lindsley, Dr. Virgil Dow, unidentified army surgeon (The New Haven Museum & Historical Society).

Surgeons try to get stoves and spend days getting signatures without approval — bureaucracy kills. Military surgeons are often saddled with administrative duties to the exclusions of scientific learning.[3]

An executive officer in another state, Dr. D. McConnell, criticized written reports submitted by his fellow doctors, a perennial problem.

It reflects sadly upon our profession as Doctors to be obliged to return so simple a thing as a monthly report for correction but in self-defense I find myself obliged to do it. The majority had some slight mistakes, which I corrected. Most however, abound in blots and erasures and to judge of the profession by appearances of our "reports" will I fear entail harsh judgment. I hope next month will show neater and more correct records generally.[4]

The Sanitary Commission suggested weekly or monthly lecture series for medical education and less clerical work. Surgeon General Hammond concurred and in addition initiated a series of sixteen pamphlets for surgeons on subjects including amputations, yellow fever, military hygiene, dysentery, malaria, fevers, soldiers' health, and venereal diseases, directions for army surgeons on the field of battle, pneumonia, wound hemorrhage, joint excisions, scurvy, cholera, vaccination, use of quinine, fractures, and water use in surgery.

Another contemporary of Jewett, just four years younger, was Dr. David L. Daggett. He graduated from Yale College in 1839 and the medical school in 1843. His grandfather, Judge David Daggett, had been the mayor of New Haven, a U.S. senator, a professor of law at Yale, and a judge of the Superior Court of Connecticut. The doctor became a member of CSMS in 1848, was president of the New Haven and Connecticut State Medical Societies, and director and consulting surgeon of the General Hospital Society of Connecticut. After the war he continued a leadership role in the various medical societies and the state hospital.

Another original member was Dr. S.B. Hubbard whose father was the first chief of surgery at Yale, the second being Dr. Jonathan Knight. He was also a director and consulting surgeon of the General Hospital Society of Connecticut. His son was Edward Hubbard, a medical cadet at age twenty who died of typhoid fever in 1863 while serving at Cumberland Hospital in Tennessee.

The youngest and brightest was Dr. Charles Lindsley.[5] He was born in Orange, New Jersey, in 1826, and later married a local girl who bore him five children. He graduated from Trinity University and attended the College of Physicians and Surgeons of New York but graduated from Yale Medical School in 1852. The committee that gave his final examination was composed of Drs. Jewett, Woodward, Knight, and Beers. His graduating thesis was entitled "Diagnosis," indicating a preference for medical rather than surgical interests. He served an apprenticeship in Cheshire, moved to New Haven, and was in a brief partnership before opening his own office. His colleagues noted that "he cared for sick in all seasons and at all times no matter how poor his patient or how inconvenient the hour. The demand for help found him ever ready and cheerful to obey delighting in the opportunity his profession afforded to relieve human suffering."

He was a tall, thin, elegant man with a full beard, an effective speaker and writer who had a host of social skills. Dr. Jewett encouraged him to present a paper to the New Haven Medical Society in April of 1858 concerning puerperal convulsions, known today as eclampsia of pregnancy.[6] His writing is crisp, modern, and honest in both analysis and treatment. "With scarcely a dissenting voice the grand chief remedy is venesection, copious depletion almost without reservation. The inference naturally drawn from this fact would be that the etiology and pathology must be as well understood and the lesions of the disease as uniform as the treatment recommended. This inference would be far, very far from the truth." The reasoning behind bloodletting was to decrease the fluid volume in a patient being consumed with congestion or excess fluid from kidney failure. He cautioned that bloodletting also causes seizures and even death and recognized low albumin in the blood and high in the urine as related to nephritis with generalized edema.

He correctly surmised that delivery was the definitive treatment. "Artificial delivery might be resorted to, if fetus is source of irritation in mother." Other options were Caesarian section, inducing premature labor by dilating the cervical os with instruments, or with douching. In 1859 he was unanimously elected to fill a vacancy due to the resignation of Professor Bronson from Yale's medical department. In 1860 he assumed the chair of materia medica and therapeutics and simultaneously was made registrar of births, marriages and deaths for the City of New Haven, where he stressed the need for accurate records and statistics. His comments on slovenly or otherwise faulty reports by those who gave impossible, insufficient, or ridiculous causes of death "may not have been relished by an unwary reporter but served the purpose in a campaign of education." Other states adopted his techniques as his work was reported in the medical and lay literature.

He was appointed attending physician to the New Haven Hospital in 1860 and became dean of the medical school in 1863, a post he held until 1885. Early in the war he was a contract surgeon in Lincoln Hospital in Washington, D.C., and later he served at Knight U.S. Army General Hospital until it closed. "In all these capacities he served faithfully and well. As teacher he was clear in his exposition of subject, as administrator painstaking and accurate. He was courteous, of good nature, and had high standards of educational work." He supported advanced teaching techniques throughout and "worked with younger members of faculty and seconded every step they took, advocating laboratory methods even though he was not a lab man himself."[7]

Financial problems were not limited to medical students but afflicted medical departments as well. Lindsley addressed these circumstances in an 1864 letter to the administration of Yale:

> To President and Fellows of Yale College in New Haven
> From faculty of the Medical Department
>   Classes in past were full but small, why?
> 1. Competition is not always the most honorable by colleges on either side of us.
> 2. Increase in city size. Students go elsewhere and graduate with ease, as the course is only 4 months.
>   Since 1864, the present faculty has been unremitting in serving a higher standard of education. Each professor has at least 100 lecture-exercises in the year. For eight or nine years our duties have been laborious but exactly and conscientiously performed, while our remuneration has been nothing worth mentioning. The income from the Fund is not equal to the expenses of a department in the care and repair of a building, and current expenses of lectures. The deficiencies are paid by ourselves. We need money for the same purposes that other departments need and receive it. The professorships of medicine and toxicology are vacant and others may resign.
>   Only money is wanted to place this school of medicine in a position of influence and prosperity second to none. How do you get money? It is suggested that, "we must go out and beg it."
>   There are personal duties and obligations to the community. How long on the present plan can the Medical Department be continued? The question is as if illusionary.[8]

He goes on to request $10,000 and recommends that schooling be held throughout the year. His proposals were ignored. Yale's medical school survived in the following decades but just barely. Dr. Lindsley wore many hats: professor of medicine, dean, researcher, public health official, writer, consultant, educator, and next-door neighbor and friend to Pliny Jewett. He taught at the free clinics, at the military hospital, and in lecture halls, and dealt with personal student problems and complaints. Lindsley was paid as a contract surgeon at Knight hospital and was credited with three surgical cases in the *MSHWR*. (See Appendix IV.)

At the war's end, Lindsley continued his role as director at the hospital and New Haven Dispensary, or free clinics. He was an authority on sanitary matters, enthusiastically tracing the sources of epidemic and contagious disease and writing many scientific papers. Like Jewett, he was a member of St. Paul's Episcopal Church and was described as a "consistent and enthusiastic churchman." He died in 1906, never having retired.

A soldier asked Dr. Lindsley for his testimony in a claim for a service-related back injury and was not disappointed by the affidavit: "I am not particularly acquainted with the soldier H.J. Thompson. He comes to me with prescription of mine given by me for a plaster and I have no doubt was given for disability. He claims pain in back and seems truthful. He claims to have been treated by me for said disability. I have no hesitation in believing such is the fact. He had prescription filled three times since 1865."[9] That would have been three times in twenty years.

By 1863, the number of sick and wounded had escalated, establishing the need for additional personnel. William Chester Minor was twenty-nine years old when he graduated from Yale Medical School in January 1863. He came from a prominent and wealthy New England family with a large business presence in New Haven. He was born in Ceylon. His father was a missionary and his mother was dead of consumption when he was only three. He lived in Asia until his teenage years and then attended Yale College. After graduating from medical school, he joined the regular army and spent the summer of 1863 at the Knight U.S. Army General Hospital. His interests were in comparative anatomy, and he was assigned to do autopsies on mostly black troops, thirty-three soldiers in all.[10]

He was then transferred to Washington, D.C., and on to Alexandria, Virginia. He claimed to have been at the Battle of the Wilderness but no such order or evidence of that exists. By the war's end, he was a captain in the regular army (as opposed to the volunteers), a position desirable for financial and security reasons, sought by many but achieved by few. He had exhibited since his teen years psychiatric difficulties, which worsened with age. Hallucinations and sexual delusions became more severe, resulting in the diagnosis of monomania, which is considered schizophrenia today. This resulted in an eighteen-month inpatient admission at St. Elizabeth's Hospital in Washington. He had claimed severe stress from undocumented battlefield exposure, and alleged having witnessed a deserting Irishman branded on the cheek with an iron, another delusion. He was transferred to New York City where a medical board confirmed his insanity and recommended discharge from the service as he was "incapacitated by causes arising in the line of duty." They declared that his illness was service-connected, resulting from psychological trauma occurring during war, thus entitling him to full pay and pension. The monetary significance was that for the remainder of his life (he died at age eighty-five) he received monthly checks, with appropriate increases, commensurate with a regular army captain's salary.

A similar case from Connecticut had a very different ending. John Henry Burnham was a captain in the Sixteenth Connecticut Volunteers from Hartford and served in the battles at Fredericksburg and Antietam where his regiment was decimated, the sights and sounds described in a letter home: "You can hear the shell and solid shot from artillery come whizzing and singing thru the air some seconds before they reach you. I think a person with acute hearing may acquire proficiency in avoiding them that would render them comparatively harmless. The bullets from musketry have a more insidious hissing sound and confound the little nasty things."

In March 1865, he was captured at the Battle of Kinston, North Carolina, and spent two weeks as a prisoner of war. By that point, his rank was lieutenant colonel. The war soon ended, and he was sent home to Coventry, where he worked in a general country store and was briefly postmaster in Hartford. The regimental surgeon, Nathan Mayer, reported that he "sustained nervous agitation" in 1863 at the Battle of Suffolk and that due to "nervous and mental troubles he was unable to perform manual work." He declined in health and was admitted to the Hartford Retreat, where he was declared insane in 1882 at age fifty-three. He was described as "five feet eight inches, weighing 135 pounds,

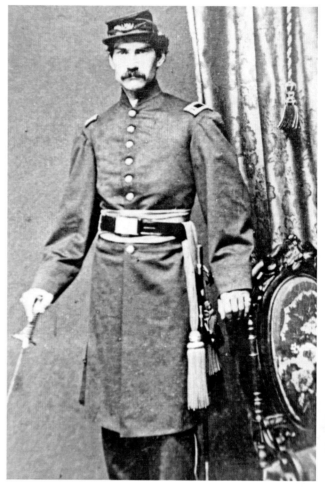

Major John Henry Burnham, Sixteenth Connecticut Volunteers (Connecticut State Library).

totally helpless and requiring regular aid and attendance of another." Dr. Charles Page, the admitting physician, rendered his opinion: "Organic brain and nervous system disease. He is insane and not likely to recover. Disease is not of recent origin. Origin is due to great hardships, exposure, privation, imprisonment, and mental anxiety during service."[11]

The government's opinion was rendered by Dr. W. W. Formain, who did not believe that Burnham's condition was service-related. He questioned whether "any long and protracted experience in deprivation of proper food and clothing may so weaken the nervous system as to render it more likely to disease." He noted the patient's attacks of moroseness, despondency, and withdrawal, in which he would sit alone for hours, silent and gloomy.

Burnham's insanity was officially designated not service-connected. Surgeon Mayer had treated a gunshot wound to the leg, and for this Burnham did receive a pension of $15 a month. Prior to the war he had been a bookkeeper and then a salesman for a general country store. He came from ordinary folks; his mother was a widow and he owned no property. Both men had the same diagnosis of monomania. Minor, a rich man's son, could provide no evidence of exposure to combat and had preexisting illness, but his condition was considered service-connected and he got a lifelong pension. The grocer's son with no preexisting illness and extensive battlefield exposure was denied.

Minor returned to New Haven and worked in his uncle's shop, Minor and Company: Dealers in China, Glass, and Crockery at 261 Chapel Street. In 1872, he traveled to London, carrying his Colt Navy revolver, and killed an innocent pedestrian, the father of a poor family of seven. Minor was found guilty of murder and spent most of the remainder of his life as an inmate of Broadmoor Criminal Lunatic Asylum. He was instrumental in writing the *Oxford English Dictionary*, using his monthly pension checks to purchase rare books that aided his research and contributions to the monumental work.[12]

Dr. Timothy H. Bishop graduated from Yale Medical School in 1860 with a thesis on cataracts. He was of slight build, stoop-shouldered, with a narrow face and handlebar mustache popular in the day. He would outlive his eighty-four-year-old physician father — another son of a Yale College and Medical School alumnus (1829) — by seven years. With the father's retirement, the job of secretary of New Haven Hospital was assumed by Pliny Jewett in 1843. Dr. Bishop the younger came in on the second wave of hospital hiring, serving as a contract surgeon while maintaining a private office practice at 215 Church Street. Along with Wilcoxson and Casey, he served on the examining board that held daily sessions for discharges and pension determinations for active-duty soldiers. One surgical case of his was listed in the *MSHWR*. (See Appendix V.)

William B. Casey was the same age as Pliny Jewett, the seventh of seven sons, from Middletown, Connecticut. He graduated from Columbia University in 1834 and the University of Pennsylvania Medical School in 1837. He married that year and had eight children, five of whom survived. He worked in New York City for two years, first at Bellevue Hospital where he gained experience with "ship's fever" (yellow fever) and then at St. Luke's Hospital. He returned to Middletown where he served as mayor for two years. From 1850 to 1854, he edited a daily and weekly newspaper in addition to practicing medicine. His first wife died in 1852, and he remarried two years later. In 1854 he joined a committee of the CMS to fill vacancies and nominate professors for the medical school.[13]

The following year he presented a paper at the CMS meeting entitled "Diseases of the Cervix Uteri." It offers a window into the gynecological treatment of that period and the experience and character of the speaker. He lectured Yale medical students on obstetrics, filling in for Pliny Jewett, who often traveled to other states as a visiting professor. Questioning well-established dogmatic treatment was not common practice for this period, as Casey's words suggest. "It is sometimes quite as useful to bring afresh before the mind well-established and important facts, as to originate new theories however brilliant and fanciful."[14]

Casey's work at Bellevue introduced him to new technology: a vaginal speculum allowing the physician to actually see the anatomy. As the house doctor in New York, he treated women working in houses of ill repute and their occupational diseases. All received speculum exams as often as necessary. Many were arrested as vagrants just so they could then be given medical treatment they otherwise could not afford. Some doctors called the speculum exam "degrading" or an "offensive professional intrusion."

The minutes of the Hartford Medical Society of the 1860s show how old and new doctors differed on this subject.[15] The senior Dr. Stanford Hunt stated he never yet had had occasion nor felt justified in making a visual examination of the womb for any instance that had fallen under his care. He suggested tonics, bathing, and passive exercise and protested severely against general use of speculum, caustics, and the pessary in uterine disease. Dr. Jackson stated that in eighteen years of practice he had used the speculum perhaps ten times, and mostly found ulcers and inflammation which he treated with nitrate of silver, perisulphate of iron, and stronger astringents. Dr. Hawley warned that because uterine disease had been neglected by the profession, quacks were becoming involved its treatment. Consequently, he used the speculum more and more for diagnosis and local applications. Dr. Jobesh of Paris, using a wooden speculum, cauterized the cervical neck with a red-hot iron for three-eighths to one-half inch and reported invariable success, especially when nitrate of silver and other caustics had failed.

Dr. Casey used oil to ease the insertion of Charrier's speculum, which was a cylindrical glass tube plated and coated with gum elastic. His treatment for acute and chronic cervicitis reflected his personal experience and general consensus: leeches for mild cases, silver nitrate for the moderate, and cautery for the severe. These treatments went on for six weeks to three months. If they failed, they would be repeated. Persistence and confidence in the treatment, it was felt, were required for best results.[16]

He felt that this disease should be fully treated because it caused 90 percent of abortions and miscarriages, all of which would therefore be prevented. Having eight children of his own plus a large practice lent experience and credibility to his remarks. Quacks and charlatans would best be defeated "when physicians see disease in the same pathological light; but when obliged to guess as to the nature and character of a difficulty or depend solely upon symptoms we shall be very apt frequently to arrive at widely different conclusions both as to disease and its remedies. Use of the instrument is a great step in advance."[17] Despite being forty-six years of age and having family and financial responsibilities, Casey enlisted on September 5, 1862 as a regimental surgeon for the Twentieth Connecticut Volunteers. He was present at the Battle of Chancellorsville in May 1863, where the Confederates sustained 13,000 casualties. He mustered out one year later, having risen to brigade surgeon. He was transferred to organize the Sloan General Hospital in Montpelier, Vermont. By 1864 he was serving as acting assistant surgeon at Knight hospital where he remained until war's end as his experience was invaluable on discharging and providing pensions for the disabled veterans. He was detailed to the Conscript Camp at Grapevine Point in New Haven to examine new recruits in an effort to weed out those incapable of performing a soldier's duties. Several of his cases are listed in the *MSHWR*. (See Appendix VI.)

After the war he resumed his large practice in Middletown, and he died in 1870. This gentleman was described as "courtly but affable, well informed, of cheerful temperament, possessing a well cultivated and practical mind, with clear judgment, and strong faith in virtues of materia medica." His judgment was incisive and sought after. "Although in every community there are those who will receive with no more implicit faith the drivel of a quack than a well-considered judgment it was comparatively seldom that the correctness of his professional opinion was called in question." Doctors with large practices work long hours. Casey reportedly "had the will to do whenever duty called. It was rare he did not leave his patients feeling better than he found them however hopeless their cases."[18] This doggedness of spirit and optimistic nature was essential in healing the broken and fevered bodies of returning soldiers.

Worthington Hooker was for many years the director and consulting surgeon for the General Hospital of Connecticut as well as a church deacon. His ancestry included the Reverend Thomas Hooker, the leader of the first colony planters of Hartford in 1636. Worthington was the youngest son of a prominent judge, born in 1806. His private tutor was the future president of Yale, the Reverend T. Woolsey, who called him "a blameless youth and one of the best scholars of his class." In 1825 he graduated with honors and began the study of medicine in Philadelphia. He won the Boylston Prize in Boston (a case of surgical instruments) for as essay and earned a medical degree from Harvard in 1829. He was professor of anatomy and physiology from 1838 through 1852, dean of the medical school from 1853 to 1863, and professor of theory and practice of medicine from 1852 to 1867.[19] Hooker was married twice. His first wife died early and childless. A second marriage produced a son.

Hooker was benevolent in appearance and in fact. He was cheerful and easy to work with, had agreeable manners and liked to talk about his personal library, 139 books of which were donated to the medical library. Despite his roots, he was a plainspoken fellow who lectured without notes. He was practical rather than theoretical, solid and emphatic rather than elegant or inspiring, and lectured five or six times a week while listening to student recitations for many years. "He was one of those classes who are accustomed to believe in earnest. He believed in his profession, the power of medicine, the stethoscope, fatty meats, three meals a day, his horse, his grapes, and himself."[20] He published a good deal in both the lay and professional journals, including *Harper's Weekly*. In 1832, he reported on a cholera epidemic, charting its epidemiology and the efficacy of his treatment. In 1839 he reviewed a paper on pleurisy by a promising young medical student named Pliny Jewett, to whom he offered encouraging criticisms.

His writing was like his lectures: practical, factual, earnest, and sometimes eloquent. Many of his remarks about physicians in 1844 are timeless and speak to the modern age. "Quackery is far from being confined to the unlearned and ill informed. Men of respectability and good sense in other matters, are not only willing to take quack medicines, but imbibe some of the wildest notions of the day and degrade the educated physician down to a level with them in their estimate of his professional character."

The causes of want of respect were many. "A popular error of the day is prejudice against use of calomel [mercury]. It is used by physicians as hobby to ride into popular favor and pretend to use drugs less than others thus by base insinuations inflict injury upon their brethren at large." He regretted that getting patients was more studied than curing them. Secrecy concerning the composition of medicines deceives and injures the community and the profession, he asserted. "Some physicians have offered medicines for sale, informing their agent that the composition can be made known to any medical man who desires it. They then flood market with ads and sell, sell, sell. The medical society's great object is to defend people against injury they are liable to suffer from quackery. It proposes to affect [*sic*] this purpose by securing the services of a body of well-educated physicians."[21]

Homeopathy was invented in the early nineteenth century and involved using medications diluted many fold, up to one-millionth the dose. Abraham Lincoln noted that homeopathic soup was so thin that it might have been "made by boiling the shadow of a pigeon that had starved to death." In 1851 Dr. Hooker summarized the medical community's reasoned opposition in *Homeopathy: An Examination of Its Doctrine and Evidences*.[22] He starts by defining this sect as "absurd, delusional, quackery. If infinitesimal doses of drugs are adequate to cure disease, then a grain of oyster shell is all that is needed to last the world."

The homeopaths recommended avoiding "coffee, tea, beer, liquors, chocolate, spices, perfumery, perfume garbs, pastry, old cheese, stale meat, pork, duck, and young veal." Missing from their list was tobacco, yet even then, tobacco was suspected of causing lung cancer, for smokers were noted to have lung diseases not previously seen. Homeopaths also preached avoiding "salt, spirituous liquors, warm apartments, sedentary life, and passive exercise, sleeping after dinner, uncleanliness, unnatural voluptuousness, reading obscene books, anger, grief, malice, and gambling. To get a cure one must avoid all these excitants."

Hooker challenged their hugely successful statistics in treating cholera, suggesting they confused it with ordinary diarrhea. A mineral spring owner kept a room full of crutches collected from those who greatly benefited from his waters so as not to require them after treatment. Over a hundred crutches were on display. A clear-eyed observer noted, "They take good care to say nothing about the heaps of crutches we burn up every year of the poor creatures that come here only to die. Dead bones tell no tales, you know."

Lack of scientific knowledge, inaccurate reporting, absence of long-term results, prejudicial and self-congratulatory evaluations, and the placebo effect all contribute to the fog of therapeutics and what actually works. The medical literature offers a litany of often contradictory studies leaving the reader bewildered. This fact of life does not escape Hooker.

> The same principles of evidence that reject homeopathic observation as inconclusive and false must reject a large portion of the observations in the annals of medicine. Too much has been taken upon trust without regard to the degree of fidelity or capacity in the observer. A sifting process needs to be applied to the recorded experience of the profession. There has been a decided movement in the profession in opposition to an indiscriminate heroic medication. The duty of the practitioner is to use in each case all the means that his judgment dictates, and learn all he can by comparing his experience with other reliable observers.

The CMS railed against nontraditional health care sects and expelled from their ranks those found guilty of practicing such heresy. In May 1852 before the same society, Hooker presented his treatise "The Treatment due from the Medical Profession to Physicians who Become Homeopathic Practitioners."[23] "Homeopathy, Hydropathy, Thomsonism and Eclecticism are upshots of the same radicalism. All are at war with general 'regular' profession. One of the expelled doctors was found to be not only an empiric but also a cheat by selling common borax as a newly discovered specific at the enormous price of a Louis d'or per ounce. Homeopathy has worn the bag and adopted the modes and tactics of quackery."

Oliver Wendell Holmes was a brilliant physician, researcher, writer, and poet. His son would become a casualty in the upcoming war, survive, and become a distinguished United States Supreme Court justice. The senior Holmes addressed the Massachusetts Medical Society in 1860 on many of these same points, setting off alarm bells to the traditionalists for whom change is always anathema.[24]

> Part of the blame of over-medication rests with the profession for yielding to the tendency to self-delusion, which seems inseparable from the practice of the art of healing. First is a natural incapacity for sound observation. Second is a singular inability to weigh the value of testimony. He got well after taking my medicine; therefore in consequence of taking it. We need statistical analysis. Lastly is assuming a falsehood as a fact.
>
> Another portion of the blame rests with the public itself, which insists on being poisoned. Somebody buys all the quack medicines that build palaces for the mushrooms, say the toadstool millionaires. The popular belief is all but universal that sick persons should feed on noxious substances.
>
> The outside pressure is immense upon the physician tending to force him to active treatment of some kind. One of the ancient superstitions is that disease is a malignant agency or entity to be driven out of the body by offensive substances. Calomel is sometimes given by a physician on the same principle as that upon which a landlord prescribes bacon and eggs, because he cannot think of anything else quite so handy!

Heroic medical therapy once popular and in widespread use during the early 19th century began to be discontinued, starting in the medical centers of Paris. Professor Louis demonstrated with statistical analysis of patient outcome studies that bleeding and the use of noxious chemicals to induce vomiting and diarrhea mostly did harm, and not much good, thus failing to justify their toxic side effects. Bleeding as a medical therapy was abandoned. Surgeon General Hammond removed antimony tartrate and mercury from the army's pharmacopeia, incurring the wrath of many physicians whose treatment regimen included the traditional running of the bowel with purgatives and emetics. Non-traditional healthcare providers along with proprietary drugs competed for acceptance among a public skeptical because of past practices.

The problems that Dr. Hooker faced in evaluating the true effectiveness of both new and old technologies are still with us. The June 2004 issue of the *Journal of Bone and Joint Surgery* notes that "many new health care technologies are adopted and used in clinical practice with little or no evidence that their use is associated with improved patient outcomes."

> The lack of published results from randomized clinical trials or other well-designed clinical outcome studies ... makes it difficult, and at time impossible to judge efficacy in every instance. Nevertheless, patients and society believe that potentially curative technologies should be made available rapidly for the public's benefit. Caught between imperfect data — clinical as well as economic, sociopolitical, and ethical and enormous patient demands, physicians must make choices about technology.... There is surprisingly little scientific or clinical evidence to support the use of many new or existing medical technologies. There is strong evidence that much of the regional variation in health care spending in the United States comes from the use of technologies and services for which guidelines based on clinical or cost-effectiveness research simply do not exist.[25]

The deans of Harvard and Yale medical schools said basically the same thing in the 1860s. Hooker assisted in the free clinic at the hospital and was likewise readily available as a contract surgeon and consultant at the army hospital. When Jewett got in hot water with Yale College over starting a new medical school at the army hospital, Hooker acted as a go-between to cool things off. In 1867 a fever proved fatal to Hooker, though it was "insidious and unsuspected." He had written a note to a friend: "I am playing ill a little ... only a trifle unwell, a good time to work."

Thirty-three-year-old Henry Pierpont graduated from Yale Medical School in 1854 with a dissertation entitled "Induction of Premature Labor." He apprenticed with Dr. J.G. Beckwith of Litchfield for a few years and then began his own practice in Naugatuck. He had to abandon practice due to recurrent illness and made several trips to Europe in an effort to gain a cure. He returned to New Haven in 1862 and was hired as an acting assistant surgeon June of 1864. He was a descendant of the Reverend James Pierpont, pastor of the First Church in New Haven from 1684 to 1714. In 1871, Henry Pierpont married the daughter of the treasurer of Yale University who bore him three children. At war's end he was a pension examiner, a post he held for fifteen years. He was also an examiner for the Connecticut Mutual Life Insurance Company for thirty years. He was described as "well-cultivated, guided by the principles of a pure Christianity, uniform cheerfulness and suavity of manner which rendered him a most welcome visitor to the sick and gave him success in the practice of his profession." He died at age sixty-one, having practiced medicine for forty years despite chronic ailments and being "never physically strong."[26] He described five cases in the *MSHWR*. (See Appendix VII.)

Frederick Levi Dibble was born in Newtown and moved with his family to New Haven at age two. He later spent seven years unsuccessfully searching for elusive riches in California's gold rush. It was then off to Australia and South America. He went on to apprentice with Dr. N. B. Ives, graduating from Yale Medical School in 1853 with a thesis on dysentery.

He married in 1861, had no children, and traveled extensively, visiting Europe five times and touring the world once. He spoke five languages and was described as kind, sympathetic, mild mannered, never in great health, and strictly temperate.[27]

He was appointed assistant surgeon of the First Connecticut Volunteers for a three-month enlistment in April 1861. He would face the Great Dismal Swamp and life in the field. "For sixteen weeks they ate salt pork, no vegetables, and hard tack full of vermin, and water that had been put in kerosene oil barrels three months earlier. Dirt and filth prevailed. The water was so thick you could lift it with a finger." And then there were "gray backs": "The lice got so big they were just like wheat." Body lice were a common occurrence, an itchy, disagreeable nuisance tolerated and taken for granted by all. The regiment was ordered ashore to bathe and wash while clothes and boats were fumigated. "Spotted fever" broke out and five men died daily.[28] Dibble's tour ended in July 1861.

On August 27, 1861, he enlisted in the Sixth Connecticut Volunteers, this time for a three-year tour of duty. He was present at the Battle of Fort Wagner, South Carolina, in July 1863; in New Bern, North Carolina, in May 1864; and later at the siege in Petersburg, Virginia. He was appointed chief medical officer at hospitals in Beaufort and Folly Island South Carolina. In May 1863 he became medical director on General Foster's staff at Hilton head. This was preceded by a reference letter from his commander to the medical director of the Department of the South. "I take much pleasure in recommending Dr. Dibble to you as a very efficient officer and an agreeable gentleman. He is the most reliable and intelligent medical officer in the department. I think you will be pleased with him."[29] He was discharged on September 12, 1864. Following his tour of active duty, at age thirty-two Dibble was hired as contract surgeon for the Knight hospital in March of 1865. Several of his cases were described in the *MSHWR*. (See Appendix VIII.) Dibble maintained a position at the General Hospital in New Haven for the next thirty years, as visiting physician, secretary, director, and consulting physician. He died in 1898 at age sixty-eight in Macon, Georgia, of stomach cancer.

Another Yale medical school graduate, W. H. Thompson, had finished schooling in July 1862. His graduation thesis was titled, "On the Use of Microscope in Medicine." Thompson was descended from other Thompson graduates of Yale who had practiced medicine in New Haven from the eighteenth century on. His family tree extended to Noah Webster and the Reverend Steele. His uncle described him as a "cheerful, constant friend and a true warm hearted man, who made a special study of gynecology and treatment of fevers, delivering lectures to Yale and other medical schools." He was discharged in July 1865 and, according to the *Record*, "having been on duty here a short time was very much liked by all."

Virgil M. Dow was an 1856 Yale medical school graduate. He was born in New Haven and named for his father, another Yale doctor who was treasurer of the CSMS for ten years but succumbed to tuberculosis at age fifty-six. The son was thirty-one years old when he became a contract surgeon and died at age sixty-two, practicing in New Haven for his entire career.

White, male, Anglo-Saxon, Protestant doctors ran this spanking-new facility. They were the offspring of the establishment, mainly Yale graduates, often with a family heritage of medicine. They helped build and maintain a city of medicine, providing state-of-the-art health care for thousands and sometimes sharing in their sacrifices and sufferings.

CHAPTER TEN

Hospital Steward

Pharmacist, record-keeper, material handler and substitute assistant surgeon were the duties of the steward. "He must have sufficient practical knowledge of pharmacy to enable him to take exclusive charge of the dispensary, be acquainted with minor surgery as application of bandages and dressings, the extraction of teeth, and the application of cups and leeches, and must have such knowledge of cooking as will enable him to superintend efficiently this important branch of hospital service." Such were the requirements listed in the *Hospital Steward Handbook*,[1] written by Dr. J.J. Woodward in 1863, inspired and promulgated by Surgeon General Hammond. No formal school existed.

They were ranked as non-commissioned officers. Pay was $30 a month with $2 a month pay increase after five years of service. An attempt by congressmen and medical officers to raise the steward's pay grade was unsuccessful. The *Knight Hospital Record* republished an article from a hospital newspaper in Virginia:

> It is a matter of rights and propriety. A steward is required to be skilled in pharmacy, minor surgery, and doses of medicine and hospital papers. They have responsibility in matter of clothing, camp and garrison equipage, medical stores, hospital fund and property. There are many incompetent stewards in the army who don't know quinine from prepared chalk and others who know nothing of these duties. The proportion is same as in all grades of officers. Due to weeding, the majority of stewards are quite fit and knowledgeable. In the absence of medical officers their position is augmented in importance. Although performing no capital operations, they dress wounds, and do other operations in minor surgery.

Hospital stewards were in charge of the dispensary and medical property. They could act as ward master and quartermaster as in issuing clothing and blankets. They could also be in charge of subsistence, special diets, ration drawing, and accounts of the hospital fund. Some found temptation from accessibility to monetary funds and services in demand.

The apothecary's primary job was to make up prescribed medications and deliver them to the wards but not offsite. Bottles were appropriately labeled with the respective patients' names and directions. Apothecaries were in charge of keeping splints, bandages, and muslin and voluminous records. Office hours were 7 A.M. to 8 P.M., but they could be summoned at any time for emergencies.

Career paths varied, with some ending in higher positions and some in jail. Frederick Treadway was a hospital steward for the Second Connecticut Volunteers from May through August 1861. He became assistant surgeon for the Twenty-seventh Connecticut Volunteers in October 1862 and was discharged March 1863.[2] He submitted a dissertation on yellow fever for graduation at the semiannual exam of the Medical Department of Yale July 28, 1863, receiving a degree of doctor of medicine.

Private Charles A. Howard deserted while in Missouri in July 1861. He disappeared and then resurfaced under a false name in Tennessee, where he performed well as hospital steward for the next three years. He was discovered as a deserter in January 1864, pleaded guilty, and was "sentenced to be confined at Alton, Illinois, at hard labor with ball and chain attached to his leg for three years and to forfeit all pay and allowance during that time and be dishonorably discharged from service." General Sherman pardoned him, allowing him to serve out his time as a steward.[3]

Nineteen-year-old Private L.H. Jones had enlisted in an Ohio Artillery battery. By August 1862, he claimed to have been an acting hospital steward. While in Memphis he worked as clerk and druggist from February until October 1863. He was then appointed clerk in the medical purveyor department in Memphis and later applied to the War Department in March 1864 for the position of hospital steward.[4] He ascribed his pleasing appearance and demeanor with "a desire to enter regular service and preference for duties as hospital steward" as reasons to be appointed. He got the job.

George Bronson was the hospital steward for the Eleventh Connecticut Volunteers from 1862 through 1865. He had some prior training as a dentist and had extensive battlefield experience.[5] "Since I have been hospital steward I have had to work more than 18 hours per day. I had to make out quarterly reports and stock of medicines ran out," he wrote. In the hot summer of July 1863, he wrote home about officers and finances.

> The hospital steward has power more than a captain or lieutenant. They can make trouble for men in camps. They are bad men to cross. I am doing surgeons duty and have for two months lived just the same as they do. I have a nice tent to myself and as good a bed. Perhaps you wonder how I live so well. I have no small amount of private practice. Many do not like having their complaints made public. Probably you can guess what they are. The men are no worse than the officers. I have both.

Some were tempted to accept financial remuneration for services rendered, including treatment for venereal disease or release from the service. "Private practice" in the army is an oxymoron and amounts to accepting bribes. Stewards could be tried by court-martial but only above regimental level and only then could they be reduced in rank.

Knight hospital began with four stewards and expanded to six. Leicester Carrington of Bristol was the first hired by Jewett for two unique reasons. First, he was a pharmacist prior to the war, an uncommon but welcome feature. Most stewards were on-the-job trainees with little to no experience in medicine. Chemists, medical students, clerks, dentists, nurses, ex-patients, and even ex-felons with some training might be considered qualified. Apprenticeship was the road taken by the majority of those entering pharmacy careers. Carrington's second attribute was being Jewett's brother-in-law. This relationship had its downside, as Carrington would find himself arrested along with Dr. Jewett. The two were arrested for unnecessarily filling hospital beds just to make the $3.50-a-week federal payments. Jewett was released in ten days thanks to the intervention of Governor Buckingham and Secretary Stanton. Carrington was jailed for three months.

By the summer of 1863, there were six clerks, some doubling as steward. The head clerk was Charles Morris who also served as steward. The clerical duties were many with reports required in triplicate.[6] (See Appendix IX.)

Two of the hospital stewards at Knight U.S. Army General Hospital underwent court-martial for "conduct prejudicial to good order and military discipline." Frank Bond was a hospital steward from December 1864 through May 1865. By 1865, he was also the general ward master, a job that included supervision of the cadets, clerks, nurses, and janitorial personnel employed on each ward. Personnel were often ex-patients, now members of the Invalid Corps with limited disability that allowed them to carry out clerical and other light-duty functions. Bond's trial was held on March 24, 1865, before a jury of seven officers, including three captains, two first lieutenants, and one second lieutenant. The first specification was that "for a pecuniary consideration paid to him, he did procure and furnish to enlisted men passes whereby they were enabled to leave the hospital grounds without the permission of their superior officer." The second charge was "appropriating to his own use $17.50 from the personal effects of a recently deceased soldier," money which should have been delivered to Major Jewett.[7]

Major Jewett testified that the duty of the general ward master was to take responsibility for the effects of the deceased and that Bond should have secured the money in a safe. The accused spent the money on a two-week trip to Washington, D.C., in February 1865, where he had been summoned as a witness for another court-martial. While the government covered his transportation costs, he claimed additional money was needed for "the maintenance of life." Dr. Jewett in addition loaned him $10 from the hospital fund, not knowing that Bond was withholding money of the deceased. Jewett called him to his office after the trip and asked what happened to the deceased's property, at which time a confession was forth-coming — albeit no funds.

A passbook was by regulation stored in the military adjutant's office, but witnesses testified it was kept by Bond. In addition, soldiers who had not been on any duty were listed as if they were, and then were given passes signed only by Bond, a violation of several army regulations. That only officers granted passes seemed news to the defendant.

For his defense Bond produced just one witness, himself. He denied all charges, claiming, "I was much in the habit of joking with the witnesses they being intimate friends of mine, therefore if I made it; it was only as a joke soon forgotten by me like any other careless remarks." Advertising the ability to give out passes was dismissed as braggadocio and innocent fool's play. He claimed ignorance about how and where property of the deceased should be handled until Jewett enlightened him regarding filling out the appropriate forms and the proper deposition of deceased property.

On Saturday, April 15, 1865, the day after Good Friday, Bond was found not guilty of selling passes, but guilty on the final charge of using the deceased's property. The sentence was reduction in the ranks to private, repaying the $17.50, and dishonorable discharge with loss of all pay and allowances that were or might become due. On the same day this case was sentenced, a court-martial began on another hospital steward, Charles Morris.

The same jury heard the case against Charles Morris, hospital steward from April 1864 through May 1865. He was alleged to have "offered and agreed to obtain description lists [duty status] for a pecuniary consideration to wit for the sum of $15." Other charges were that "without authority [Morris] detained in his custody discharge papers" of several soldiers from the possession and custody of Major Jewett without his knowledge or consent. And

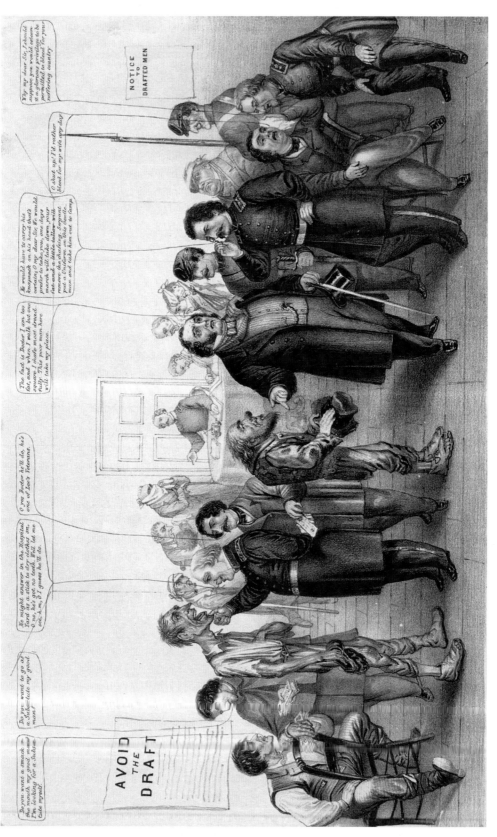

"Offering a Substitute—A Scene in the Office of the Provost Marshall," 1862. Doctor taking bribe, "He might answer to the Hospital Yard as a stick to dry clothes. Oh no, he has no teeth, I guess he'll do" (The Library Company of Philadelphia).

finally that he "did for a pecuniary consideration recommend to his superior officer names of enlisted men for passes." The charges amounted to accepting bribes to facilitate both medical discharge and unwarranted passes.[8]

Two witnesses testified that Morris offered descriptive lists for the right sum. Other witnesses claimed passes were sold as well as claims for state bounty. The trial was postponed for three days because Major Jewett was unavailable "on account of physical disability," a reference to a serious knee injury on Good Friday, the same day Lincoln was assassinated. Upon return, Major Jewett testified that the steward's "duty was to make out the final statements and discharge papers and prepare them for my signature." He did not know if the steward retained them in his own custody without his knowledge or consent.

A discharged soldier testified he paid Morris $10 for services rendered. Another denied making any payment, although others indicated that they had been present when the bribery transpired. Morris claimed that charging $30 or $15 or $10 to get descriptive lists had been made purely in a "joking" way. He described the sergeant who testified against him as a "court jester, a professional mimic with a distempered brain, whose speech no one interprets literally, asks a silly question and elicits an extravagant reply." He admitted that issuing the passes had been done to allow soldiers to "draw an installment of the state bounty. Surgeon Jewett on handing me each batch of papers when they came, ordered me to make them out immediately, and has never expressed any dissatisfaction at my management of them." Morris was found guilty of receiving money for obtaining descriptive lists, and received the same sentence as Frank Bond. On review, the decision was dismissed on a technicality because one of the judges was absent from the first part of the hearings, and Morris was returned to full duty. The trial had been interrupted three times due to Major Jewett's injury and the Lincoln assassination and subsequent funeral.

The charges against both stewards centered on bribery. The highly desired passes enabled the pursuit of happiness for soldiers in downtown New Haven while receiving bounty payments from the state. That money changed hands is clear: several witnesses gave unshakable testimony on that point. That it represented the tip of the iceberg is likely.

The Medical Department's sensitivity to bribery is illustrated in the case of Surgeon Ferris Jacobs, who held the rank of major in the Third New York Cavalry. He was in private practice for twenty-five years when appointed brigade surgeon in April 1862, and built from scratch a sizable convalescent hospital in Alexandria, Virginia. Private William Kellogg had a "decrepit" or club foot, although Jacobs described him as "quite ill." Kellogg wanted to apply for medical discharge but, according to his brother Myron, claimed that he could not get an examination to evaluate his condition. Myron Kellogg offered the doctor $10 to arrange an exam, which was accepted in front of two clerks. Declaring the money "a present and nothing else," Jacobs found Kellogg disabled and recommended that he be sent home.[9] Surgeon General Hammond was asked to review the case and concluded: "The explanation of surgeon Jacobs appears lame and unsatisfactory. This is the first case of the kind that has been detected and I think it cannot be too promptly punished. I recommend that Surgeon Jacobs be dismissed from the service of the U.S."

Secretary of War Stanton received the following letter from Ferris Jacobs, a captain of the Third New York Cavalry and the doctor's son:

> Should a morally innocent act of impropriety and imprudence (already terribly punished) forever deprive him of a long history of faithful and honorable efforts? Shall this follow him to the grave, and pursue and humiliate his family for years to come? I am his son. I have served continuously since the first outbreak of the Rebellion. I respectfully ask that justice may be

done and that my family be saved from further sorrow and suffering and that I may again stand without shame among gentlemen and my comrades in the army.[10]

The chief clerk and orderly gave corroborating evidence and support for Surgeon Ferris in a January 1863 affidavit. In no other instance had the surgeon accepted money; they had heard the doctor actually refuse money under similar circumstances. He had said only that he would help papers along. "We knew from our observation that Dr. Jacobs could have received amounts of money on various occasions and that he refused them." In December of 1862, six doctors and eight clerical workers separately declared loyalty and appreciation of his efforts in building the new hospital, affirming Dr. Jacobs' accomplishments while saying nothing about the actual charges.

Supportive letters were sent by a U.S. senator and other doctors from his hometown. The secretary of war revoked Hammond's order, allowing reinstatement following which the doctor voluntarily resigned. The charges of bribery and fraud were used to destroy the military careers of both Surgeon General Hammond and Major Jewett. The strategy fully succeeded in the former case and largely failed in the latter, but left perpetual and undeserved stains on both.

In December 1862 the Connecticut legislature on a motion by Dr. Grant of Enfield formed a committee of three to investigate Dr. Hubbard of New Haven in his capacity as assistant surgeon at Camp Rendezvous. The charge was "taking of fees beyond what are allowable by law for examination of persons claiming exemption from military service under any pretext or circumstances whatever."[11] This was extended to include "any individuals ... accessory to the fraudulent and improper obtaining of certificates of exemption." Dr. Nicol was added to the list and both were eventually acquitted, but the House censured them "for improperly charging extra fees for examinations made as surgeons of the post." The Senate tabled the motion and it died. Dr. Grant had applied for the position of regimental surgeon to the Medical Board earlier in the year but was denied and without an examination.

The public was made aware of physician bribery with reports in the mass media. The cartoon of "Offering a Substitute, A Scene in the Office of the Provost Marshall [*sic*]" portrays two doctors; one in military uniform and another in civilian clothes. The first doctor is reviewing a wealthy and obese gentleman who, to avoid draft induction, has procured an obviously defective man as substitute. Nonetheless, he is denied by the incorruptible army surgeon. The second doctor, the civilian, takes the bribe from an agent who recommended an emaciated spit of a man for service.

For each soldier excused from duty, another took his place, and the consequence becomes the defining question, whose son is the replacement? "Do not take bribes, for bribes blind the clear-sighted and upset the pleas of those who are in the right" (Exodus 23:8).

CHAPTER ELEVEN

Nurses

In the nineteenth century health care was principally delivered at home with family members providing nursing care. The destitute and indigent were treated in hospitals that were sometimes referred to as "pest-houses." Most hospital nurses were from the lower classes, since taking care of men who were strangers was not thought fit for a "lady" in the Victorian era. Some questioned whether any proper woman would take such a job. In the South slaves often filled the role of nurse, orderly, or grave digger.

Florence Nightingale opened the first school of nursing in London in 1863. There was no formal nursing school in the United States until Bellevue Hospital in New York opened one in 1872. Medical forces in Connecticut considered creating a nursing school in 1872 but "declined to do so as other organizations were going to do the same and they would generally support them."[1]

Dr. MacLeod's experience with nursing in the Crimean War was given credence by the work of Nightingale. "They must combine a vigorous body with a well-balanced mind un-tinctured by vain 'romance.' Be subservient, without fussiness or nervousness; act calmly while facing danger and have lots of common sense and cheerfulness." Their "kindly sympathy and gentle care" were most needed in human sufferings and especially at the sickbed.

Dorothy Dix was hired by the U.S. government to recruit and supervise female nurses but was unable to overcome the male-dominated system that severely limited her power and authority. Her requirements were that nurses be over thirty and plain "almost to repulsion" in dress and devoid of personal attractions, know how to cook all kinds of diet, renounce colored dresses, hoops, curls, jewelry and flowers on their bonnets, look neat themselves and keep their boys and wards the same, read and write for the boys, be in their room at taps, not go to amusement places in the evening and be paid 40 cents and one ration daily.

When the war started, the only trained nurses were nuns. Male convalescent soldiers filled those positions, making up most of the nursing staff. Experiencing and surviving injury or disease provided on-the-job training on how to render care to fellow soldiers. Deserters and stragglers accepted the job just to avoid trial and punishment. Some doctors preferred female nurses rather than "rough country crackers who did not know castor oil from a gun rod or laudanum from a hole in the ground."

Because of the constant hemorrhaging of manpower the partially disabled were allowed to serve as nurses or in other supportive capacities. Wounded or ill soldiers in recovery were transferred to the Invalid Corps or, as it was later called, the Veterans Reserve Corps, and put on "light duty," which often meant serving as cook or nurse. Quality varied; some patients described their nurses as "feeble, weak, stiff, decrepit, debilitated, emaciated, or broken down." Others felt that "the nurses knew as much about cleanliness as did the surgeons," a conclusion not necessarily meant to be an endorsement. The Sanitary Commission rendered an early review of army nursing in *Hospital Transports*.[2] "The male nurses are of all sorts. The convalescent soldiers have been the most satisfactory. The process of taking on hundreds of men, many of them crazed with fever was quite difficult for anyone to deal with." Dr. Tripler's handbook held that the medical officer should select nurses with approval of the commanding officer. Nurses were to be from the privates of the regiment who would then be "exempted from all other duty except parades and weekly inspection and may be excused from this if the sick need them."[3] Having specific soldiers assigned strictly as either nurse or ambulance driver was a new concept not accepted by most of the regular army.

The *Record* reported on a need for criteria as to who amongst disabled soldiers should be sent home "to plow and to mow and to reap and to sow." "Those cripples are now in the country, in hospitals, and demand every attention that can be paid them. To be sure, glory is in every scar, and homage is theirs from all for their deeds of valor and their sacrifices. Let them be helped on and cheered through life and then their sacrifice is worse, perhaps than death to them."

A poem from the *Record* poignantly illustrates the painful dilemma of many returning wounded soldiers. Simply entitled "The End," it discusses the loss of comradeship and glory, isolation, and a dark, cloudy future.

> Crippled, forlorn and useless,
> The glory of life grown dim,
> Brooding alone o'er the memory
> Of the bright glad days gone by,
> Nursing a bitter fancy,
> And nursing a shattered limb;
> Never again to dream the dream
> That young ambition weaves.

Peer groups could offer hopeful encouragement from an insider's perspective as to what was possible. Amputees could speak to those who already had their prosthesis and were functioning members of society. They could see from others with the same condition that it was possible to perform activities of daily living and a meaningful occupation without an arm or leg.

The Invalid Corps was established to keep the disabled functioning in some capacity as soldiers. General Order No. 36, issued in 1862 and reinforced a year later, stated that the chief medical officer in each city should "employ as cooks, nurses, and attendants, any convalescent, wounded, or feeble men who can perform such duties, instead of giving them discharges." Service in some capacity would be enforced. Soldiers unfit for battle were made into guards, clerks, hospital attendants, orderlies and nurses.

In another poem from the *Record*, a just salute to the Invalid Corps is offered from a grateful nation.

They're serving their country as faithfully still,
They have stood by the guns where the shell and the shot
Fell thickly around them yet faltering not.
The arm, that's now shattered, our banner once bore
The foot that now limping ne'er faltered in fight
Nor ever turned backward in cowardly flight.
Good order and peace in the rear to preserve
Oh, soldiers, we're proud of the name that you bear!
And we honor you more for each scar that you wear.

Many could still serve their country while maintaining a sense of self-worth as a man and contributing to society despite physical disability. The assistant provost marshal of New Haven County, Angel Putnam, recognized possibilities in June 1863: "There is a desire on the part of the disabled soldiers here to raise an invalid corps. What steps should be taken in the premises?" Civilian labor was scarce and salaries were high, making manpower limited. According to headquarters there were "no applicants" for the Reserve Corps in the summer of 1863.

There are great numbers of soldiers in this district who have been discharged but those who are well enough to do anything prefer to go into the manufactories where at light labor they can earn from five to eight dollars per week and remain among their friends than to become privates or NCOs in the "corps of honor."[4]

At the Knight hospital, doctors and nurses dined in their own mess hall. Separate living quarters for male and female nurses were provided. The head nurse was responsible to the doctors for care of the sick and wounded and directed ward housekeeping. Female nurses were paid 40 cents a day or $12 a month plus rations, with quarters and fuel provided. Causes for dismissal were drunkenness, use of profanity, neglect of duty or gross misconduct. Posted prominently were rules for patients and functioning of the wards.[5]

Patient Rules
1. Wash from head to foot.
2. If can walk comb hair in morning.
3. Take off hats in wards and boot and shoes before lying down.
4. No profanity or indecent language, no immoral or infidel sentiments, no gambling, no smoking.
5. No books or pamphlets of immoral or indecent nature.
6. No male in female ward and vice versa.
7. No patient in dead house, kitchen, or theater without permission of superintendent or other officers of house.
8. Expose to outside air daily. To leave hospital grounds need written permission.
9. Do not walk on grass when exercising.

Ward Rules
1. No bundles, carpetbags, or baskets.
2. No clothing under pillows or tucked in beds or windows.
3. No packages lying about or old newspaper.
4. No littering.
5. Those rags used for dressing wounds which are too much soiled to go the laundry, are to be buried or burned in open air.
6. No ward will be left unattended.
7. Night watchman tour is 9 P.M. to 6 A.M.

Leaving no doubt as to appropriate behavior on government property, visitor rules were posted prominently.

Notice to Visitors — Knight Hospital
1. Hours. 10 A.M. to 4 P.M. Wednesday.
2. Under no circumstances take articles of diet into wards. Give to medical officers of the day who will distribute them to those intended.
3. Visitors will observe the utmost quiet and decorum.
4. Observation of rules is essential for the welfare of the patients and provides Discipline for the hospital. If fail to comply, will be denied admission in the future.
      P. A. Jewett
      Surgeon U.S.A. in charge

All levels of society were prepared to make sacrifices to get the job done. Miss Emily Sedgwick, for example, was the sister of Major General John Sedgwick, who was killed at the Battle of Gettysburg. After his death she served as nurse at Knight hospital, leaving in June of 1865 due to ill health.

Ms. L. Hanfour of Granby had nursing experience in London and in the U.S. She was especially keen on doing her part, applying in April and again December 1861. "I will spend my time and my life if need be in the hands of liberty and right and also to try to help those who are suffering for that cause."

J. Huberny of Waterbury asked the governor to hire his daughter in August 1861, if not as a rifle toting volunteer, then as nurse. "Is it your intention to send any female nurses connected with the hospital department with the new regiments now being organized? I have a well-educated daughter who because she would not be permitted to shoulder a musket is anxious to become a volunteer nurse for the sick and wounded and if female nurses are to be sent I will forward such recommendations as she may be able to obtain for your consideration."

Sylvia Houghton of Woodstock applied to Governor Buckingham for a position in nursing, offering recommendations of Drs. McGregor and Holbrook. "Knowing you have taken an active and deep interest in the suffering of our brave soldiers who have laid all, even life up on the altar of our country. I have taken the liberty of addressing you, to ask the favor of your assistance that I too may contribute the wide mile, to do something for those noble men who sacrifice so much. In the capacity of nurse hope I could alleviate their sufferings, cheer the discouraged and really make myself useful in the government service if I knew where to apply for the situation in our own state or elsewhere."[6]

Dr. Robert Ware (a bachelor) filed this report on men and women nurses while working for the Sanitary Commission:

The country should be proud of those faithful men who labored day and night to alleviate the sufferings of battle without the hope of honorable mention or a brevet in this world. May they have their reward in the next world.

If women comprehended their true work and had the patience to show that they do so comprehend it, the deep prejudice against them, in the minds of the army surgeons, would be removed. But women have not as a general thing, seen their place or duty. Benevolence must be obedient. Sisters of Mercy are the preferred nurses. Women would be more useful than the sisters if they would learn their true place.

A year later, the same doctor was an assistant regimental surgeon stationed in New Bern, North Carolina, with the Forty-fourth Massachusetts Volunteers. He had acquired a different view of the fair sex and nurses in general.

With us are engaged several New York ladies who are most useful and efficient. I should not have supposed that women of their breeding and habits could go through with so much and such fearfully disagreeable work, but they are untiring, always cheerful, ready, and uncomplaining; and by their very presence, apart from the actual assistance in nursing soften the treatment which, at the hands of the best intentioned men, is somewhat rough and harsh. They are charming company, and I am rapidly learning to eat with my fork — when I can get one.[7]

In Woodward's *Manual of Hospital Steward,* the subject of nursing is defined: Thou shall not talk back to the surgeon or challenge his authority, whether you wear pants or dress.

Absolute obedience in these respects is their military duty and ... every time he disobeys or neglects the surgeon's directions as to the care of patient in any particular, he risks unnecessarily the life of a fellow creature. It is not for him to judge the propriety or importance of the measure directed: for this the surgeon is responsible. Blind and complete obedience is necessarily required of him and for this he will be held strictly responsible.

Surgeons who felt their authority threatened by civilian nurses had an easier time with subservient women of the church who were absolutely obedient and hardworking as well. Dr. Silas Weir Mitchell was chief of staff at Turner's Lane Military Hospital in Philadelphia. Despite his advanced thinking on many issues, however, Mitchell had distinctly paternal and condescending views about female nurses, consistent with the times.

Some were terribly earnest, utterly ignorant and quite incapable of discipline. Others if more efficient were not punctual and came and went as they pleased. A large proportion was early credited in the papers for patriotic services and was seeking that notoriety which is the motive force of so many of the aspirations. The best nurses were catholic [*sic*] sisters.[8]

Dr. Simon Baruch, a Confederate surgeon and father of the financier Bernard Baruch of the Franklin D. Roosevelt era, described nurses as "fussy female notoriety seekers, quarrelsome, meddlesome, busybodies, and wretched females."[9]

Acting Surgeon General Barnes, in a report to Secretary Stanton after Gettysburg, was critical of newly arrived nurses and doctors.

Experience has proven that many of the physicians volunteering their services were worse than useless for field service and for this reason the surgeon generals of each state have been invited to select physicians of reputation and ability who will voluntarily hold themselves in readiness to proceed to the positions where their services would be most demanded upon notification of this office. By telegraph and railroad the services of over 100 experienced surgeons can thus be almost immediately available upon an emergency such as Gettysburg.

The presence of females and female nurses on the battlefield causes great inconvenience if not absolute injury to the wounded. They require the shelter and transportation that of rights should be devoted to the hospital purposes and in their ministrations are extremely adverse to discipline, control or advice from proper authorities.[10]

Male nurses could be just as difficult, as witness the lawsuit filed by Edwin Bennett against Pliny Jewett in July 1863. He signed a one-year contract in April to serve in the U.S. Army as nurse and perform duties in connection with sick and wounded as required by medical authorities and obey all orders emanating from them for a period of one year. He had left the hospital without a pass and refused to return. He was found guilty of disobedience of orders and other misconduct and was confined to the hospital guardhouse to be relieved from confinement when he returned to duty. The petitioner claimed no such authority over him existed. The judge disagreed, claiming it was "absurd to suppose a nurse in military hospital could be permitted to refuse at his own caprice to aid in amputation of a limb or relieving himself from labor to leave a sick man to die for want of attention."[11]

American women made essential contributions while enduring hardships and succumbing to diseases contracted while caring for loved ones in distant locations. They too offered painful and sometimes fatal sacrifices. Attention must be paid to their energy, persistent devotion, nobility, and quiet personal heroism. At the war's end, the *Record* certified the thoughts and hearts of its patients and staff.

> The patriotic fire has glowed nowhere with a truer brighter and steadier radiance than among the women of our country. What flocks of Florence Nightingales have cheerfully left their happy homes and flown to the distant hospitals to cheer with their songs of kindness the sick and wounded soldiers of the country? What tender care and nursing have their willing hands afforded? What words of cheer and Christian counsel have they given to the sorrowful and dying?

An article in the *Record* in January 1863, "At Hospital Grounds," described the atmosphere at the new army hospital.

> The wounded soldiers are getting along very comfortably under the care of the physicians in attendance, Drs. Knight, Hooker, Jewett, Daggett, Hubbard, Peck and Lindsley. Several nurses and many male assistants are doing all in their power to minister to the comfort of the invalids. The large tents have a pleasant look and the disabled men speak in terms of the highest praise of the kindness shown them. In a neat tent in the foreground, Dr. Jewett presides and here an ample supply of stationary [*sic*] is kept and soldiers' letters are forwarded with dispatch. Many are not able to write but dictate to others who kindly do it for them.

CHAPTER TWELVE

Provost Marshal and the Patient

Getting men to the battlefield was critical and retaining them equally so. As early as July 1862, the War Department appealed to Governor Buckingham and others to return their volunteers to the battlefield.

> There are no doubts a large number of soldiers absent from the army on sick leave who are abundantly able to rejoin their regiments but who are neglecting their duty and spending their time at home among their friends. The penalty of being considered deserters is in many cases insufficient to induce these men to come forward and report themselves. It has been thought necessary to ask the vigorous cooperation of the governors of states in finding out and sending these men to join their comrades in the field. I am directed to request your Excellency to adopt such measure for this purpose as it may seem to you most efficient and proper.

In March 1863, Congress passed the Conscription Act in answer to the Lincoln administration's call for an additional 300,000 troops. In the popular song, "We Are Coming, Father Abra'am," patriotic passions were stoked "amidst bayonets gleaming" and "spangled flag in glory and in pride … marching to face the foreign foe." The enforcer of the draft was the Provost Marshal Bureau, a division of the Department of War whose primary goal was to register every male citizen, including all immigrants who had filed for citizenship, between the ages of twenty and forty-five. The quota for each district's draft would be based on this enrollment. The bureau would be a combination police department and magistrate authorized to conduct military tribunals, including suspension of the writ of habeas corpus. The consequence was the arrest without charge of over 4,600 people, among them newspaper reporters, the editor of the *Chicago Tribune*, a congressman, and members of the Democratic Party. Some called the Democrats "copperheads," likening them to a deadly venomous snake lurking in the high grass whose bite could be fatal to limb or life. The only sensible recourse was no compromise and extermination of the evil reptile to protect decent God-fearing folks. The Peace Democrats saw the phrase differently. They decided that the copper "head" was the image of Liberty on copper pennies, and they used it as a proper badge.

The bureau's responsibilities included suppressing marauders and gambling houses; protecting private property and preserving good order; supervising and disciplining hotels, saloons, and places of amusement; conducting searches, seizures, and arrests; preventing straggling; assuming custody of deserters and POWs; and issuing passes to citizens and

149

hearing their complaints. Their most important function was to get and keep soldiers on the field of battle. The interaction of provost marshals, medical personnel, and patients is illuminated by the Draft Registration Records, which for New England are kept at the National Archives in Waltham, Massachusetts. It is from this repository that much of this chapter is derived. Letters sent and received by the surgeons at Knight U.S. Army General Hospital, medical registers of those examined for exemption, medical records of enlisted and enrolled men, and letters received and sent by the provost marshals and military commanders relating to sick and wounded soldiers highlight this relationship.[1]

By June 1863 anxiety about the draft was coming to a boil and especially in the immigrant precincts of Connecticut. The draft enrollers were paid for each person identified as eligible for the draft. Padding these lists with fictitious or real names, eligible or not, was thus financially rewarding, particularly in parts of towns lacking political clout and without ready access to justice. As the draft lottery of July 1863 approached, many of those registered left for Canada and parts unknown. Lieutenant August Putman, deputy provost marshal of New Haven County, reported to Colonel Pardee about struggling mightily against "defectives," "copperhead justices," and "copperhead lawyers." He was aware of the public's sentiment and those who practiced "rascality"[2]:

> In the 5th district which comprises one of the most thickly populated Irish Wards of New Haven and in some of the dark places of our rural districts, reports have been made of obstacles to enrollment. I am happy to report that a visit from one of my deputies with a copy of the law in one hand and a force of unarmed Invalid Soldiers from the U.S. Hospital to support it has invariably resulted in a peaceful obedience to the law.
> There are lots of deserters about the Country but most of them have left off their uniforms and it is difficult to find them out. The Irish are in great distress. They call upon me all times day and night Sundays and all. The Copperheads fill their head with all sorts of stories. Among those in circulation I give two specimens. First was that the draft has been made and all the Geeks are drafted and second that I had eight hundred handcuffs come to take them off with. We shall have trouble with them, but it will have to be met firmly in the outset and then I apprehend the whole crowd will simmer down immediately.

Guns and troops were at the ready in Connecticut as the resentment in the immigrant quarters was palpable. Unarmed Invalid Corps troops who were not likely to be attacked were used as guards to accompany these officials who canvassed door to door. New York City was not so prepared. Lieutenant Putnam's warnings of June 1863 became reality in July with draft riots in New York leaving over 1,000 dead, fifty-two buildings burned to the ground, blacks lynched, and a black orphanage destroyed. Thousands of Union troops were brought in with fixed bayonets and live ammunition, and they fired on civilian mobs armed with fists, knives and clubs.

Single and married men between the ages of twenty and thirty-five were considered Class I while those married and over thirty-five were Class II and exempt. In the second district, out of 1,460 examined by a surgeon, 846 received exemptions because of physical disability. By furnishing a substitute soldier, 580 were excused, leaving just 34 drafted men entering service. Businesses existed whose sole purpose was to provide such replacements. Substitutes came from the ranks of those who had already served a tour of duty or foreigners who had no obligation to serve. Another means of draft avoidance was paying a $300 commutation fee. Those who could afford it readily paid and suffered no stain on their escutcheons. Although this practice might be called "poor men fighting a rich man's war," most of society accepted the transfer of responsibility.

An objection to that concept was raised by the editorial board of the *Record*, which declared that those who failed to serve, even when providing a substitute, were a disgrace in the North or the South.

> In the South those between the ages of sixteen and fifty who do you not serve are considered a miscreant and fall into disgrace. In the North if of suitable age and not physically disqualified, he must have a very low estimate of the duty he owes his country if he can satisfy his conscience by paying a few hundred dollars to send a substitute to the army instead of going himself. Hordes of hirelings are not a sign of strength to south. We cannot avoid a feeling of shame and humiliation at the sight of a body of recruits setting out for the army under a strong escort of soldiers with loaded muskets and fixed bayonets. Do your duty before it is too late.

By December 1864 the call was for even more men to advance a spring offensive. The same newspaper editors continued to urge young men to join, emphasizing romance, if not patriotism, as reason for enlisting.

> What will be his chance with a sweet, pretty, enthusiastic girl, if some scarred soldier, even though wanting a limb, should enter the lists against him as matrimonial prize? How ashamed would he be when her pretty mouth asks, "what corps did you belong to, and in what battle did you participate?" to answer, "None." Go yourself and do not send substitute.

E.D. Townsend, writing for the War Department, issued General Order Number 301 in December 1864. The purpose was to stop the leakage of troops and bolster the army's numbers. The *Record* trumpeted the headline "Every Man to the Front — strengthens the victorious armies" and announced:

> Every officer and soldier capable of duty is wanted in the field and if not on duty is ordered to their respective organizations. All Provost Marshals and Board of Enrollment are instructed to employ most diligent exertion in forwarding soldiers to the front and arresting deserters, shirkers and all fit for duty that are absent without proper authority. Surgeons in charge of hospitals are directed to send forward all who are fit for service, taking care not to expose any who are unfit. Every effort must be put forth to fill up the ranks, strengthen our armies and aid the patriotic and gallant troops now smiting the reeling enemy with victorious blows.

The question "Are your brothers to go to war while you stay here?" was just as vexing an issue in biblical days (Numbers 32:6). Some northern states and even townships offered to pay the $300 commutation fee by raising funds through taxes or bonds for those without financial resources. Manufacturers and other business people offered to cover that cost and thus retain skilled labor.

Over half the available inductees failed the preinduction surgeon's exam (the same rate as draftees in World War II). Some were exempted because of social factors, such as being the sole means of support for a widow, orphan sibling, motherless child, or indigent parent. Nationwide, of the 207,000 men drafted, 87,000 paid for exemption. Only 46,000 of the drafted actually served; the rest were excused for the reasons elucidated above.

Between December 1864 and April 1865 in New Haven County, 102 recruits were exempted for physical reasons. The examination record consisted of the following categories: name, age, nativity, occupation, height, complexion, eye and hair color, chest expansion, and physique, which was recorded as "good" or "bad." The last column was for "remarks," which declared whether a recruit was accepted or rejected and, in the case of the latter, the reason. Early in the war, the average age for Connecticut volunteers was twenty-six. By 1864 and 1865 the range in age was twenty-one to forty-four, averaging thirty-six years. Eighteen through thirty-five was the accepted age for the draft with exceptions for musicians.

Heights could range from four feet, seven inches, to six feet, though the accepted range was five feet, three inches, to six feet, three inches. Medical texts declared that "the proportion of men six feet and upwards in our hospitals suffering from disease such as dysentery, diarrhea, and hemorrhoids is much greater than men of medium height."[3] The maximum weight allowable was 220 pounds. In this same group, twenty-three were unmarried, and seventy-nine married or at least claimed to be. Those married and over thirty-five were exempt, a fact well known to the public. Not all these guidelines were scrupulously followed, however, as the need for warm bodies trumped all.

Occupations were far-ranging: reporter, teamster, seaman, printer, railroader, druggist, clerk, shoemaker, cigar maker, cabinet maker, carpenter, raftsman, baker, painter, mechanic, box maker, stableman, mason, laborer, stove keeper, machinist, boatman, farmer, joiner, grocer, photographer, farrier, blacksmith, saloon keeper, student, waiter, truckman, coal dealer, plumber, seaman, cook, bookkeeper, furniture dealer, inspector, livery manager, pattern maker, gunsmith, tailor, merchant, manufacturer, hatter, boat cutter, and unemployed. There were medical cautions stressed by the experts: "Certain kinds of mechanics are objectionable, especially tailors and shoemakers. Men, who have followed these professions uninterruptedly for fifteen to twenty years, if they have entered them early in life, are commonly unfit for soldiers. Permanent flattening of the thorax and gibbosity with diminished vital capacity occur in these occupations."[4] Those under twenty-five were thought susceptible to disease and deformity from backpacks and prolonged marching.

Complexions were described as dark, ruddy, fair, or black. The eyes were black, blue, gray, or hazel. The hair was brown, black, red, blond, or nonexistent. Chest expansion was thirty-two to thirty-nine inches upon inspiration and twenty-nine to thirty-six upon expiration. A chest measuring less than thirty inches was grounds for rejection. Aside from being too short or tall, having a deformity of the chest, back, or extremity would lead to rejection if the physical trait was thought likely to interfere with carrying a knapsack or firing a weapon.

By 1863 the volunteers had been used up and Main Street had precious few bodies to offer the war machine. A popular song of the time was "The Captain of the Provost (A Parody)," which deftly and with humor summarizes army life and those who avoid serving in it: skedaddlers, bounty jumpers, medical and social exemptions, conscription buyouts, and sunshine patriots.[5]

The skedaddlers from the draft are trying every plan,
No one now 'bove thirty-five but is a married man,
The young men too, are all at once, taken very ill,
And nothing can affect a cure but an exemption bill.

Oh the country now is thick, with lame, blind and sick,
None stirs about without a crutch or a stick.
I haven't got three hundred, what will become of me
When the Captain of the Provost takes a sly glance at me.

Uncle Abe is full of jokes, for he takes poor white and black
And packs them off for Dixie to keep the Rebels back,
In battling for the Union I think it is but right
To let them all, rich and poor, smell powder in a fight.

Oh! Round each big hotel lounges many a gay young man
Who can wink at the ladies and punish juleps well;
If they'd only put them through how tickled I would be
When the Captain for the Provost takes a sly glance at me.

There were several reasons for being exempted from service, including medical, social and economic. General disqualifications included feebleness, scrofula, syphilis, cancer, intemperance, and solitary vice. Convicted felons were exempted. Alcoholism was considered a social vice rather than a disease and was a disqualifier only if chronic. Physical ailments thought contraindicated for the life of a soldier could be obvious. He had to carry a knapsack, withstand prolonged walking, and fire a weapon, which required eyesight, the ability to hear an order and flex the appropriate fingers. Physical grounds for exemption included the following.[6]

1. Poor vision.
2. Deafness.
3. Loss of arm, hand, leg or foot.
4. Anchylosis shoulder, elbow, wrist, hip, knee or ankle.
5. Total loss of thumb, loss of distal phalanx of right thumb.
6. Loss of any two fingers one hand.
7. Loss of index finger of right hand.
8. Loss of first and second phalanges of fingers of right hand.
9. Permanent extension or flexion contracture of any finger except little.
10. Total loss of great toe.
11. Varicose veins with chronic swellings and ulcerations.
12. Abnormal mobility and luxation (voluntary and involuntary) of bones.
13. Overriding of toes, great toes crossing others. (Bunions).

A major cause for exemption was absence of teeth. Biting off the end of a powder cartridge was necessary to load a rifle. While there were edentulous people who could do so, it was felt too difficult for most. Advanced caries or poor dental health was associated with nutritional deficiencies, which in turn often signaled poor general health. Deformity or ulcerations of the lower extremity would make marching, walking, or climbing a hardship if not an impossibility, and accounted for over half the cases. (See page 140.)

Below is a sample list of causes for rejection or exemption in New Haven County December 1864 through April 1865. The numbers are from averaging lists of one hundred consecutive examinations.

Hernia	15	Deformity of foot	5
Entire loss of upper teeth	11	Deafness	4
Loss of all teeth	9	Knee contractures or ulcerations	4
Shortening or deformity of leg	9	Loss of right eye	4
Varicose veins with ulcerations	6		

The reasons for rejection in the musculoskeletal area were "club feet, bad feet, loss of all toes right foot, toe contractures, extensive bunions, extensive necrosis of right tibia, ankylosis [stiff] hip, leg 1½ inches short, leg 2 inches short, leg 4 inches short, leg 5 inches short, ankylosis knee, ankylosis shoulder, ankylosis elbow, ankylosis little finger, chicken breasted, large tumor right side of spine, loss of right thumb, loss of ring finger, loss of distal phalanx right thumb, permanent extension of left index finger, permanent extension of two fingers left hand, injury hand, injury both hands, rheumatism." A deformed lower extremity would severely limit marching and make running impossible. Ankylosis, or joints that do not bend, had the same effect, and when involving the upper extremity meant inability to fire a weapon.

In the neurologic arena were "paralysis agitans, mental and physical debility, drunk, general debility, curvature of spine with spinal irritation, permanent deafness, epilepsy, fits, non-compos mentus [dementia], excessive stammering, and depressed skull fracture." Rounding out the list were "hemorrhoids and stricture of urethra, partial loss of penis, gonorrhea, syphilis, retraction of right testicle, enlarged heart, cleft palate, scabies, skin disease, weak lungs, obesity, cataracts, nearly total loss of vision congenital, and anasarca."

Total baldness was considered incompatible with wearing a soldier's headgear and therefore grounds for exemption. Some of these gents must have been sorry spectacles besides the absence of hair: "Too old and bald" age forty-two, "bald" age thirty-six; "too old and broken down" ages thirty-nine, forty, and forty-five. "Not acceptable morally," "no consent of parents" (underage), "under criminal charges of robbery," "knew nothing of the genuineness of his certificate," "backed out because companion was rejected," "lied so unreasonably that no reliance could be placed on what he said," were deciding factors noted by the examining surgeon.[7]

If one failed exemption for the usual reasons, one could claim to be a member of the Confederate army. Announcing provenance as a Confederate veteran or deserter was thought by some to be a sure ticket out. They might offer to serve in a "safe" place such as the western frontier or even Connecticut. Private Charles Williams of the Fifth Connecticut Volunteers announced his little-known Confederate pedigree and decided to become a hometown Yankee in February 1865.[8]

> I am from the Rebel lines as you already know and I have no desire that I should be sent anywhere where I would be in danger of falling into their hands. Put me on duty here at this camp and I promise to do my duty upright and faithful. For my wife and child for their sake I would rather be retained here.

Private John Knost professed to have served with the Confederates in Louisiana, Alabama, and elsewhere, preferring "to be transferred to the frontier if possible." He was mustered in November 1864 and mustered out August 1865 with the Sixth Regiment. Private Charles Granbosy claimed to be twenty-two years old, born in France, and having spent three years as assistant surgeon in the Magruder Division of the Confederate army in the Peninsula and Seven Day Battle and in a general hospital in Richmond. In March 1865 he "now respectfully requested to be transferred if possible to another regiment doing duty in the west." He was examined on January 24 and 25, but on each occasion was "so much under the influence of liquor as not to be fit" and was "sent away to get sober." On the third try he was accepted. These three cases bespeak the desperation to get warm bodies in blue uniform. How effective the men were as soldiers can be surmised.

In December of 1862 *The Hartford Times* described the "Beauty of Drafting," citing statistics from Governor Buckingham's address to the legislature that after two drafts 4,212 men were called up and only 76 were mustered in. For New Haven County, out of 312 draftees, 194 were rejected by county or post surgeons, two were over forty-five years old, forty-six were in jail or did not report, thirty-five deserted, twelve more detached by the secretary of war or selectmen, and eleven had substitutes, leaving only twelve who actually mustered in.

Some lied about their marital status, age, medical condition and past history to avoid the draft and service. The 1863 song sheet "How Are You, Exempt?" summarizes in rhyme what most knew about dodging the draft:

How are you, Exempt?
I s'pose you feel "all right"
As the Surgeon said you'd never do
To take your gun and fight.

What did he say the matter was?
The trouble man with you?
Did he say you'd got the heart complaint,
And test you through and through?

Did he say that that was all?
Did he say you were too short?
Or too slender or too tall?
Was your case one of debility,
Once caused by a fall.
Did he say you could not see, sir.
With but one eye at all?

Tell us what the doctor said,
Did he say non-compos mentis
Which means weakness of the head.

Or did he say your back and legs
Were shaped so crookedly
That you'd never do to take your gun
And go along with me?[9]

A more pressing issue for the provost was the medical furloughs which permitted twenty days of leave and required official renewal extensions. Numerous furloughs from reputable and not-so-reputable sources were issued, making them difficult to supervise. The furlough required a sworn statement by a physician in good standing certified by a magistrate. One copy was to be sent to the issuing hospital, one to the nearest military facility, and the third was to be kept by the soldier. The document was supposed to state the nature of the disease, the extent of the disability, the length of time sick and under the physician's care, and the length of time before being able to travel. Pleas for transfers, medical discharges, release from arrest, and a host of other earthly requests were sent to Dr. Jewett as chief of Knight U.S. Army General Hospital. Letters from civilian doctors revealed an uneven expertise and sometimes shading of the truth. The provost's approval often reflected the credibility of the signing doctor and the patient's background, rather than the diagnosis or prognosis described.

Dr. Curtis was a respected member of the Hartford Medical Society who wrote concerning the health of a new recruit:

Chronic catarrh is increasing in the mucus membranes of the lungs and is likely to eventuate in "catarrh consumption." It is unjust to this soldier to keep him longer in the service. He will become less competent to perform his duties and I am quite sure that he has prospects of having induced incurable disease. I think the good of the service and the soldier requires his discharge.[10]

Dr. W. Joule of New London wrote this note to Dr. Jewett for Joshua Dyer, of the Colored Troops:

He was visited at home and was house confined due to nephritis and spinal irritation, and was unable to return to the hospital. He resides in New London and was out for two months.

Numerous other letters requesting extension of their furloughs were sent by physicians on behalf of sick or wounded soldiers. They were addressed to the post of the soldier's origin, be it the Knight U.S. Army General Hospital, Fort Trumbull, or Camp Rendezvous, and were reviewed and evaluated by the provost marshal. The following excuses were "disapproved."

Acute tonsillitis.

Chronic inflammation in side, with bloated bowels and tumor on testicle and is wholly unable to rejoin his regiment.

Suffering from disease which makes him wholly unfit for duty and unable to travel.

Suffering from slow or continued fever of mild form.

Suffering from diarrhea and debility and will not be fit for duty in less than 20 days more. Has already gone one month.

Diarrhea.

Acute dysentery.

Vomiting and diarrhea which has weakened him and produced disturbances of his systems.

Chronic diarrhea and heart disease.

Sick with chills and fever and a bad diarrhea and suffers from wound in left leg.

Sick for five months with diarrhea and has had convulsions but is much better.

Feeble, debility caused by scurvy. He has chronic diarrhea.

Sick for two days, pneumonia.

Rheumatism.

Is very weak and in low conditions and is unable to travel. Dr. Austin. [The Provost concluded that] "this signature is thought not genuine at this office."

Suffering from paralysis and diarrhea — is in his opinion *able* to travel to the field but would be of no use after arriving there.

Severe lesion of the spinal column.

Unfit by reason of partial paralysis of the right arm with general debility. [Had been at Turner's Lane Military Hospital in Philadelphia].

All patients suffering from gunshot wounds were approved for furlough extension. They were often described as confined to bed, unable to travel, and suffering with general debility. Some recovered nicely and lived a long life, and some died at home. A description of such patients follows:

Unable to report to hospital by reason of gangrene from gunshot wound in left hip and great general debility, confining him to his bed. Wound nine by four inches.

Lost his left leg, is confined to his bed, has spasms and is unable to stand on his crutches more than five minutes, has great irritability of nervous system.

Painful stumps.

William Tryon of Hartford was examined in November 1864 by Dr. Ellsworth. He described a "bullet wound through stomach, liver and lung. Each hand lost fingers, two gone on one hand, unable to travel." A thoughtful and compassionate provost wrote, "The man had no intention of deserting from hospital or even absenting himself without authority. Evidently unable to travel but has no evidence of authority for his absence and cannot give him permission to remain. If returned as a deserter I recommend charge be removed and he permitted to remain at his home until he is able to return to hospital."

A special category was returning prisoners of war who suffered from malnutrition often aggravated by traumatic and infectious diseases. In May 1865 Major John Henry Burnham of the Sixteenth Connecticut Volunteers was stationed in New Bern, North Carolina, having survived the horrors of Antietam and a yellow fever epidemic, but he was unprepared for returning prisoners of war.

Quite a number of our boys who were prisoners have returned to us not looking very well but alas, they are but a drop in the bucket to the great number of those whose bones are lying under the sod in Dixie. Somebody must have a terrible punishment in store for themselves for treating our men with such horrid brutality.[11]

The environment and conditions of prisoners of war were often desperate, even fatal, as these statements requesting medical furlough indicate.

Patient is from Libby prison. Severe and constant cough and hurried inspiration forty per minute. Rapid pulse and every afternoon followed with profuse perspirations, expectoration tinged with blood. Emaciation and is constantly growing worse rather than better.

Patient is a war prisoner. Not only emaciated and debilitated but a completely used up man. He is suffering from the effects of starvation and is hardly able to walk across the room.

He is suffering from cruel treatment in rebel prisons which caused emaciation, general debility, coughs, chronic diarrhea.

Greatly emaciated from violent cough and dysentery which may be killing him.... Kept alive until January 3, 1865 when he died.

In the public's heart there was no more incendiary subject. Arrangements were made after the battle of Winchester between Stonewall Jackson and Union forces to quickly exchange doctors for humanitarian reasons. With Grant taking command, exchanges were discouraged since the discrepancy of manpower meant greater pressure on the South, whose diminishing personnel could not be replaced. The consequences were ill-fed, ill-clothed and ill-housed prisoners who died by the thousands. Connecticut agents reported in 1863 that Union soldiers who were released had "no clothing, no place to stay, little and yet unhealthy food, little transportation home and no back pay to get there."

Agent Robert Corson listed eighty-three paroled Connecticut prisoners transferred from Baltimore to Philadelphia in April 1864.

Most of these soldiers are in the same condition which I found those at Annapolis last fall. Many have lost their limbs by being exposed to the cold storms on Belle Island. Starvation is to be seen in their faces and it makes us heart sick to look at these brave boys and think that they should be returned to us in this condition and that there are still many others in the hands of those bad men. I understand that these men are to be sent to this city as soon as they are able to be transported. Very few of them will <u>ever</u> be able to enter active service again.[12]

He reported in October 1864 on twenty-four men paroled from Richmond. "These poor fellows tell the same sad story of the brutal treatment they have received while in the hands of the rebels. Some of them are from Andersonville and report that within the last seven months over 12,000 Union soldiers have died at that place."

Agent Almy was offered a listing by state of those buried at Andersonville that contained 300 Connecticut men just from February 1864 through 1865. "Atwater desires to dispose of these lists by states and receive compensation for the same. The risk which he assumed in the copy of this list was great and endangers his life if detected. I think this is the only list in existence and will be very valuable to those who have lost their relatives in adjusting claims for pay with the government." As late as March 1865, released prisoners were presenting with scurvy, chronic dysentery, and even frostbite.

John Allen of Plymouth joined the Ninth Regiment in August 1861, was discharged disabled in December 1862. Later, he joined the First Connecticut Cavalry, on December 10, 1863. He was captured in June 1864 at Ream's Station and died in September 1864 at Andersonville Prison in Georgia. A list of nineteen other cavalrymen who had died there found its way to the governor, who registered his disgust. "Sergeant Gusley states that a man by the name of Allen belonging to the Cavalry received a cut on his foot, that gangrene settled therein but the surgeon refused doing anything for him until the lower part of his leg had literally rotted off, when it was amputated but in such a manner as to require a second amputation from which he died."[13]

Mrs. Alfred Chappell had asked the governor for her husband's back pay, without which she and her two children were destitute. In August 1863 she wrote the "Surgeon in charge of the hospital" at Camp Parole, Annapolis, concerning her husband, a resident of Norwich and member of the Eighteenth Connecticut Volunteers who had been captured at Winchester and was paroled four weeks later and transferred to Annapolis. He and others of his regiment were sick paroled prisoners, and, she wrote, "I am of the opinion that it would be better for the service if all such should have furlough or be permitted to return to Connecticut and will be obliged if you can consistently with your duty and aid in receiving this object."[14] Chappell died just six weeks after this request was made. His regiment's casualties were fifty-two killed, 656 captured, and ninety-one died in prison or later of disease.

The fate of prisoners was a heavy personal weight for Buckingham, who had witnessed the consequences of his constituents' prolonged confinement. In a letter to President Lincoln dated November 18, 1863, he vents his anger over a meeting with the Reverend H. Farnsworth of the Eighteenth Regiment, who had taken part in an exchange with Libby Prison while leaving seventy-two soldiers still in captivity.

> Colonel William G. Ely of the 18th Conn Vol. was held in the hospital about ten days. One infirmed private was brought from Belle Isle and was thoroughly worn down with a degree of emaciation making him unable to mend his broken foot and suffered amputation as a result. Those who must wait until the next exchange are facing a prisoner's grave. There are more now dying than were being released. If included in an exchange they would be unfit to participate in service hereafter. I might add the statements from the tormented I have heard and fully endorse all which show the persecutions and suffering of the most diabolical treatment. As President I know that you cannot condemn or sacrifice your honor for this entire neglect which you cannot reprieve over principle which is well established. I wanted to write and ask if you could review the subject and see if in some way our soldiers could be secured from want and the integrity of the government be preserved. I know you will do this if at all possible.[15]

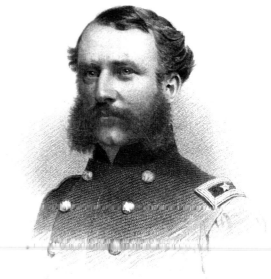

By March 1864, with no release in sight, the governor appealed to the district commander, General Ben Butler, with better results. "Colonel William Ely and most of the officers of the 18th regiment have been in Libby prison.... If you could see the rebel colonel and get a parole extension for Colonel Ely or in any way better his situation (others officers are also important), your efforts will be highly appreciated by the citizens of Connecticut and especially by this department."

Colonel William Ely of Norwich joined the Eighteenth Connecticut Volunteers in September 1861 and was captured along with 656 others in June 1863 at Winchester, Virginia. Forty-

Colonel William G. Ely, Eighteenth Connecticut Volunteers (author's collection).

three died in prison. The rations were meager, the water foul, blankets absent and men herded like cattle. Officers had the same lack of necessities as the privates. Ely was paroled in March 1864, along with others from his unit, in time for the spring election. They were photographed posing with the governor on a second-floor veranda during the coming-home festivities in Norwich. Ely was again wounded, in June 1864, in Lynchburg, Virginia, and was promoted to brigadier general by brevet in March 1865. He was discharged disabled on June 27, 1865.

The fall of 1864 meant the presidential election. Family and friends of prisoners used the occasion as leverage for their release. Josiah Peck, from Bristol, was chairman of the Union town committee, and warned the governor of the consequences of "not doing all that duty and humanity would seem to require to exchange our men. Unless something is done soon many who have been Union men will with-hold their votes in the upcoming presidential elections and a few of them will vote for General McClellan being made to believe he will be able to bring about an exchange." On October 5, 1864, he posted the following to President Lincoln.

> Members of the 16th Conn are prisoners in the hands of the rebels, captured last April at Plymouth N.C. An entire company making up that regiment came from Bristol. Some are from business and property families who came out from a sense of duty for their country. Nothing definite has been heard from them since their capture until recently that several of our brave men have died from the terrible treatment they have received from the hands of the rebels at Andersonville Georgia. Our community is filled with sad grief of the sad news carried by the death of so many of our beloved men and that so many are suffering in such wicked and terrible manner according to all accounts. The anxious inquiry is asked almost universally now why does our government now not affect [*sic*] an exchange with the rebels whereby our men be extracted from their hands. Mothers who have given their sons, wives who have parted with their husbands, feel deeply upon this subject. They sent out our men expecting they might be killed in battle and were prepared for such news. But can hardly be reconciled to think our friends must starve to death in rebel hands when it seems they might be exchanged for their men we have in our possession. Can that be brought about in some way and soon?[16]

Franklin G. Peck was captured on April 20, 1864, at Plymouth, North Carolina, and pardoned on November 30, 1864. He was mustered out on June 24, 1865. Fred H. Peck was pardoned on February 28, 1865, and mustered out on June 24, 1865.

Two weeks later the War Department replied, "The department is using every means in its power to affect [*sic*] a general release of prisoners with the rebels and it is hoped that a release will be obtained soon." The department also responded to the governor's separate inquiry concerning "the petition of certain citizens of Connecticut asking that measures may be taken for their relief." Major General Hitchcock, the commissioner of exchange, advised: "The poor condition of the prisons at Andersonville is the subject of correspondence between General Butler and the rebel agent of exchange. The contents of the Richmond papers inform us that the barbarian General Winder who has abused those prisoners has been dismissed by his own government for 'incompetency and inhumanity.' The best relief must come through the Union army." Left unsaid was Grant's policy on exchanges.

Another Bristol resident, W. H. Nettleton, wrote Lincoln on behalf of his brother and others in the same circumstances with the same regiment.

> Six of them have died at Andersonville and many more at the point of death, a lingering suffering death, ten times worse than the death on a battlefield. I am sorry to say that the fact of our soldiers being permitted to suffer and die instead of being exchanged is having a very bad influence here and elsewhere upon our coming election. The copperheads have a great deal to

say about it and to my certain knowledge gain converts through that instrumentality. I feel the importance of the coming election, everything is at stake and I am laboring hard for the Republican cause. And I feel for our prisoners, especially my only brother who enlisted out of pure patriotism notwithstanding he was in poor health and leaves a family to mourn his hard fate not knowing whether he is alive or dead. I hope and pray if there is any possible way to affect [sic] an exchange that it may be done speedily for humanity sake.[17]

George E. Nettleton of Bristol died two weeks after his pardon, Christmas Day, 1864. Dennis Nettleton of Guilford died in prison on February 25, 1865.

Helen Scott of Delaware, Ohio, proposed yet another solution in December 1864 to the secretary of war: provide Union nurses with appropriate supplies to relieve the sufferings of Union prisoners.

If the plan is practical (consent of the Confederacy obtained) I propose in company with some true women to be selected by you to visit all the hospitals in the confederacy containing union prisoners distributing goods furnished by the United States or the Sanitary Commission. No compensation is required. All that is expected of the government is to furnish supplies necessary and to pay transportations and other expenses necessarily incurred. You are well aware of the desperate conditions of those prisoners now being exchanged. What must be then of the suffering of those still in the hospitals. I am willing to have all of the danger of abiding in the malarious prisons of the south if by so doing well lessen the sufferings of our country's defenders.[18]

While many prisoners died in captivity or shortly thereafter, others suffered the consequences of that experience over a lifetime. Pain, suffering and personal indignation followed. Tuberculosis was the "white plague," with no effective treatment until the antibiotics of the twentieth century. Some soldiers' symptoms and physical appearance suggest this highly fatal scourge. The malnourished and chronically ill from other causes would be particularly susceptible.

Chronic affection of the lungs and affection of the brain which will probably cost him his life.
Chronic diarrhea, incipient tuberculosis, scurvy, and starvation. Inflammatory rheumatism of the knee, elbow and shoulder.
Profuse night sweats and discharge of matter from the lung of the affected side.
Discharge of blood from the lungs, shortness of breath and profuse perspiration.

Most patients had their medical furloughs approved with ailments ranging from malaria, pneumonia, and bowel infections to trauma and neurological disorders. Below are diagnosis "approved" for medical furlough extensions:

Suffering from chills.
Miasmatic fever.
Hernia and inflamed testicle which renders any kind of motion almost impossible.
Disease of spine caused by his horse falling on him.
Hemorrhoids and prolapse of rectum.
Hemorrhage of the stomach, alcoholism.
Chronic diarrhea and debility from intermittent fever.
Home sick with chronic diarrhea and unable to travel.
Diarrhea [many cases].
Chronic affections of the liver and is much reduced in physical strength.
Disease of the kidney, irritation of the stomach and constipation of the bowels.
Hypertrophy of the heart and general debility.
Acute bronchitis.
Diphtheria.
Typhoid.

Sub-paralytic condition of the flexor muscles of both upper and lower extremities.

Unable to leave his bed by reason of paralysis of one of his legs from sun stroke. Hearing
entirely gone and is reduced in every particulars. Dr. Curtis, Hartford.

General debility and derangement of the liver and digestive organs, palpitations of the heart
and difficulty breathing.

Affection of the head and general debility.

Rheumatism.

Most requests for extension were approved, the most common condition being diarrhea. A furlough that was approved despite no documentation provided was the note by Dr. Coggs-well which simply stated the patient was "sick." Approval depended on who signed the report and sometimes the circumstances.

The provost marshal of Connecticut, General F. Lemay, issued guidelines designed to improve soldiers' battlefield availability. The deserters would be renamed "stragglers" to remove any stigma and fear of trial. The role of civilian doctors was to be suspect and could be overruled by a military commander. The hometown doctor supported the home team, his patient, unlike the army surgeon, who primarily supported the government.

The furloughs of most of the soldiers now in the State will expire on or before the 20th. It is desirable that all should be returned speedily to their commands. There will probably be many who will delay not with the intention of deserting, but will remain at their homes on various pretexts and excuses. All such should be looked up and returned as stragglers. It is distinctly announced on orders from the War Department that no plea of sickness or other cause not officially established, and no certificate of a physician in civil life unless it is approved by an officer acting as military commander will relieve a soldier from charge of desertion. In the absence of a certificate the soldier is to be considered absent without leave.

It has been the practice of some physicians in this State to give certificates stating that soldiers were unable to travel when such was not the fact. Such cases coming to the knowledge of his. General Order 92 of 1862 provide that any officer or Private whose health permits him to visit places of amusement, to make social visits, or to walk about the town, city or neighborhood, will be considered fit for duty, and as evading duty by absence from his command. Arrest deserters and return all stragglers to the nearest military post.[19]

Just down the road from the hospital was the U.S. Draft Rendezvous Camp, which processed new recruits, both volunteers and drafted. A disillusioned army surgeon described "another shirk and deadbeat. Should be sent to duty and forced to do it. On the list sent I should write malingerer opposite his name." The difference between those slow to return to duty, those absent without leave, and those who had deserted was often subject to interpretation. The reasons for desertion were many, though most were for the bounty. Bad news from home, the absence of social outrage or peer pressure, absence of pay and poor officers were often in play. Many found camp life and the general life of the soldier difficult, dangerous, boring, or unprofitable and sought to improve their lot through other means.

During the entire war, out of 249,000 desertions, 103 white and 39 black soldiers were executed in the Union army. There were 4,720 desertions from Connecticut, and 33,430 desertions from the U.S. General Hospital System. Deputy Provost August Putman suggested a more lenient and humane approach to keep soldiers in the field:

There are a number of deserters at large who after months of service either from homesickness while in a state of intoxication or some other cause was induced to desert and who are now thoroughly sorry for it and would be glad to return if they had not the fear of death before them. Should we not allow some deserters to surrender voluntarily and just reduce them in pay?[20]

Those caught deserting, being absent without leave or committing criminal or other unsocial acts in violation of the military or civil code could face "riding the horse," a punishment of sitting on a wooden beam for long periods of time. This was not conducive to a healthy or happy prostate, much less the rest of the soldier's behind, but it was better than jail time or being shot. Peer pressure had some effect, though the public had mixed views on the subject and did not consider taking "French leave" a treasonable offense.

The *Columbian Register* printed a letter to the editor in November 1864, just prior to the presidential election, the following complaint:

> The *Record* noted "large board fence" built around hospital grounds to the chagrin of the "fence Jumpers." It is to the shame of those who built it. The Hospital should give the soldier patient's rights, not given in the field. In no regiment are they hampered and fettered as in the Knight U.S. Army General Hospital located in the enlightened city of New Haven. Mr. Merchant needs be more truthful with his statements and more impartial.

L.J. Merchant was the editor of the *Knight Hospital Record*, which indeed described the erection of a fence ten feet high and fifty feet long as well as a building for the guard and drummers. Parties of armed guards, composed of convalescents, patrolled the hospital perimeter and attendance was taken twice daily. Even though the fence was erected while Dr. Jewett was under arrest and out of state, the blame for its construction would be laid at his feet. The perimeter works were recommended by the War Department to discourage unauthorized departures. The desertion rate at Knight hospital for three years was 4 percent, about average for a state hospital.

The desertion rate for the North was one out of ten and for the Confederates one out of nine. Many communities did not consider deserting to come home and take care of the crops and family matters a disgrace, but the right thing to do. In both North and South execution was a desperate attempt to set an example with the ultimate goal of maintaining the respective army's manpower. Ending the war was the real solution.

Diagnosis number 152 was added to the medical register as "death due to execution." For the soldiers and their families, the finality and harshness of this diagnosis only hardened existing sentiments. There was a remedy for virtually all ailments, but not for this. As a soldier from New Haven put it after having witnessed the event, "We are not dying fast enough, so they have just started shooting us."[21]

The whereabouts of soldiers was a continuous source of bedevilment for both North and South. Keeping accurate records as to the state of health and whether a soldier was even alive required a keen administrative apparatus aided by the new telegraph and cooperation between government agencies. A cordial relationship with the provost office and Knight U.S. Army General Hospital is suggested in a series of letters with Major Jewett. In May 1863 the groundwork for an exchange of personnel is prepared in this letter to Captain Benjamin Pardee about processing deserters.

> The patients in this hospital are under my command. In addition I have what is called the Invalid Detachment who are under my immediate command but are subject to the order of the Military Court of the State. Are you authorized to take care of and to arrest deserters?[22]

The impending draft resulted in a sudden demand for additional clerks, met by personnel from the Invalid Corps under the command of Jewett. He won the gratitude of Provost Colonel Terry: "I desire in this connection to express my appreciation of the promptness with which Major P. A. Jewett Surgeon in charge of the U.S. Hospital in this city has met all my requisitions for squads of men for this and other purposes."

In July 1863, fearing that the conflict in New York City might spread to the hospital, Jewett asked Captain Pardee for arms: "I request that you send me, for the men at this hospital, eighty muskets and accoutrements. I should be glad to receive them as early as 5 o'clock P.M."

A year later he was again asked to loan experienced clerks, this time to the Provost Marshal's Office. His letters on the subject hint at quid pro quo.

July 7, 1864
I do not well see how I can spare a single clerk, at present. I have my post return to make out and several special reports. I am also receiving men frequently and also am giving a large number of furloughs. All this gives my clerks full employment. Several will return early next week from furlough. I shall then be able to send you the men.[23]

July 30 1864
General Orders forbid my detailing convalescents for duty except at the Hospital. I will give you two good men from N.R.C. the first of the week.

A week later three clerks were transferred to the provost. Two months later, the doctor was arrested and briefly imprisoned on charges of keeping patients in the hospital for personal financial gain. Two months after Jewett's release from prison, the same Provost Office beseeched Jewett to allow it to keep two of his clerks as they are "honest and know their business." He magnanimously consented to his recent jailer.

Not all cases were clear-cut. On June 12, 1863, the War Department showed a list of 175 men from five Connecticut regiments who were considered deserters. Of these, fourteen were from Knight U.S. Army General Hospital.[24]

Sir,
George M Loomis company B, 10th Regiment returned to this hospital from desertion on 24 August 1863. When he deserted he was on the list of men to be returned and was arrested and handed to the provost marshal.
Respectfully yours,
P. A. Jewett

2 Sept. 1863,
Major Jewett,
Walter Fish Company D of 10th Regiment Connecticut volunteers was reported from your hospital as being deserted 10 April 1863 and still remains so reported. The selectman of his town and the man himself who writes from your hospital on 30 August, deny the desertion. Will you report the facts of the case?
Adjutant General Office , G. Morrow

To Adjutant General Office
2 November 1863,
Sir,
John W. Smith Company D, 11th Regiment is now in this hospital. If he has been reported as a deserter from this hospital, it must be a mistake.
Very respectfully yours,
P. A. Jewett

27 November 1863
Private Enoch Powers was a patient August 1863 and *not* deserted as reported.
Respectfully yours,
Pliny A. Jewett.

The census of April 10, 1865, listed twenty-one deserters from Connecticut regiments who were assigned to Knight hospital. One such soldier on this infamous list was Thomas

Muldoon of the Fifteenth Connecticut Volunteers, Company C. He was actually a prisoner of war as a result of the Battle of Kinston, North Carolina. He sustained a spinal injury and paraplegia, which proved fatal. He was paroled March 26 but died on April 9, 1865, and was buried in Kinston, never to return home. The obvious clerical error was corrected. It didn't do Muldoon much good, but perhaps avoided needless embarrassment for his grieving family.[25]

Even the hospital cook John Grant deserted, prompting this suggestion from Acting Assistant Surgeon Blake on an appropriate replacement from the Reserve Corps:

> Sir, I would respectfully request that Private David Eastern a colored recruit for the 11th Rhode Island be detailed as cook in the hospital at this post.

Doctor Jewett wrote to the Provost Marshal's Bureau in December of 1863: "I wish to hand these men [deserters] over to you." In May of 1864 he added, "There are several men now in my Guard House who have been reported or received as deserters. I should be glad to 'get rid' of them as soon as possible. Please send for them at your earliest convenience." Lieutenant Stearns of the Reserve Corps sent another letter on Jewett's behalf on the same subject next month. "I am directed by the Surgeon in charge to inform you that there are three deserters in the guard house at this post, of whom he would like to have you take charge."[26]

Missing from statistics were those who went home either on furlough or without approval who never returned because they could not. Dying at home rather than in a hospital was sometimes the choice made by returning veterans. Such a tragedy is illustrated by this sad tale about a widow and four fatherless children.

> 23 May 1863
> Adjutant General
> To General Williams,
> Concerning the widow of Edward Dunn of Company K 24th Regiment, a man who was reported as deserter; he was home with a permit and overstayed his time. He was arrested and sent back to his regiment. He then became ill again and went home to his wife. He did not improve and was sent to a military hospital and per Dr. Jewett's certificate died 13 February 1863. Now under these circumstances could he be called a deserter? He did not run away from service but left with a written permit on account of a sickness contracted in camp. His widow is poor and sick and has four young children and needs immediate relief. Cannot the money be allowed to her?
> John D. Landis[27]

Private John Sawyer of the Eleventh Connecticut Volunteers was found guilty of desertion despite being a hospital patient, as reported by the local provost marshal. Bureaucracy can be an ass.

> The fact that he is now in Knight Hospital does in no way clear him of the crime of desertion. If a man deserts his regiment and afterwards delivers himself up at a military post or reports himself at a hospital and is received, the commandant of the post or surgeon in charge of a hospital reports the fact to his company commander. If the officer asks for the soldier's return then the surgeon or other officer need deliver him up. It may be a man is reported as a deserter when in fact he is not as in being detained at a hospital by continuance of illness. But his company commander receiving no report of the fact believes the man was discharged from the hospital and not having joined his company therefore is a deserter.[28]

Bounties were offered for information on deserters. One marshal noted a recent trial of boardinghouse keepers accused of helping deserters who were tried and found not guilty.

He describes the Irishmen as "keepers of grogshops and persons of influence among their countrymen." The verdict emboldened the secession sympathizers and those who actively assisted conscripts and substitutes to escape. "We should be allowed to make summary arrests of all such persons and transfer them with written charges to custody of the U.S. marshal in the same way as when a person obstructs the draft. Many of the substitutes have turned out to be deserters."[29]

The hiring of substitutes encouraged the lame, halt, blind, deaf, and dumb to enlist. From the start, many could not fight because of physical or mental handicaps. Once a soldier was mustered in, the state was liable for his pension regardless of preexisting conditions. This obligation constituted a large financial drain that the nation could not endure. Money changed hands and fraud was committed to fill quotas and pockets. Recruits who had already received a pension for disability tried to reenter the army surreptitiously by hiding a disability (assuming it was real) or recreating the "ailment" artificially when it was convenient in order to get another paid medical discharge. This offered a reliable source of revenue for unscrupulous agents who provided replacements whose sole virtue was having a pulse. Draft avoidance was considered a legitimate and honorable thing to do for those who could afford the fee, which rose to $750 towards the war's end.

The Hartford Daily Times
September 1864

SUBSTITUTES

Now is the time to get your substitutes and be clear of the draft, for the next three years. Aliens and those who have served three years in the army are the ones to get. No others except these are furnished.

 178 State Street
 Headquarters for Volunteers and Substitutes
 George W. Pomroy
 Authorized recruiting agent, first district
 Hartford, Ct.

Early in the war, most recruits listed Connecticut as their place of birth, but by 1864 fewer than half did. A quarter of the examinees were natives of Ireland; fewer came from Germany, England, France, and Canada. Nativity was considered important, for medical textbooks and other sources attributed personality and character traits to race, color, or nation of origin. The lack of industriousness, intelligence, cleanliness, and morality were ascribed to immigrants as hereditary. Many considered the newly arrived as "not real Americans."

Most of those being examined as substitutes were foreign born, with half from Ireland and the rest from Germany, England and Canada. The provost felt that the majority of substitute recruits were actually deserters.

In his text *A Manual of Instructions for Enlisting and Discharging Soldiers* and in his other writings for the Sanitary Commission, Robert Bartholow described behavior patterns believed due to racial or ethnic origins.[30] He was a native of Maryland and had practiced in Philadelphia and Cincinnati. He was known as a chemist, army surgeon, sanitary reformer, and writer as well.

Celtic races have less tenacity of purpose and mental hardihood. As mercenary soldiers they did not exhibit the same zeal, energy and power of endurance. They submitted less patience than the Americans to the requirements of discipline, were frequently turbulent under hardships and given to complaints about the rations and fatigue duties. Irish laborers were especially notorious for their dislike to fatigue duties.

Concerning Germans, there are certain defects of structure, common in a greater or less extent to all Germans, which impair their powers of endurance—a predominance of the lymphatic temperament; a patulous or unusual weakness of the abdominal rings; a flatness of the feet, and a tendency to a varicose condition of the veins of the inferior extremities. They are also noted for thrift, fondness for good living, and a love of ease and enjoyment.

Concerning the Negro, his chief physical defects are small, ill-developed calves and bad feet, and a proneness to disease especially of the pulmonary organs. Unquestionably less enduring than the white soldier; less active, vigilant and enterprising and more given to malingering. The Mulatto is feebler than the Negro, invariably scrofulous, and more frequently the subject of pulmonary disease.

Surgeon Nathan Mayer, a recent German immigrant himself, had a more positive view of substitutes. "The conscripts themselves or rather the substitutes for there is hardly a drafted man among them, truly comprise all sorts and conditions of men. Fully half of the consignment has served before in our own or in European armies. We have quite a number of English, Irish and German regulars who came to this country for the purpose of enlisting. They have taken the substitute money and entered the army at better wages than they ever received before. They esteem their bargain a good one and intend to do good service." He found them reliable and honorable men, noting that many saved their money and sent it to their homes in New York and elsewhere."[31]

The governor described the issue to Secretary Stanton from a different perspective. "This office has been besieged by a rash of substitute brokers who have been making a large amount from their rascality."[32] The whole lot was nothing more than "vagabonds and thieves."

In November 1863, the following edict by Assistant Adjutant General George Rubbles offered a caution and proposed a solution.

On re-enlisting men who were discharged from service with physical disability in 1861 and 1862: if they lost the disability, they will be considered only as a new recruit not as a veteran. Thus the person who brings him in gets $15 and not $25. Great care must be taken in the physical examinations of all men of this class.

The same "rascality" was denounced by Provost Marshal August Putman, whose savvy and experience is reflected in this communication of February 1864.

Both of these men sent for examination for enlistment have been drafted and rejected by the Board. Both were arrested also as draft deserters by me. Thomas Slack was accepted as a recruit. He had already been in the service and discharged for disability and has been in the work house all last summer as a common drunkard. He took the bounty, deserted and then was arrested by me, sent to Fort Trumbull and discharged from the service by a Surgeon on account of disease of the heart. He is not a fit man to enlist. None are fit for the service.

Who was disabled and who was not? Gamesmanship was rife and the system easily manipulated. Bribes and bounties, absence without leave, desertion and malingering were costly distractions but not determinant of the war's outcome. In June 1863 another provost marshal sought to make things more efficient by red-lining the obviously unfit and the repeaters:

I have written "not subject to military duty" or specified the disabling circumstance where the disability is *very* apparent hoping that when the Board of Enrollment meets they will see fit to strike such names from the enrollment without the necessity of their having to be put to the trouble and expense of a surgeon's examination.

General Lew Wallace, who would later write the biblical novel *Ben Hur*, reported to General Lorenzo Thomas on eight soldiers who were dismissed as disabled and wrongly allowed back into the service:

> The circumstances attending the reception of these men into the service under the present high sale of bounties now being paid seem to disclose a condition of inattention to proper duty if not gross faithlessness to the government on the part of recruiting officers and examining surgeons so extreme that I consider it my duty to present these papers to the War Department for proper consideration due them.

Dr. J. Curtis, the surgeon for the Board of Enrollment at Camp Rendezvous, agreed with this assessment in a whistle-blowing statement concerning fraud to Pliny Jewett.

> I am satisfied that fraud is being practiced upon the government by these discharges. This Board of Enrollment had for a long time been corresponding by letter to the Provost confident that worthless men had been substituted for good after examination. If the Board considered these men disabled and clearly worthless they should not have received their discharges but punished them. I did not mean the word defrauded applied to them and by that the Board of Enrollment.

Perhaps in retaliation, Dr. Curtis was accused of approving damaged goods in the form of recruits found to be disabled only after being mustered in and was forced to defend his actions. An eighteen-year-old developed ulceration of his leg and dysentery just three weeks after induction, requiring dismissal from the service. "He was more than fortunate in the cultivation of ulcers. I have no doubt they were finally produced by the applications of some escharotics." Another applicant denied epilepsy and after induction had fits. A forty-year-old with callused hands thought due to lifelong labor became stricken with "general debility," and also required discharge. A scrofula patient, another with acute rheumatism and a third recruit with political connections who developed chronic swelling of the heel all were released post-induction.[33]

Dr. Curtis defended his positions by pointing out, "I have never received a word of instruction upon the subject of these examinations and have supposed that I had no decision in their cases." Self-inflicted wounds from escharotics, tourniquets, or needles can fool even the experienced. Feigning diseases physical or mental can be an art form. Young doctor Curtis spoke the truth and discovered that challenging entrenched power has its consequences.

Medical discharges early in the war were sometimes conducted without involving the Medical Department. This practice was corrected by strict changes in the chain of command. Regimental and departmental medical evaluation became mandatory. For those partially disabled, transfer to the Veterans Reserve Corps was considered. The following letter illustrates disputes that can arise.

> On 13 Feb. 1863 I was discharged from the U.S. Hospital in New Haven on account of permanent injuries caused by wounds received at the battle of Fredericksburg, 13 December 1862 in the hand and hip which unfitted me for service in the field. On the same evening I received a notice from the Commander of the 14th Connecticut Volunteers that I was promoted to 1st Lieutenant of my own company by his Excellency the governor. Knowing my condition and that I could be of no use but rather add to the list of incompetent officers, I thought best to take the advice of my attending surgeon and declined the position that the place might be filled immediately. This I did but my letter was either mislaid or discarded. I was ordered 1 March to report to the regiment without delay. I replied that my injuries were such as to oblige me to not report. I trust this explanation will be satisfactory to you and at headquarters and that nothing detrimental to me either as a soldier, officer, or citizen will arise from it.
>
> Edmond A Fox
> Late orderly sergeant Company I, 14th Connecticut Volunteers.[34]

He was twenty-one years old at the Battle of Fredericksburg in December 1862 when a gunshot wound of the right index, middle and ring fingers resulted in stiff, painful digits, making him unable to fire a weapon. His medical discharge was signed by Dr. Jewett on February 14, 1863. Fox received a pension for many years and ended up with fingers "exquisitely sensitive, tingles to touch on pressure like an exposed nerve. They are worse than asleep."

An anguished parent leaves no stone unturned to save his or her child. In October 1864, Jeremiah Tifft of Hamden, Connecticut, wrote three letters to the medical authorities about his beloved son and why he should be discharged. They apparently agreed, complying with the father's request a few weeks later.

> My son was enticed from his home and *drugged* and brought to first Rhode Island and then to Massachusetts. He was made to enlist in the Second Regiment Connecticut Artillery and they robbed him of a large amount of bounty money. He is not able bodied, nor fit to be a soldier from the fact of his being in habit of having fits from his childhood up to the present time. He is sure to have more fits when any excitement around him. He has lost part of his teeth and has sore jaws and tonsils in his throat and cannot masticate hard food. Also he has a weak leg, he is of unstable mind and a *perfect coward* and is simple in many things as a child and that he is incapable of supporting himself. To the above and I solemnly swear, so help me God. His mother is nearly insane and wishes to see him (she is 150 miles away). I have no doubt his mother would become immediately a raving maniac if he should have to go. My son has not the judgment enough to know what ails him and never has had the sense enough to support himself as a jeweler at 22 years of age. May he be immediately discharged?[35]

Invoking another medical opinion about a son's total incapacity to serve, Mr. T. E. Doolittle predicted catastrophe if his partner's son was mustered in.

> Mr. Weaver has been drafted from Hamden and I have no doubt but that he is absolutely incapable of labor. He has suffered from severe stroke and Dr. Lues has told this boy that any labor would probably produce certain death. He is too ambitious and has suffered several relapses from attempting to work. You should give him a chance like he got one from Dr. Trues who told him before he went away that if he was drafted he would give him a certificate that would discharge him at once, as he can neither read, write or labor.
>
> P.S. He is definitely over thirty-five.[36]

War does have its moments of honor and glory when men can achieve that which they could not in civil society. Of course, there is a seamier side as well, and not all men in blue were noble or patriotic. The newly inducted soldiers of Connecticut — volunteers, substitutes, and drafted men — were at Camp Rendezvous in New Haven. The substitutes were "men of almost every nation under heaven." A newspaper article entitled "Stampede at Rendezvous" described the attempted escape at dusk of 100 recruits who tried to rush and scale fences guarded by two men. An editorial in the *Knight Hospital Record* pointed out, "The men who were mostly recruits threw away their knapsacks and overcoats. Two men were wounded one in the chest. If the officers in command would make a severe and summary example of a few of the deserters, we think the crime would speedily go out of fashion." Two of the officers were incapacitated by inebriation. Little wonder the inmates decided to leave the asylum.

Casualties from the southern battlefields were appalling enough. Connecticut soldiers being killed by Connecticut soldiers added another wicked ingredient to this deadly brew called civil war. The treatment for this condition would not come from the provost but from the war's end.

CHAPTER THIRTEEN

Medicine and Politics

By the spring of 1864, the Union army was under the command of an aggressive westerner, a West Point graduate and uniquely successful general, Ulysses S. Grant. He won battles decisively, eliminating Confederate armies at Fort Donnellson, Tennessee, and at Vicksburg, Mississippi. Unconditional surrender was his calling card, indicating that this hard war would be finished by hard men doing whatever was required. He devised a three-pronged attack on the Army of Northern Virginia and the seemingly invincible Robert E. Lee: surround them and shut off their oxygen and lifeblood. There would be no retreat. The public and Congress were hopeful but skeptical, while Lincoln was determined and unwavering. Battlefield victories were required; no substitute would do.

The quiet courage shown by Grant was also reflected in the enlisted man. They were portrayed by the *Record* as self-reliant, durable, and able to survive deprivation in silence like a long-suffering widower. Building a lodge with an ax, he makes himself comfortable in the southern fields. Mud fills the cracks of his living quarters formed with white pine logs and its branches providing protection from wind, rain, and snow. He warms himself with a chimney built of sticks and mud. The window space is covered by a piece of tent, and hinges are placed on the door. This is the abode of he who will be asked to make the ultimate sacrifice.

The reason for continual prolongation of the war, according to the *Record*, was "overestimated strength of the Union army and underestimated Confederate army." Lincoln had not won a majority vote in 1860 and faced a difficult reelection in the fall of 1864. He and his supporters realized that every vote would count and that soldiers favored their commander-in-chief. Defeat on the battlefield or even a poorly timed setback could eliminate hopes for the November election. The persistent and increasing numbers of sick and wounded were fuel for the opposition. The Democrats underscored this with a peace alternative: end the conflict and leave the Confederacy in place. This was a rich man's war being fought by the poor. The vital interests of the North were at risk from a debilitating and catastrophic war, and not from the institution of slavery or the Confederacy. Benjamin Franklin's argument that there was never a bad peace or a good war made sense. The choice became McClellan and division or Lincoln and union.

The soldiers' sentiment was to finish the job so that their efforts and suffering would not be in vain. Early in the war, field conditions and hospital care was wanting, as described by a soldier in the Sixteenth Connecticut Volunteer Regiment. His letter was published in the *Hartford Daily Times*, on December 9, 1862.

Suffering Soldiers — anonymous letter.

Our brave Connecticut soldiers are suffering greatly, sadly neglected. Our wants are uncared for. Regiment was rushed off to start, poorly organized and equipped. Most of the soldiers were ignorant of muskets. In Washington, we were turned out like animals with no shelter, no food for two days, and then sent to fight with veterans at Antietam. Now troops are in graveyards and hospitals. We are dirty, ragged, shoeless, with no knapsacks, and lousy. No wonder our hospitals are full. Greatest wonder is that we are not all dead.

Do we have a Governor?

Criticism of health care delivery was not always fact-based but often reflected political or financial interests. The *Hartford Courant* ran an editorial on July 8, 1863, about Knight U.S. Army General Hospital in answer to remarks from correspondent "W."

Why is it soldiers are kept in the hospital at New Haven and other hospitals when they are able to return to their regiments? Had the persons in charge of the hospital rather have the pay kept for such soldiers than to return them fit for duty?

Why is it when a soldier is sick or wounded and wishes a furlough to go home and will bear his own expense his people being willing to take care of him that he is not allowed to go?

Editorial Comment. The correspondent claimed no less than 100 men in the New Haven hospital who are able to return to their regiments. We cannot explain the reasons why Dr. Jewett does not arrange for their return. The same is true of other hospitals. Men are kept in positions there that ought to be in the field. The acting adjutant, the ward master, the surgeons orderly and soldiers holding other positions are strong robust fellows and could better serve their country before the enemy than hanging upon the skirts of a hospital. The position they hold should be filled by soldiers who are unable from debility or disability in consequence of wounds. We believe Dr. Jewett if he will move on the matter, can muster from his wards over 100 men which nation-wide is 25,000 more men to the front. Men who are able should go back and not be kept at nursing and other duties of a menial character. The Knight Hospital is one of the best conducted in the country and the remarks above may not be applicable to its Surgeon in Charge for he has to be governed by the orders of those above him.

Armies cannot allow soldiers to write their own furlough. That civilians should not practice medicine was equally obvious. Editorialists and peace party partisans could not determine who was medically fit for duty. Both Jewett and the governor promulgated policies whose goal was full occupancy for this hospital. That was how the bills would be paid.

Sending sick and wounded soldiers home to vote was a bipartisan event. Colonel Almy, the agent in New York City, wrote a letter to the governor marked "Private" in March 1864 just prior to the gubernatorial race. All patients in Baltimore and Annapolis hospitals or invalid corps of any state were furloughed home until April 7. The entire Eighteenth Regiment and all clerks were furloughed. This came to over 2,000 voters. "If there are any doubtful towns where a few votes from those regiments will secure our representations I can probably obtain them. Secretary Stanton has advised 'I do not care to know the particulars, but just tell me what I can do for you and it shall be done.'"[1]

Colonel Almy had a different explanation for the public concerning transfers home. His opinion was published on March 23, 1864, in the *Palladium*.

All Connecticut Soldiers are to be transferred to New Haven hospital as per Colonel Almy. "I know well these homes out of which two three or four go willingly to battle and to death, and how darkly the shadow rests on the hearts of many mothers, sisters, and wives with no murmur or complaint for the dead but sadly watching the destiny of the others yet living. Never have Connecticut "boys" failed to face their foe while living or died showing their backs to the enemy. Connecticut mothers should be rest assured that her son in New York or here is looked after and cared for at home and in the field by both State and National authority. Each soldier is kindly and constantly watched over.

For the election on April 1864, Governor Buckingham had some help from furloughed hometown soldiers. New Haven's regiment, the Fifteenth, was stationed in New Bern, North Carolina. Only individual companies of that regiment known to be of Republican sentiment received twenty-day furloughs and traveling money to return home and vote. Those known to harbor Copperhead sentiment were delayed or prevented from returning north altogether. Articles in the *New Haven Palladium* orchestrated some administration-friendly notes and rang the bell of "patriotism":

March 1864
General Dix ordered furloughs for hospital soldiers. At the Knight Hospital 114 furloughs were issued from a bed census of 300 men. All Connecticut men in the east are ordered transferred to Knight Hospital.

April 1864
The Fifteenth Connecticut Volunteers and Governor Buckingham.
A soldier writes, "I am left almost alone, as all of our company officers and nearly half of the company have gone home. They will vote for Buckingham who is the man for us. The right man is in the right place. I am really glad for the country's sake that Buckingham was heartily reelected. It must aggravate the Copperheads very sore at being so badly beaten. My only desire is to crush out this rebellion as effectually and easily as Connecticut Union men have in opposing and defeating rascally copperheads.

Private Charles Foote of the Fifteenth Regiment described the practice in New Bern, North Carolina, on April 1, 1864. "They have sent home voters who came from country towns to secure them. 160 voters were sent on the L.R. Spaulding to vote in Connecticut. New Haven is considered safe and no voters from here were sent home. But Wallingford, Meriden, Durham and Branford were not thought to be safe and most sent home were from there."[2]

The *Columbian Weekly Register* published a letter from an anonymous private on April 23, 1864. "About 180 of our boys went home last week to vote. Of course most of them were Republicans, for the names were sent on here from Connecticut. We were all glad they got a chance to go home but thought it a very mean trick for any party to resort to. It is outrageous for if a man's family were all dying he could not get a furlough to go home and visit them but when a party wants 180 voters, they furlough them all at one time, 150 voted for Buckingham."

Major Eli Osborne, whose father was the tax collector for New Haven, expressed his Democratic outrage from New Bern, April 3, 1864. "Have been busy due to the departure of the Republican voters. It is an outrage. We are veterans too! If needed to elect Buckingham, furloughs are available. It's 'damnable.'"[3]

Every successful politician knows how to count votes and if necessary how to procure them. Both sides practiced exclusionary politics. In May 1863 the legislature decreed that soldiers could vote without returning home, but this was ruled unconstitutional by the State Supreme Court on the grounds that absentee ballots required an amended constitution. Not to be undone, the governor issued a proclamation in September 1864 stating that any soldier drafted or volunteered "shall when absent from this state because of such service have the same right to vote in any election." He did not extend the provision for those in the regular army, and with war's end the edict expired.

The presidential election in November produced wholesale furloughs. J.L. Cooley was a clerk in the ordinance office in Washington who proclaimed in October 1864 that he did not expect to be allowed home to vote as he was a McClellan man and would vote and do what he could to elect him. He did not see how an honest man who loved his country could support "Lincoln who violated the constitution, his oath of office, and was trying to enslave the white man and free the niggers."[4]

An agent from the U.S. Sanitary Commission while visiting Brown U.S. Hospital in Louisville, Kentucky, on October 9, 1864, noted that the agent for New York "would give no paper or stamps to those who would not vote for the little McClellan."

Private John Filus, a clerk stationed in Virginia, reported in November 1864 that "only those who talked about going home to vote for Little Mac got a free pass. So far I have done my duty getting rid of men always finding fault, cursing the administration, cursing Mr. Lincoln, stylizing his supporters as nigger lovers, nigger on the brain, and black Republicanism sons of bitches. Now that I have been discharged, the copperheads crow and chuckle."

City councilman L. Thattlemen wrote to Republican headquarters in Boston on October 31, 1864, warning that their candidate was going to lose and that "every man entitled to vote in the third district should be sent home. The opposition is bringing every exertion to defeat our man. 1300 names have been added to the list, mostly opposition in that district. Need to send home those who are entitled to vote. Arrangements will be made to send home those who can vote for us."

In the presidential election of November 1864, agents in Philadelphia gave furloughs to Connecticut soldiers in hospitals. "The men are going off in large numbers. I am sending to the hospitals today to see that no one is over looked as I am sure every man is wanted," one wrote.

Governor Yates of Illinois solicited Stanton's assistance to curry his soldiers' votes. "I would like to call your attention to the importance of immediate action in granting furloughs to sick and wounded Illinois soldiers in hospitals. If an order is issued to medical officers having charge in general hospitals that the furloughs are granted immediately. It would be the means of giving them a choice of using their right of suffrage to many who would otherwise be deprived of it without just cause. Please let me know immediately what steps will be taken and if it is necessary to appoint agents to procure the names of those soldiers entitled to furlough."[5]

Governor Bradford of Maryland asked the surgeon general for the same. "There are at present in hospitals in different states a number of Maryland soldiers many of whom are voters able and anxious to return to the state and vote in the coming Presidential election. I respectfully ask that such an order be issued from the office of Surgeon General as will secure to such soldiers the ability to vote at that election."[6]

One of the furloughed soldiers deserted, continuing on to Canada with his wife to visit his mother, whom he had not seen for three years. This desertion was reported in the *Record*.

> While in Canada the mother and wife persuaded him to become a deserter. Respectable men desert often through the influence of their wives and relations at home. There are of course numberless bad men in the army who seize upon every opportunity to leave the service.[7]

Soldiers individually suggested extension of furloughs and transferring sick or wounded from out of state hospitals to "help the cause of liberty and the restoration of the union by voting for Mr. Lincoln." A letter signed "A Connecticut Soldier" pointed out that "many sick and wounded soldiers are not ready for duty for thirty to sixty days. Why not send them home to vote and recover with healthy air of New England to invigorate our fallen energies so that upon our return we could enter upon our duties in the field with better feelings. Other states are doing the same."[8] Some soldiers refused to vote at all unless permitted to go home.

Joseph Petit of the Second Connecticut Heavy Artillery spent four weeks in a hospital before requesting transfer to New Haven. "I am a poor Irishman. I voted for Lincoln unlike the very few of my own countrymen nearly all democrats as you know. Why did I go and fight for the Negro after electing old Abe?"[9] He got his wish, was promoted to lieutenant and mustered out in August 1865.

A hospital patient in Portsmouth, Rhode Island, had a similar sentiment. "We would show the copperheads and traitors that soldiers from the front think that 'Peace' on any other terms than that offered to the South is not the kind of Peace that soldiers from Petersburg Virginia want. Give us voters a chance at the coming election and we will show copperheads that although we are weak in Body we are Union at Heart."[10]

On election eve in November 1864, the provost marshal advised the governor that Connecticut soldiers dispersed across the country realized they would be "in every way greatly benefited by being transferred home and will all understand they are indebted to you for what seems to them a very great favor." The governor needed no encouragement. He wrote in November to the surgeon in charge of a general hospital near Philadelphia, "Hiram Johnson of the 21st Regiment is a patient having a flesh wound in the arm. His friends here are desirous that he should have a furlough until after the election and fear that he has been overlooked in the application of the general order granting furloughs to men in the hospital. They will appreciate anything you may be able to do to facilitate his obtaining a furlough to New Haven."[11]

With the end of spring 1864, the fighting in Virginia took up in bloody earnest. In May came the Battles of the Wilderness and Spotsylvania, followed by a brutal campaign at a town called Cold Harbor. Despite 44,000 Union casualties and 25,000 Confederate, no resolution of the war was in sight. Unlike those generals who preceded him, Grant plowed forward into the headwinds of protest and disappointment. Summer would percolate with siege warfare along the lines at Petersburg.

Medical professors and students from Yale played important roles in the delivery of health care for the local citizens as well as returning Union soldiers. The political fabric at Yale was intricately woven, painstakingly maintained and virtually impenetrable. The president of Yale L.D. Woolsey ruled this roost for thirty years, leaving his mark on the college. (Eventually an imposing commemorative statue of Woolsey was erected at its center.) Major Jewett sent a supplicating letter concerning their torn relationship and the proposal of a second medical school in New Haven. It is said that rubbing the toe of the right boot of the Woolsey statue brings good luck. We have no evidence that Jewett tried that on the living specimen.

New Haven June 20th, 1864
Rev. L. D. Woolsey D.D., L.L.D.
President Yale College,
Dear Sir,
    My respect for you personally and officially is my apology for sending you this note. I am

glad to hear from Dr. Hooker that he has explained to you some matters, in connection with the Medical Institution and me. I fully endorse all that he said to you. I entertain great respect for my old associates in the Medical Faculty; and for their good if no other consideration influenced me. I trust the Medical Institution of Yale College may prosper. I should regret doing anything to prevent its prosperity. I have no desire to again become a candidate for any chair in the Medical Faculty. My present position alone, if there were no other reasons, would prevent it. It is true at one time I should have been disposed to press my claims for The Chair of Surgery; but that time has long since passed by. I beg to assure you that I shall not object to a provision in the charter of the Surgical and Pathological Society preventing said Society from granting Diplomas or teaching any of the branches of Medical Science; or doing anything that may conflict with the Medical Institution of Yale College or any other Medical College, in this State or any of the States of the Union; or of the so called Confederate states. The idea of making a Medical College of that Society never entered the brain of one of the signers of the petition. It undoubtedly originated with someone who has procured admission to the honorable position of professor in some underhanded way, hence his suspicion with reference to others.

    Very respectfully

    Your obedient servant

    P. A. Jewett[12]

The writing of this letter was no doubt painful. Jewett acknowledges on bended knee that he would not become chief of surgery at Yale. In 1853 Dr. Knight addressed the medical school's relationships with local and state organizations like a wizard in his kingdom having waved his wand making all happy and prosperous.

> The result of this arrangement has been eminently happy; all unpleasant feeling was at once and forever allayed; the members of the Society became interested in the school; we have at all times had the benefit of their counsel and support ... and no instance of disagreement has ever arisen among the members of the board, between the School and State Society; each has regarded the other as a fellow laborer in the endeavor to promote and advance the interest of medical science.[13]

Dr. Knight believed he had chosen his replacement, Jewett, a man who lost the keys to the throne and became involved with a competing medical school. Doctor-owned and -run proprietary schools were locked in the past. Hospital-based treatment and hands-on training was the new gold standard, but two medical schools at the same military hospital were not sustainable.

The following announces the proposed new medical school to be based at the military hospital.

Prospectus

of the

"Knight" Medical School

    The undersigned, in view of the unusual advantages offered at the Knight U.S. Army General Hospital for clinical instruction, have decided to open a private Medical School, and in connection with the two daily recitations to study disease at the bed-side.

    We cannot conceive a surer and more rapid manner for the student to become thoroughly acquainted with the profession, associating intimately, as he must, the Principles with the Practice of Medicine.

    In connection with the above the various Post Mortem examinations and surgical operations will be conducted under the direction of the teachers; thus affording to the pupil the advantage of viewing disease from its outset, through its several stages, and in all its Pathological characteristics.

    Buildings are in process of erection for the additional accommodation of 500 patients making in the aggregate 1,000 beds.

The summer course will commence February 15 and conclude July 15, with a vacation of two weeks in the month of May.

Students will have free access to the Wards at all times.

Terms — $40.00 for the Course payable in advance.

Lectures on Military Surgery will be given during the Course by the Surgeon in Charge.

Instructors

W. B. Casey, M.D.	Theory and Practice of Medicine and Obstetrics
L. D. Wilcoxson, M.D.	Materia Medica
T. B. Townsend, M.D.	Principles and Practice of Surgery
T. H. Bishop, M.D.	Anatomy and Physiology
L. D. Wilcoxson	Secretary

TEXT BOOKS	For Recitation	For Reference
Surgery	Druitt	Gross, Erickson
Medicine	Watson	Wood, Bennett
Materia Medica	Beck	Pereira — U.S. Dispensatory
Anatomy	Wilson	Gray, Sharpey, Quain
Obstetrics	Tyler Smith	Ramsbotham, Bedford[14]

The lecturer for military surgery — the "Surgeon in Charge" — was Pliny A. Jewett. He concedes that only the Connecticut Medical Society in conjunction with Yale College could issue diplomas. But what if this new federal institution was not bound by local rules but by Washington's? The Knight U.S. Army General Hospital served perfectly as a hands-on teaching facility offering medical and surgical conditions not seen in a civilian hospital. The lecturer on surgery was to be Jewett's thirty-year-old former junior partner, T. B. Townsend. The others were in private practice and on the staff at Knight U.S. Army General Hospital.

The founders of this new medical school might have considered first defeating the Confederacy before taking on the bulldogs of Yale. The medical school prospectus was a declaration of war on Yale with the winner in no doubt. Yale was to New Haven what the Vatican is to Rome. The long knives would be out in retribution for this original sin and hospital antagonism against the Democratic Party and those supporting its presidential candidate, General George McClellan.

Dr. Francis Bacon was appointed the new chief of surgery at Yale in September 1864. He graduated had from Yale Medical School in 1853 and served as assistant surgeon for eight years, suffering exposure to yellow fever epidemics while stationed in Galveston, Texas. He enlisted in the Second Connecticut Volunteer Regiment and served at the battle of Bull Run. He became brigade surgeon in July 1862 and was recommended by General Foster to the secretary of war for promotion: "He is in every respect most deserving, his moral and professional character is all that can be wished and his zeal and devotion to the service is most honorable. I commend him to your most favorable consideration."[15]

Bacon was placed in charge of the U.S. General Hospital at Harpers Ferry, Virginia, with orders to "break up the hospital without delay" in August 1862. The hospital surgeon was relieved of command. "I have this date taken charge of this hospital. The imperfect state of the hospital books rendered the earlier execution of the necessary receipts impossible." Major Bacon became the medical director for General Casey's division in Washington in August 1862, serving through May 1863 when he assumed the same position for Major General Banks in the Department of the Gulf. He was placed in charge of St. Louis U.S. General Hospital in New Orleans, Louisiana, in June 1863, serving until March 1864, and was president of the board of examiners for surgeons and assistant surgeons for the Gulf department.[16] He had just passed the medical boards himself in July 1862. His treatment for secondary wound hemorrhage stressed direct pressure rather than exploration in a swollen and perhaps infected wound and the benefits of getting a consultation when any doubt arose, a conservative and correct response typical of his demeanor.

In July 1864 he applied for a twenty-day leave of absence, claiming he had "private business of the greatest importance urgently requiring my personal attention necessitating my asking this favor. I may add that during the whole term of my military service beginning in April 1861 I have neither asked nor received any indulgence of the kind." He left for Washington and resigned in August 1864. The following month he began his new job as chief of surgery at Yale College, having been unanimously elected to fill Knight's position. The vote included six physicians of the Connecticut State Medical Society (C.S.M.S.) and the Corporation of Yale.

He seemed the ideal candidate with his extensive military and especially hospital experience. If the current chief at Knight U.S. Army General Hospital needed replacement, they were ready. He was professor of surgery from 1864 to 1877. He resigned in 1881 and began receiving his army pension the following year. He published nothing, was described as having "inflexible honesty," and lived to a ripe old age, but was unnoticed by the new generation of surgeons.[17] The better man did not get the job, and the consequences adversely affected all parties involved.

On July 7, 1864, New Haven's Fifteenth Connecticut Volunteers marched from New Bern to Kinston in effort to cut off the railroad, but ran into a guerrilla force, sustaining a few casualties. New Haven's sons and husbands often appeared in print in the local newspapers. Being listed as a casualty was one way. Another was letters describing living conditions, food quality, health care and officer efficiency. "We suffered terribly on account of the heat, want of water and blistered feet," reported one private. The *Hartford Times* editorialized in November 1864 on the wisdom and honor of continuing the war:

> War patriotism, what is it? If it had been made a rule from the beginning to send every man to the field that declared him in favor of the war, and no other, no state in the Union would have furnished a single regiment. If it had been made the rule to divide the cost of the war among those who urged its prosecution, not one man in one thousand would open his lips to speak of war but to advice [sic] against it. If all the leaks in the treasury and avenues to illegitimate profit were this day closed up, the mouths of nine tenths of the war patriots of this country would be shut up at the same time.

Certain to agree was William Bigelow of the Seventh Connecticut Volunteers. He wrote home in November 1863, "I do not believe there is enough patriotism left in this regiment to keep a mouse alive." He was captured in Charleston five months later and died in Andersonville in April 1864.[18]

The chicken hawks and antiwar opposition were outraged by a list of two hundred newspapers muzzled by Lincoln. The editors were arrested and sometimes imprisoned, their papers suppressed, their offices mobbed by hooligans, and their equipment destroyed. The writ of habeas corpus and freedom of the press supposedly guaranteed in the Constitution was suspended. All these newspapers were of the "conservative" bent, according to the *Hartford Times*, which on September 18, 1864, published the names of those drafted. Eighty-two out of 310 seemed destined to serve from Hartford County. On October 1, 1864, the *Times* published a list of Connecticut soldiers who were patients in New York City hospitals. There were 295 names in all, a list covering most of the front page and part of a second.

On September 21, 1864, the *Times* announced the arrival at Knight hospital of the steamer *Cosmopolitan*. The cargo consisted of 150 sick and wounded Connecticut soldiers, mostly from the Seventeenth and Twenty-ninth Volunteers. The patients' names were listed along with some diagnoses. There were seven cases of chronic rheumatism, two of chronic diarrhea, two of syphilis, one each of fractured femur, inflammation of the liver, inflammation of the tonsils, acute diarrhea, jaundice, consumption, typhoid malignant fever, acute dysentery, dropsy, and anemia. Here was a partial list of what the draftee could look forward to! One could contemplate the odds of winding up an inpatient or corpse.

The West Haven Fair, one of many run by the U.S. Sanitary Commission, raised $1,000 as Connecticut's civilian population mobilized to help the war effort. Exhibits included Indian life in a wigwam with arches made of colorful flower bouquets, the nursery rhyme's lady in the shoe with her many children, a fishpond, fortune-tellers, old folks at home with a most bountiful table, black Aunt Jemima and attendants sitting around a spinning wheel serenaded by singing men and women. Refreshments, kisses from young ladies, knick-knacks, and other souvenirs were offered for sale.[19]

A cautionary tale had just been told in the nation's capital. In August 1864 the thirty-five-year-old Surgeon General William Hammond was found guilty in a court-martial and ordered "dismissed from the service and to be forever disqualified from holding any office of profit or trust under the Government of the United States."[20] The charges were purchasing poor-quality blankets, favoring a drug company that supplied inferior products, removing a medical purveyor from office illegally and the unlawful purchase of medical and general hospital equipment also of poor quality. His real crime was firing corrupt politically appointed contractors and replacing them with honest and knowledgeable individuals.[21]

Hammond had removed calomel from the drug tables, having seen firsthand the severe side effects of gangrene of the face and other complications. He weighed the limited benefits with known toxicity of medications considered a mainstay of traditional American therapeutics. Some resented the implication that they did not know their craft by using such harmful agents. Opposition to his order was spearheaded by the American Medical Association in a scathing letter to Secretary of War Stanton on August 7, 1863. They described the removal of calomel and tartar emetic (antimony) as "maniacal and unnecessary," and "an indignity to the military surgeon while it is in direct opposition of the opinions of the regular profession of medicine." In addition, they wrote, it "implies a lack of confidence in those skills as a body," "is unjustifiable," and is "impolitic and prejudicial to the interests of the service." The better approach was to hold "each surgeon individually responsible for the proper discharge of his appropriate duties."

Hammond required army surgeons to pass written and oral exams. This was fully supported by the Sanitary Commission's report on surgeons. Senior doctors worried about passing exams on the latest in book learning and viewed this as yet another challenge to their competency. As a response to political pressures, some were passed in spite of their exam results on the basis that experience will likely produce good judgment and on the insistence of Secretary of War Stanton.

Of greater importance was Hammond's perceived failure to support the Lincoln administration and give wholehearted support to a government under siege. Evacuation of the wounded often took several days. Hammond's public statements indicated that had he warned Secretary Stanton of the need for an independent ambulance system but was denied because of lack of money and support by regular army officers. Henry Bowditch, a prominent medical professor of Harvard, lost his son at a skirmish in Virginia and leveled charges of incompetence about an ambulance system without dedicated drivers or nurses which was under the command of the quartermaster corps rather than the medical department. His son, a lieutenant, was shot in the abdomen and found by chance a day later. He had received no care or attention whatsoever.[22] Arguments softening the blow and defending the administration could have been made to assuage the grieving father. Intestinal wounds were 100 percent fatal because there was no bowel surgery. There were not enough ambulances in the entire world to evacuate in a timely fashion the enormous numbers of casualties occurring in so many battles. Given the circumstances, they had done their best. Instead, Hammond was critical of the administration and indirectly of Stanton, who was blamed in the press for the lack of an effective evacuation system. Hammond was right medically and logistically but not politically, and in Washington, the only business is politics.

Another example of political naïveté was his reply denying Governor Buckingham's request in July 1862 to transfer home patients of his state:

> In reply to your communication to the secretary of war asking transfer of sick Connecticut troops to New Haven. In the opinion of this office great confusion and inconvenience to the service together with much suffering to the sick and wounded result from the unnecessary transfer of sick and wounded from the hospitals to which originally sent and in some instances even the deaths of men so transferred has resulted. Inasmuch as no exceptions could be made without seeming invidious, the general rule has been adopted by this department of sanction no transfers that cannot be shown directly to benefit the public service.[23]

The governor repeated this request in May 1863 to the newly appointed Surgeon General Barnes. "Could you make an adjustment in the transfer of the sick and wounded soldiers of our regiments to recuperate in their home state? The transfer to home surroundings would be of great benefit for the troops and would cause great gratification in the people of the state." The immediate reply was, "The surgeon general directs me to acknowledge the receipt of your communication of the 20th relating to the transfer of sick Connecticut soldiers in South Carolina to northern hospitals and to inform you that orders will be at once issued on the subject in conformity with your request."[24]

Doctor Hammond's crime was political, and so was his trial. His chief supporters, the McClellans' and Democratic Party, were out of power or intimidated. He was offered a quiet release out of Washington with pension intact but he refused, demanding complete exoneration, which required an open trial and court-martial. Secretary Stanton handpicked his jury. None of the judges were from the medical corps, a clear violation of regulations. A reporter cautioned one judge during lunch not to have extra beers that might cause him to sleep through the proceedings. The judge remarked, "asleep or not, it matters not as we are going to find him guilty." The charges were false, and the witnesses against Hammond were crooked contractors or outright incompetents whom Hammond had fired or testified against previously. The trial started on January 30, 1864, and lasted four months.[25] He published at his own expense a sixty-one-page booklet explaining the charges and his innocence. He was found guilty in August 1864 and departed for New York City disgraced, nearly bankrupt from legal fees, and without a pension.

Another changing of the guard occurred in New Haven with the resignation of Dr. Knight on May 28, 1864, ending a fifty-one-year career. He died on August 25, prompting Major Jewett to issue Special order No. 137 the next day from the Knight hospital.

> In addition to his exalted reputation as a Physician and Surgeon, Dr. Knight stood pre-eminent for urbanity of manners, genial social qualities, and that great moral excellence which adorns the Christian gentleman. He has left behind a character worthy the emulation of his brethren in the profession. As a tribute to his memory the Officers of this Hospital will attend his

funeral in a body, and wear the usual badge of mourning for thirty days. The Flag will be displayed at half-mast until Sunday evening, the 28th.[26]

This was front-page news for the *Register*, which declared on September 3, 1864, the death of "one of our great men, a pre-eminent practitioner especially in surgery, in acuteness, accuracy and breadth of his observations, and in judiciousness of his practices. He was a counselor in cases of difficulty, luminous, impressive and honest, teaching for fifty years."

The people of New Haven had other bad news to digest. Their own Fifteenth Connecticut Volunteer Regiment stationed in New Bern, North Carolina, was struck by a yellow fever epidemic, leaving many dead and a massive quarantine closing off the area to commerce and travel. A summary of the event was printed in the *Palladium* on October 28, 1864:

> The disease started early September. Early cases were listed as "congested chills." Cases sprung up all over town. Panic seized all the inhabitants of this town as the disease hit merchants, soldiers, civilians and government clerks indiscriminately. All who could leave have done so and with haste. Due to the rapid spread of this disease in the regiment, they were replaced by Negro troops. A black skin has proved not as susceptible to this disease as white. The disease is abating, and hospital patients are all recovering. We have had a severe frost and several cold days, something we all prayed for. The number of deaths of soldiers and civilians will probably exceed 1,200. Some of the scenes here were terrible. God has visited us with a terrible scourge. For His favor in abating the disease, we are grateful.

On November 5, the newspaper listed the names of fifty-five dead from the Fifteenth Regiment alone. The explanation for the epidemic was "the fever originated from the ship at the foot of Craven Street, New Bern, which was filled up last June by Provost Marshal Captain Bradley, with manure and barrels of rotten beef." Some southern doctors with long experience surmised that infected ships were the cause, not local sanitation deficiencies, and that quarantine for at least three weeks was essential to keep it out. The cause of "Yellow Jack," or the "Saffron Scourge," was attributed to "perfidious effluvia," or decomposing animal or vegetable matter, prompting concern over dumping garbage in stagnant water. The actual cause is a virus transmitted by mosquitoes and introduced by visiting ships.

In their Sunday prayers, some southern ministers beseeched their Eternal for a blessing in the form of yellow fever epidemic against which true southerners would have natural resistance from previous exposure and invading northerners would not. They reminded their flock that if they faithfully observed the commandments, "The Eternal will ward off from you all sickness; He will not bring upon you any of the dreadful disease of Egypt, about which you know, but will inflict them upon all your enemies" (Deuteronomy 7:15) and "God will also send a plague against them, until those who are left in hiding perish before you" (Deuteronomy 7:20).

What the "Yellow Jack" failed to kill, Confederate bullets would. The fear of this disease cannot be exaggerated, as the mortality rate sometimes exceeded fifty percent. This was the "newcomer's" or immigrant's disease that would not afflict true southerners.[27] Their protection stemmed not from superior morality or physical prowess but from immunity produced by previous contact with the same disease. Being native-born did not protect 1,200 civilians along with many Union soldiers who would fill the local cemeteries.

Death from disease, death from battle, stalemate in Virginia, more men needed in a draft, graft and corruption — these were the news items of the day. The *Register* gave illustrations of what it considered to be widespread corruption, especially in Washington:

Contractors have carried on this war. The blood of our men, the groans of our wounded, the tears of orphans, and the wail of the widower have been coined into money. They have swindled the government out of hundreds of millions. They have plied fortune on fortune. Corruption runs riot in Washington. Even senators have acknowledged taking bribes of half a hundred thousand.[28]

On the heels of the Hammond case in Washington, another medical corruption story was reported by the *Register* in mid–October 1864. The Western Sanitary Commission and its secretary Dr. J.S. Newberry were compared to "the recent arrest of another doctor and the 'irregularities.'" The commission listed a financial statement totaling $321,065 with salaries of officers at $60,721 and other exaggerated expenses, leaving only 25 percent of the monies actually going for materials sent to the soldiers. Most of the funds went to overhead and not to suffering and needy soldiers. "No reports will follow. Those getting all this money won't issue more reports for perusal of honest men. Our conclusion is that the soldier's friend will give him money or aid through another channel. Give your money to another charity."

Presidential politics in New Haven drew blood, as reported by the *Palladium* on September 9, 1864:

> The soldier, who was beaten by the Democrats at the Music Hall last evening for calling for Lincoln and Johnson cheers, was Sergeant Braman of the Rendezvous. He was severely beaten and it is since reported that he has died.

The Music Hall was near the post office in the center of town and was the place to be for concerts, demonstration meetings, operas, and minstrels. Nearly all the great actors, singers and orators appeared there. It seated 2,500 but could hold over 3,000. It was described as roomy and plain. There was poor egress in case of fire or altercations and the stairs were very narrow.

The *Register* editorial on October 1, 1864, was titled "The Hospital Soldier" and discussed unfair practices against the supporters of "Leetle George" McClellan and the Democratic Party.

> Dr. Wilcoxson, Surgeon in charge at Knight U.S. Army General Hospital said "there was *not* a double guard posted on the hospital grounds on the day of the Democratic Convention and the men were not marched to the Republican meeting." Almost all the men were denied a pass last Thursday. A few braved the guardhouse to be present. Dr. Wilcoxson refused to allow the drum corps to play for McClellan Club stating it was not allowed in a political function. It was however at the Lincoln meeting; though under orders soldiers marched behind the bands run by sergeants under orders as well. Men in the hospital ought to think as they please as to who the next commander in chief of the army should be. There are differences of opinions and a large proportion of soldiers support McClellan. Will Dr. Wilcoxson send soldiers to attend the next McClellan meeting? Soldiers have the right to hear both sides.[29]

A week later, Wilcoxson was no longer in charge, and Sergeant Michael McConnell sent a letter to the same editor:

> Those cheering for Lincoln were D. B.s At the McClellan meeting, a sharp lookout was kept. At the Lincoln meeting gates were thrown open for those who wished to remain in the hospital. Five hundred soldiers attended the Lincoln meeting and half were for McClellan who just went to have a good time. If there is any soldier with the D. B. stamp capable of contradiction of these assertions, I am happy to hear from them.

The answer came in the first issue of the *Hospital Record*:

We noticed in Saturdays *Register* a letter by a patient in this Hospital who calls himself a true soldier and says that those men that cheer for Lincoln are what he calls D. B.'s. Now, any true soldier would not call another a D. B. unless he was positive that he really was. He says that those that vote for Lincoln have left the front without cause. This we know to be a lie. He then asks the following questions:

First. How many men are there in this Hospital?

Second. How many men had the privilege of voting?

Third. Why were the gates not open on night of the McClellan demonstration?

For the first he shall find out himself. For the second, all had the privilege of voting. For the third, no person asked to have gates opened, and that more passes were given out that day than generally. We are not of the D. B. stamp, nor do we believe that all the soldiers that vote for Lincoln are. But we do believe that Sergeant McConnell will keep away from the front as long as he can and that all the brave and true soldiers are not to be found in the 4th U.S. Artillery.

Not to be outdone, McClellan supporters gave their own political banter and spin with these comments from the *Register* a few days later:

The *Knight Hospital Record* misrepresents the hospital and is hardly worth notice. The bad grammar and unintelligent expression so constructed are slurs on soldiers or portion of them. To go to the McClellan meeting one needs submit a list of attenders and get passed by three officials.

On October 5, 1864, the *Knight Hospital Record* trumpeted uncompromising political positions that did not reflect the views of half the Union's citizens. The *Record* was unabashedly pro–Union, pro–Lincoln, pro–Republican, and fiercely against Copperheads and other "traitors."

On October 19, 1864, a grand Union rally was held, generously supported by the Knight U.S. Army General Hospital. The gates were thrown open; armed guards stood at attention and drum and fife corps at the ready; glee clubs sang, and a team of horses was draped with the red, white and blue. The proposed parade route was outlined in the local newspapers, street by street. Vehicles and houses were covered with bunting and dried floral decorations. Veteran soldiers and hospital patients marched or were carried in carriages in the procession. There were fireworks and rousing speeches. Refreshments were served for the collective gathering, estimated at 10,000. The *Record* editorial declared,

Let every soldier that believes in closing the war, and putting down the rebellion at the point of the bayonet, join in the grand rally for Lincoln and Johnson. Let us show that the majority of the soldiers do not believe in giving up now, after so much blood has been spilled in so good a cause. It has been asserted that the soldiers will accept peace on any terms, and that the majority of them are for McClellan. Let us show today, that this assertion is not true. The soldiers want peace, but not a peace whose terms would be dictated in Richmond. Grant, Sherman, Sheridan and Farragut are the soldier's choice for Peacemakers. We speak this, knowing how the majority of the soldiers here in this Hospital feel. Let every man turn out and swell the ranks to such an extent that it will astonish the Copperheads and those men who believe in accepting peace on any terms. The old battle-flags of the different regiments will be carried by the soldiers. Then "Rally round the Flag, Boys!"

While the procession was passing up State Street, a stone was thrown by one of the McClellan brats, which struck a discharged soldier over the eye, inflicting a slight wound. A soldier, employed in this office, was struck and slightly cut on the wrist, at the same time, by a piece of iron. One of the boys was immediately arrested and locked up. A transparency carried by one of the soldiers, bore the inscription, "Bullets for our enemies in the field, and ballots for our enemies at home," and we hope there will be plenty of the latter for them on the eighth day of November. There will be not less than 100 from this Hospital in the procession. Rally, boys! For Lincoln and Johnson and show that soldiers can whip traitors at home, as well as in the field.

On October 22, 1864, the *Register* accused hospital officials of deliberately sequestering eligible hospital voters out of state. "Among soldiers sent away from Knight U.S. Army General Hospital to Massachusetts were many Connecticut voters who were perhaps sent to Readville Hospital in Massachusetts by express train, to deprive them of their voting rights." A train derailed that was transferring 400 patients from New Haven to a town in Massachusetts resulting in twelve deaths and many injuries. (See page 34). That such a disaster was fodder for the cannons of political warfare indicates the pervasiveness of bitterness and hatred.

Out of 1,000 patients and a few hundred employees, only twenty-six men went to the McClellan procession, held in the evening. "The gates were thrown open and all who wished to go went," claimed the *Record*. This was disputed by the Democrats, who once again charged the hospital with unfair practices. When Lincoln rallies were held, the gates were left wide open, military bands played patriotic popular songs, torchlights for the procession into town were provided, armed guards kept the peace, and no formal permits seemed required. The McClellan forces claimed that just the opposite rules applied to them. The gates were closed, and special permits were required to get them open. No musicians were available, and the procession proceeded in pitch darkness. Guards were accused of accosting rather than protecting the demonstrators, as were other citizens not wearing uniforms. According to the *Record*, this was not the case.

The *Record* asked, "Can you tell the difference between a copperhead and a rebel?" One week before the election, their editorial warned of "domestic traitors and foreign enemies," the "so-called peace party of McClellan," "armed murderers and incendiaries," and "most stupendous frauds." They were not describing marauding rebel army units or the violence of pro-slavery militia. They were describing the Democratic Party. The epithet "traitors now in arms" applied to both Confederate rebels and fellow northerners. This sentiment was reflected in Governor Buckingham's response to congratulations on reelection from Secretary Stanton: "The copperheads have sunk into their holes and hiding places and I only hope that whenever they make their appearance again they will receive the indignation and contempt which treason merits." The country was divided and each state was divided with no middle ground for compromise after four long years. Those who disregarded this sentiment did so at their own peril.

Lincoln was described in glowing terms: "God Bless our Noble President, an honest upright man, for he will put rebellion down, deny it ye who can." On the wards were large pictures of Lincoln and the favorite General Grant. Signs proclaiming "the Union forever" and "Ward 2 will never surrender" were appropriately dressed with garlands, wreaths, and decorations made by patients and family members.

On October 16, 1864, Governor Seymour, the New York Democratic gubernatorial candidate for reelection, claimed, "After the election Lincoln will ask for another draft." In New Haven, the *Register* on October 18, 1864, prophesied endless drafts and longer enlistments.

How Many More Years of War!
"Four more years" says Lincoln.
"20 more years" says Butler.
"30 more years" says New York Times.
"An interminable conflict" says Thurlow Weed.

"The war is a permanent institution" says Jim Lane, and then will follow drafts and drafts and drafts. What say the people?

The birds of this flock were all lined up on the same tree, singing the same song at the same time. The *Hartford Times* proclaimed "Estimate next draft at 500,000." Two weeks before, the same newspaper had estimated a draft of 300,000. There would be not one- or two- but three-year terms of enlistment, this time with no substitutes permitted. On November 2, 1864, a headline read:

A Wholesale Draft Coming!
A peremptory draft without power of substitution
More men and more conscripts.

A poll taken in the hospital wards in New Haven showed Lincoln with two-to-one edge. The First Connecticut Artillery called the "McClellan Regiment" voted Lincoln 260, McClellan 226, and doubtful 2. In Pennsylvania, the official soldier vote was 68 percent for Lincoln and 32 percent for McClellan. The army of the Potomac and the army of the James voted two to one in favor of Lincoln. Sheridan's army voted three to one and Sherman's four to one. A newspaper account of a visit to the Armory Square Hospital was indicative.

And how the boys would rally if we told them "Uncle Abraham" was coming. He would go down one side of the ward and up the other shaking hands with every one and speaking a kind word. I have often seen the tears roll down his care worn cheeks while he was talking with some wounded soldier.

Provost Marshal Colonel Sewall placed an ad in the *Register* October 26, 1864, entitled "To soldiers at home or on furlough." He extended furloughs of all soldiers who could vote in the presidential elections. The *Record* ran its own poll in October to determine the popularity of the Lincoln administration among its many patients (see Table 4).

TABLE 4. THE *KNIGHT HOSPITAL RECORD* PRESIDENTIAL ELECTION POLL

Ward	Lincoln	McClellan	Doubtful
1	58	8	
2	64	26	
3	35	7	
4	38	26	
5	30	17	
6	43	38	
7	49	27	
8	32	11	18
9	61	30	
WARD TOTALS	410	190	18
Duty Men	55	8	
One hundred fifty-ninth, Veterans Reserve Corps	50	4	
TOTALS	515	202	18

On November 4, a grand torchlight procession was held in Hartford from 7 P.M. to 4:30 A.M. Trains arrived overflowing with Lincoln supporters, along with hundreds of horsemen and thousands of torches and displays such as "One government, one flag, one Union, now and forever," and "Our hearts are with you." There were tricolor banners, flags and wreaths on every building, post and factory with portraits of generals, naval officers and President Lincoln in the windows of every house, hotel, shop, and office.

Military and civilian bands, soldiers of all ranks, glee clubs, and carriages marched in a blaze of glory illuminated by torches, Chinese lanterns, and fireworks before candlelit homes and businesses. The posters and illuminations were new and old in the largest political demonstration in state's history. "Hurrah for Abe and Andy," "We trust in God, Grant and Gunpowder," "The secession will soon go Down," "Little Mac is Ready to Surrender," "Undivided devotion to our adopted Country," "When Men are men and all are free, then will our country peaceful be," "Our Brave Volunteers: the Country must reward them," "No middle ground; you are for this Government or Jeff," "Fear God and Hate Snakes," "The War a Failure? No, Sir!" "No compromise with traitors," a soldier putting a bayonet through a copperhead snake with the motto "There is a band of Copperhead snakes," "Shenandoah Harvest — reaped by Early, threshed by Sheridan," "Our way to peace — crush the rebels," "Be men and fight it out — Sherman," "This rebellion is tottering, Phil Sheridan — God bless him!," "Keep your Eye on the Flag boys," "A true democrat is a loyal patriot," "To stop the war — whip the rebels," "Hope of the rebels — a divided North," "Our peace Commissioners — Grant, Sherman, Sheridan, Butler, Farragut," "Our country — those who don't like it may move out," "The left wing of Lee's Army — the copperheads," "It won't do to swap horses now," "Victory with us is Peace," "Our cause is just: In God is our trust," "Abe is able to save the Union."[30]

Just weeks prior to the presidential election, prompted by an anonymous letter, a War Department official from Washington visited the Knight U.S. Army General Hospital. Based on this investigation by one man lasting a few hours, Chief of Staff Pliny Adams Jewett and Chief Hospital Steward Leicester Carrington were arrested and transferred to Governors Island prison in New York. The only account of this episode came from the *Register* (a Democratic Party newspaper). The charges were "keeping sick soldiers longer than was necessary in that hospital, and charging at the same time the daily allowance for their care and board." The paper went on to say that "irregularities" in Knight hospital had attracted the notice of the department in Washington. A special agent was sent who, after a single day's investigation at the hospital, found the irregularities so flagrant that the two men were immediately arrested and sent to prison. The notion that "disaffected and disappointed persons had caused the arrest to be made is all moonshine," quoted the news source.[31]

The arrest was not mentioned in the *Palladium* (a Republican Party newspaper) until a month later, when Jewett was returned to duty. He was released within the week of arrest "pending a court martial" and allowed a visit to New York City with General Dix, who was the commander in charge of the Department of the East. Dix was well informed about Knight U.S. Army General Hospital. In the spring he had ordered furloughs for 114 patients out of 300 patients, allowing them to vote for governor. On November 2, 1864, he ordered the clerks to work double overtime, ordering 500 furloughs for patients to be sent home to vote for the right candidate.

On November 5, 1864, just in time for the election, the *Palladium* triumphantly published an order from the Adjutant General's Office of the War Department in Washington that had been sent to Major General Dix. A week later the *Hartford Daily Courant* published the same item.

Sir: The Secretary of War directs in accordance with your recommendation of the fourth, that Surgeon P. A. Jewett formerly in charge of the Knight Hospital at New Haven be restored to his position.

Both newspapers left out the final sentence of this letter, which cautioned that the order was "subject to a trial and when the interests of the service will permit." This admonition was repeated on the cover envelope of the report, emphasizing the contingency of Jewett's reinstatement in case it was missed the first time: "He still is subject to trial, when the interests of the service render it necessary."[32]

In confirmation of this decision, surgeon William Sloan, medical director of the Department of the East, located on Bleecker Street in New York City, wrote on November 9, 1864:

In accordance with instructions from the Secretary of War, Surgeon P. A. Jewett U.S. Volunteers is restored to his position, subject to trial, and is assigned to duty as Surgeon in charge of Knight General Hospital, New Haven Ct. and will relieve Surgeon G. O'Leary U.S. Volunteers.[33]

Dr. Jewett confirmed his return to duty to Surgeon General Barnes on November 30, 1864, on stationery engraved "Knight General Hospital, New Haven Connecticut."

I have the honor to report that I am on duty as surgeon in charge of this Hospital and acting under special orders dated A.G.O. Washington D.C. Nov 5th, 1864.
   Very respectfully
   Your obedient servant
   P. A. Jewett
   Surgeon U.S. Volunteers[34]

After two months' imprisonment, hospital steward Carrington was released from Fort Columbus in New York Harbor, one day before Christmas. General Dix restored him to full duty as chief steward at Knight hospital since according to the *Record,* "upon investigation ... the charges against him were false and malicious."

After just a few hours of investigation, what evidence could have been discovered that justified the arrest of a Yale professor, a distinguished surgeon and head of a thousand-bed hospital? The federal government penned the contract, paying $3.50 per patient per week. Maintaining full occupancy was an economic necessity and was obsessively promoted by the governor. Stanton intervened likely due to his requests. The presidential election was just a couple of weeks away. With the arrest of Jewett, the decks were being cleared for a possible new administration at the army hospital and in Washington.

Lincoln certainly got Major Jewett's vote. He escaped the ignominy and financial drain that Surgeon General Hammond had endured. There was no court-martial and thus no formal written statement as to charges made or evidence submitted. Those favoring prosecution would continue to lurk in the dark, knives at the ready to slash with the same charge no matter how false and unfair that might be. For hospital patient Joseph Vail of the Eighth Connecticut Volunteers, the episode was over. Railway ties were placed in the center of the kitchen to facilitate movement of food to the eating areas.

I arrived Saturday evening. Most of the boys were out, as usual. Dr. Jewett came back. He has been at work on improvements in great earnest. I cannot tell you what he has done, for I had not the time. He is now building a railroad from the kitchen towards pavilion one and two for conveyance of diet for those unable to leave their beds.[35]

A headline in the *Hospital Record* hailed Jewett's resurrection:

Return of Major P. A. Jewett

Major Jewett arrived here this morning and immediately took charge of the Hospital. The news of his arrival spread through the Hospital like wild fire, and a crowd soon collected in front of the Office and gave him three rousing cheers. The boys feel that no better surgeons could be appointed to take care of sick and wounded soldiers than any at present in this Hospital; and we say welcome to the old Commander of Knight General Hospital.

The effects of his arrest would linger, as so-called irregularities were intimated by the Copperheads of New Haven. The *Register* displayed sour grapes after the election in this "anonymous" letter to the editor.

Political influences were brought to bear in the Presidential campaign and arguments made by some of the Doctors friends to have him reinstated without examination or trial was well known. But no steps were taken by the friends of the sick and disabled soldiers to counteract them as they deem it an affair of the department and not of our citizens, not one of who would willingly pluck a single leaf from the laurel that encircles the brow of the worthy Major. May we inquire of the courier what has become of the doctors worthy associate, who was arrested with him and whether he too has been whitewashed and honorably reinstated. A Citizen.

The storm clouds lifted and a ray of sunshine broke through with the fall of Atlanta, a prize for President Lincoln brought about by General William Tecumseh Sherman: "Atlanta is ours, and fairly won." The people then spoke, giving Lincoln a second term of office. He was elected without a majority in 1860 and would win reelection four years later by a hair's breadth. Out of 85,443 votes cast in Connecticut, Lincoln's majority was 2,427. He carried Hartford County with its 17,300 voters by only 9 votes. He lost in New Haven with its 18,155 voters by 921 votes. McClellan, the little general who won no major battles as a soldier, was good enough for the citizens of New Haven County, a Democratic Party locality in perpetuity.

On October 23, 1864, Lincoln proclaimed a day of national thanksgiving, for the last Thursday of November. This would be a day for family, community, and nation to unite in prayer and feast. Knight's hospital fund was used to finance a gala affair on Thanksgiving Day as reported in the *Record*.

Many passes were given to visit friends and family, while the larger portion preferred to remain here. At 3 P.M., the drum sounded dinner call. Men marched to the dining room where a splendid dinner [was] prepared for them. Major Jewett made a few remarks, telling them to eat all that was on the tables, and if they wanted more to call for it. With three cheers for the Major they charged the works like veterans and in a few minutes almost everything had disappeared. Everybody was satisfied. The articles received from citizens were thankfully received.

Dr. Jewett issued formal thanks. The source of funding and other financial transactions would be transparent and meet all army regulations.

In behalf of the "Sick and Wounded soldiers," I would thank those citizens who contributed articles for a dinner on Thanksgiving Day. Arrangements have been made with the Commissary to purchase all necessary articles for a good dinner from the Hospital Fund.

They consumed 100 turkeys, 100 chickens, fifty geese, 800 pies, two and a half bushels of cranberries; 125 bunches of celery, two bushels of apples, twelve sides of spare ribs, forty puddings, and one barrel of cider. For Christmas the Hospital fund provided yet another "splendid dinner" for the troops. There were 594 pounds of turkey and geese, 160 pounds of chickens, two bushels of apples and 200 pies served, among other delicacies. A banquet with the best of food and drink soothes the most savage, and pays appropriate tribute to those who suffered most from the bitter diet of the past four years. Men could swap stories, feel good about them, and amiably chart the future while burying animosities and petty disputes.

The evening entertainment was a concert by the hospital choir and band. "The Post Band brought smiles on all. Only the appearance of the paymaster would complete their happiness." The band's primary purpose was to play at sporting and social events and offer general entertainment. On solemn occasions, the band played the *Dead March* while guards kept time to the music. A separate fife and drum corps played at military functions such as parades and formations. On the battlefield, musicians served as stretcher-bearers, as did other noncombat personnel. The importance of the bands is highlighted in an exchange of letters by Major Jewett and an off-post officer, D. D. Perkins, on October 1, 1863. The doctor pointed out that two of his musicians were unfit for duty and asked for replacements. He was referred to Captain Remington who emphatically promised to "make and unmake musicians in his company whenever required to improve its efficiency. The muster roll of the company will show who the musicians are at the time of muster and from what date."[36] A drummer was later transferred from a nearby post.

The Union Soldiers Glee Club was formed by six of the hospital clerks, some recuperating patients from the Invalid Corps. They gave free concerts at 8 P.M. in the gaily decorated chapel. The *Record*'s music critic gave rave reviews to the well-attended concert: "Singing and instrumental music was good. The club need not be afraid to perform before any audience, for we think they would give satisfaction anywhere." When weather permitted, they performed atop the roof of the original state hospital building, and could be heard on all the wards, which was especially appreciated by the bedridden. On a summer evening overlooking the bay, convalescing patients would be left to their own thoughts, as the popular music of the day filled the air, reflecting common personal experiences and feelings.

On December 30, 1864, a social hop was held in Smith's Hall with music provided by the Thomas Quadrille Band. Entrance into this Friday evening bash cost fifty cents. Two weeks later, a grand masquerade ball was held in Exchange Hall, this on a Thursday evening. Attendance was considerable despite the inability of the sicker and seriously wounded to attend. A brass band played as hopes of interaction with the fair sex was rekindled for these veterans.

Band concerts, solo performances, a quintet of singing clerks, and the Union Soldiers Glee Club all provided entertainment for throngs of patients, their families, and visitors, ladies and otherwise. They sang in the chapel, beautifully decorated with the Star Spangled Banner, where a "trumpet imitation by Mr. Rowe was well done and drew forth the loudest applause." The songs delivered that evening to an appreciative audience were: "O hail us ye Free," "Come where my love lies dreaming," "Wake Nicodemus," "Eight dollars a day," "Do they pray for me at home," "There's beauty everywhere," "Let me shed one silent tear," "Mother kissed me in my dream," "You don't know how we miss you dear," "Napolitaine," "Alleghenies Mountain Home," "Happy be Thy Dreams," "Zula Zong," "Keep this Bible near your heart," and "Good Night." These tunes are not household favorites today, but at the time were high on the hit parade and reflected the moods, beliefs, hopes and aspirations of their listeners.

Nicodemus is a black slave from Africa whose sole wish is to be placed in a hollow oak tree to be awakened at the Grand Jubilee as prophesied in the Bible when slaves were to be freed. He cries out, "The good time is almost here, it is a long, long day on the way." "Zula Zong" is also from black culture and represents a mythical beauty, an angel in a fairy tale, a dream of a departed love. The music and lyrics, however, were written by white men and performed by white men before mostly the same. Other songs reflect dreams of love left behind, either romantic or maternal, and whether the dreamer will be remembered alive or dead.[37] "She will watch o'er thee from the radiant skies" implies the certainty of motherly comfort even in the hereafter. "Mother kissed me in my dream" is about a young soldier who was severely wounded at Antietam lying in a hospital at Fredericksburg. A sergeant passing by his bed and seeing his boyish face light up with a peaceful smile, asked how he felt. "Oh I am happy and contented now," the soldier replied, "Last night Mother kissed me in my dream!" He did his duty, fell in the fighting, but knew no peace until the maternal kiss. "Keep the Bible near your heart" gives a mother's advice and prayers to her son on patriotism, duty, country and the ultimate sacrifice of death.

> All's well, he sleeps, the orange flowers bloom at his grave
> Sadly she weeps for him who died upon the battle field
> Her own loved soldier boy so brave
> Your country's voice is calling
> Stood forth the patriot's mothers boy
> Fatal ball came swiftly slowly he sank upon the sod

"Eight dollars a day" was written during the Mexican War and illustrates a comparative and critical point that soldier's pay was $7 a *month* while the "Washington politicians" was $8 a *day*:

> And next in order of the day comes the mad cry of war.
> While very few of the longest heads can hardly tell what's for.
> But "war exists" all parties cry and the enemy we must slay.
> So congress backs the President at $8 a day.
>
> Then the cry of war runs through the land for Volunteers to go and fight in the war for slavery on the plains of Mexico.
> $7 a month to be shot at that is the common soldier's pay while those who send the poor fellows there get $8 a day.

On January 11, 1865, the *Knight Hospital Record* began a three-part story on a patient's journey from battlefield to hospital.

> As the ship docks, the work of debarking commences, and men long associated with rough surroundings of war are suddenly brought in contact with the busy life of a city, the wonderment depicted in their countenance, is as believable as if awakening from Rip Van Winkle sleep. We are now in the Hospital that is to be our home until our wounds heal and we are again fit for service or if permanently disqualified to receive discharge and return proudly to open arms of dear ones at home. But in the meantime many, very many have received a final discharge and await the reward of all their heroism and sacrifice in another world. May it be ample.

A smallpox epidemic broke out in January 1865, and a handful of those patients were still in the hospital weeks later. The *Record* issued this report.

> As several cases of smallpox have made their appearance in this hospital, the Surgeon in charge has ordered no more visitors will be allowed on the grounds. The public need entertain no fears of its spreading; they have all been properly attended to. Every case as soon as discovered is removed to the smallpox ward.

Initial indications were that the four cases were fine: "none are dangerously sick, and all are doing well." On February 1, 1865, the first patient died. Typically, an isolation ward was a tent placed at a distance from the main hospital. This could be a tent on the other side of a river or on a boat docked downstream. For large numbers of smallpox patients, separate hospitals were temporarily erected.

Francis Bacon, who had replaced Jonathan Knight, described the facts known about smallpox in his qualifying exam for surgeon. He described it as "a general vice of the blood with the virulence of morbid poison." The size, confluence and configuration of the pustules were considered prognostic: the more lesions and the more pus the worse the outcome. Extensive lesions meant troublesome fevers. He noted that the very young and the debilitated fared the worse. Those with "extreme nervous depression or pulmonary complication" had a bad prognosis. Those who survived the initial prodromal usually survived. As for treatment, "little can be done except to correct as gently as may be disturbances of particular functions." Mild saline cathartics, opiates for restlessness and Dover's powder were best. Frequent spongings with warm water alleviated burning and uneasiness for the skin. He cautions against chilling the surface. "After eruptions apply cerate or some non-irritating unctuous substance to shield pustules from air, it is soothing to the patient and may prevent scarring." For stomach irritability he used hydrocyanic acid, and for back pain hot fomentations and local anodynes. Diet should be encouraged as failure to eat was a bad sign. "Stimulate with alcohol and camphor or carbonate of ammonia only if shows signs of depression."[38]

The *Register* of New Haven weighed in with its editorial in favor of vaccination on March 4, 1865.

> Smallpox and vaccination. What security is afforded by vaccination? To half of mankind, a single successful vaccination is absolute and perpetual protection. To another it is absolute for a time. A small number loses its power and needs revaccination. The scar of vaccination is not proof of permanent protection. A person once attacked can get a second attack. Cases are known of two or three attacks per patient. One is noted to have had seven attacks. Fifty-seven percent are liable to get it again. Forty percent have absolute protection with a scar; sixty percent are susceptible to re-infection. The vaccine is immediately effective in preventing disease. The death rate in those vaccinated is one per 330. The death rate in those with disease is one per four. Thus, there is a marked decrease in fatality. Vaccination does not endanger life, does not engender scrofulous disease, nor cause deafness or blindness. We are lost wondering why there are men carping, dissatisfied, and querulous, who insist vaccination is only the invention of doctors, by which "they kill more than they cure." [The British Parliament, as a result of his great discovery gave 53,000 pounds sterling to the general practitioner Dr. Jenner.]

On March 14, 1865, the second case occurred at Knight hospital and was dutifully reported in the *Record*: "Theodore Bradley a Private of Company H, Seventh Connecticut Volunteers died of smallpox." In a week there were only six patients on the smallpox ward, which was about to close. A month later, a "colored man was brought in having caught the disease outside the hospital. He is on the gain. Two deaths occurred from the disease owing to the excellent care and attention which they have received from the surgeon in charge of them." No additional cases occurred at the hospital. The vaccination program worked.

Smallpox was a fact of life. Vaccinations were mandated by the Union army and were generally successful. The Sanitary Commission supplied vaccines for civilians and contrabands. They noted that with cowpox vaccine, revaccination was necessary, but they downplayed any complications from the procedure. A successful vaccination was defined as redness and a vesicle on the sixth day. Fever, systemic rash, and vesicles were a possibility but of no great concern. Surgeon Hubert Vincent Holcombe reported several systemic reactions in the vaccination program which forced cancellation of his regiment's marching orders in Virginia. The Medical Department was eager to learn more about this complication and sent this inquiry. "Medical officers vaccinating soldiers, contrabands and citizens since the recent smallpox appearances should list the following: source of virus, how preserved, markings if any, comparative values of each kind, number of vaccinations performed, and results."[39]

Blacks seemed more susceptible to the disease but had the same mortality as whites, 25 percent. Dr. Page of the commission noted in 1863 in Port Royal, South Carolina, that "smallpox broke out amongst those Negroes not vaccinated giving a frightful glimpse into what might have happened without fore thought of the commission." He reported from North Carolina a similar problem among Negroes thought due to the "imperfect character of vaccine matter received in that department." The mortality rate there was 37 percent.[40]

Dr. Newberry, also of the Sanitary Commission, reported from the South that Negroes and contrabands were escaping from plantations and infiltrating Union forces, spreading this disease to those not vaccinated: "A great number of troops are suffering seriously from the effects of inoculation." George Champlin, a private in Hartford's Sixteenth Regiment, described the local false gossip claiming "one of the hospital nurses said that twenty men had died from the effects of vaccination and that was more than had died of smallpox." William Abernathy, a private from New Haven's Fifteenth Regiment, wrote about his experiences with vaccination: "I have a very sore arm where the Doctor vaccinated me which I suppose makes me invulnerable against smallpox. The boys who have it, about 70 of the 500 who were vaccinated are all complaining about it like me."[41] Local and transient systemic signs and symptoms caused by the vaccine were a very small price to pay for the consequences of getting this dread disease.

Magical cures with proprietary "medical" liniments were often touted in advertisements in journals, newspapers and minstrel shows. The *Record* noted that the British army had reported on a "cure for smallpox" discovered in its practice in China:

> The English army in China has made a great discovery in the way of effectual cure of small pox. The mode of treatment is when preceding fever is at its height and just before an eruption appears, the chest is rubbed with croton oil and tartaric ointment. This causes the whole eruption to appear on that part of the body to the relief of the rest. It secures a full and complete eruption and prevents disease from attacking internal organs. It is regarded as a perfect cure.

The poultice left a scar and was commonly used as a counter-irritant for treating a host of conditions, including pneumonia, cancer, migraine, and consumption. Private William Abernathy of the Fifteenth Connecticut Volunteers described his experience with this treatment.

22 Jan. 1863
> Went up to the surgeon again and got excused. Don't know exactly what is the matter with me only that I feel bad. The doctor covered my chest with croton oil and gave me some medicine, which made me sick all afternoon. Our tent is very wet inside and everything is damp. No wonder a man does not feel very well.

23 Jan. 1863
> My lungs or chest are covered with little blotches from the effects of croton oil. It resembles the measles. When a man makes up his mind he is going to be sick, he generally is. I have not had anything to eat for the last two days except crackers, coffee and a little pork. Hope for a box from home.

24 Jan. 1863
> My chest is a mass of blisters and is so sore it hurts me badly to stand. The doctor is sick and I don't know what I shall do for it. There has been no mail in 15 days. The doctor hasn't been able to do anything today and of course has let me go with the rest. I went to the hospital and a worker there says blisters saved me from lung fever.
> The doctor was so sick no one went up to him.[42]

During the Civil War, there were 12,000 cases of smallpox in the Union army with 4,000 deaths. Some of these failures were from ineffective vaccines. Often crusts used were dried out or otherwise useless. The South had a much less successful vaccination program, a deficiency that endured for years and was affected only with the start of World War II. Opposition to vaccination existed then as today because of ignorance, prejudice, and religious extremism. As late as 1880, eighty percent of the population of some southern states were still not vaccinated.

By March 1865 five new pavilions were whitewashed, eliminating the need for tents and greatly expanding capacity. The dispensary was remodeled and "new bottles with fine gilt labels adorned the shelves." Grained shelves and cabinets were built, making it equal in appearance to the privately owned pharmacies in the city. For the month there were 225 admissions, 45 returns to duty, 16 discharges, 15 desertions, and 3 deaths; 563 remained in the hospital. More were expected with the spring offensive.

CHAPTER FOURTEEN

Private Pliny Adams Jewett

By the spring of 1865, Richmond was starving; Confederate desertions were on the increase, replacements nonexistent, and supplies dwindling along with the will to fight. The feared and elusive Confederate armies were dispersed, defanged, and defeated through large swaths of smoldering ruins. On April 4 headlines trumpeted "Richmond has fallen!" Lee surrendered to Grant at Appomattox Court House on April 9. A *Record* editorial on April 12 proclaimed "The End Cometh," describing a hopeful, benevolent future where "man's inhumanity to man" would cease and festering wounds heal.

> The States lately in rebellion will again be gathered back into the fold, and the citizens of our common country again meet together as friends and wonder that anything could have so long widely estranged them. Let us do our utmost to hasten and consolidate our glorious re-union. Let us bear no grudges and indulge in no sneers or revengeful feelings. Let us welcome back our erring brethren and show them that we don't hate them for all the misery and suffering they have inflicted upon us. Let us imitate our noble Chief and honest, kind hearted President and concede that with all their sins and faults, our late enemies have some qualities to admire and for which we are proud once more to hail them as our fellow countrymen.

This tone of reconciliation and forgiveness lasted forty-eight hours. On the evening of April 14, Good Friday, Lincoln was shot in the back of his head and died the following morning. The mood, intent, and direction of the country abruptly changed, leaving basic issues unresolved for a century. The reconstruction of the Union would be long, painful, and incomplete. Some wounds neither heal nor kill but fester, fouling the air and draining the body of strength.

It was the worst of days for the country and especially so for the Jewett family. "The Assassination of Our Noble President," screamed a *Record* editorial, reversing the generous attitude and hope for the future expressed just days before. At first there was disbelief as a nation's collective heart was plunged into woe. The sheer wickedness of this foul deed brought forth an eruption of anger fueled by frustration and war weariness: "A wise states-man, great patriot, noblest citizen, and charitable and generous Father" was gone leaving a dark abyss. The ship of state was rudderless and in danger of floundering. A very different editorial blazed from the pages of the *Record* on April 19:

We have no heart to give utterance to our feelings over this sad and terrible calamity which has come so unexpected upon the Nation. But the people cry aloud for vengeance. The spirits of the departed heroes, who have fallen in this war call for justice; and the maimed and crippled soldiers now swarming the country, demand it. Let every traitor now beware of the vengeance of an outraged people. Let every sympathizer with this accursed rebellion be marked and no mercy shown him. Let there be Justice for the noble man who has just fallen by the hand of a traitor. Let the Traitors be exiled.

On the afternoon of Good Friday, Dr. Jewett was driving home in his carriage when he was struck by a New Haven Fire Department hose cart, which destroyed his carriage while severely and permanently injuring his knee. But for the Jewett family that was the least of it.

Major Jewett's brother Henry Hatch Jewett was five years his junior and died at age twenty-seven in 1849, followed by his wife the following year. They were survived by a nine-year-old daughter, Elizabeth, and her eleven-year-old brother Pliny. The responsibility of raising these orphans fell to the Jewett clan, the grandparents and especially the uncle. The boy was named, after all, Pliny Adams Jewett.

Jewett the Younger was just twenty-three years old when he enlisted in the First Connecticut Cavalry Volunteers in April 1863. He was captured at Bolivar Heights, Virginia, on July 14, 1863, just a few months after joining the unit, and paroled from Belle Isle Prison six weeks later. He survived a most difficult time, unlike many of his comrades who were imprisoned for up to nine months. Rather than enroll in college or seek employment back home, he reenlisted for three more years of battlefield duty, eventually becoming quartermaster sergeant.

His letters home give an insider's unvarnished view of soldier's life — an eyewitness account, fresh, unflinching, and uncompromising about war's smells, sounds, sights, and hardships. Pertinent parts of his letters to his cousin Steve, his sister Lizzie, and Uncle Pliny follow.[1]

April 5, 1863
Virginia,
Dear Steve,
There is a dead man lying outside of my tent shot through the head by a bushwhacker last night and four horses came in last night without riders, one saddle covered with blood. This country is full of bushwhackers. In the daytime they work on their farms, but after dark they slip out and sneak around behind the fences and in the woods shooting every stray soldier that they meet.
I sat down by the tent cold and hungry, no rations, thinking how I ever would get my tent up when I heard "Hello Pliny." There stood Joe Ellis [a friend from New Haven], and the first thing he said was "Had any breakfast. I said, "I haven't had my yesterday's dinner yet." He made some coffee and pulled out some bread, butter, chunk of pork and helped me pitch my tent. [He shares tent with four others.]
I wish that you would ask Uncle Pliny to get me a map of Eastern Virginia compiled in the office of the Coast Survey and printed by W. H. Morrison in Washington. It looks like a book and can be sent by mail very easily. It contains all the crossroads and lanes about here and way to Richmond. One of the boys had one sent to him. It is very useful on a scout.

Asking Uncle Pliny for material support, usually in the form of money, was routine and guaranteed success. Grandmotherly advice was also of great value, as the letter on page 195 might indicate.

Knight Hospital Record.

TERMS $1 50 A YEAR, IN ADVANCE.   VOL. 1.--NO. 29.

NEW HAVEN, CT., WEDNESDAY, APRIL 19, 1865.

ANSWER TO "JUST BEFORE THE BATTLE MOTHER."

No, I'll not forget you, darling,
Though the cruel chance of war
Leaves you on the field of battle,
Where I'll never see you more—
Leaves you where the cry of "Onward!"
Troubles not your slumber deep—
Leaves you where the din of battle
Cannot wake you from your sleep!
No, I'll not forget you, darling,
Though if one fond pressure, more
Could be granted to me, darling,
'Twould not leave my heart so sore.

No, I'll not forget you, darling,
O, 'tis strange that you should ask,
When my thoughts from morn till even'g,
Round your very soul are clasped;
Let it ever like a halo
Round your rugged pathway shine—
The love of Mother, God and Heaven,
Let it round your soul be twined.
No I'll not forget, &c.

No I'll not forget you, darling,
But oh, the time has been so long
Since the morning that you left me
To defend the right from wrong.
Till now I feel my sad heart sinking,
While I think you may not come,
When this raging strife is ended,
And your comrades reach their home.
No, I'll not forget, &c.

No, I'll not forget you, darling,
Be thou always brave and true,
God will guard you there as safely
As beneath my roof he'd do.
And perchance, when all is over,
You with others, too, may come,
Crying—"Victory is ours,"
While we give you welcome home.
No, I'll not forget you, &c.

For the Record.

CAMP REMINISCENCES.—NO. 1.

BY G. N.

Through the wild and mountainous region of the Old Dominion State, there has existed an element containing a vein of anecdote and story, which only need to be woven together to form sketches of a very interesting and entertaining character. In Harper's Magazine, a few years since, appeared the writings of Port Crayon, giving personal experience of the rough, wild scenes of the dense forests, almost limitless mountains and craggy mountains occasionally he meets a gouty and grouty one, and tells funny things about him and [illegible]. But these sketches were written [illegible] ago, before the red island of treason

has so long floated like an evil spirit over the land, excluding, for the time, our boasted peace, happiness and prosperity. In our connection with the armies of Virginia, since the summer of '62, we have necessarily become familiarized with the country and the people, and have had an experience among the natives, whites and blacks, containing a spice of humorous interest. We have seen the F. F. V.'s flying from their homes before our advancing legions, while their slaves have been suddenly transformed to masters and mistresses, and transferred from meagre huts to gorgeous parlors, from bare floors to Brussels carpets, from pots and kettles to sofas and pianos, from stinted fare to sumptuous repasts—but without further introduction, inviting you, dear readers, for companions in arms, we will sling our knapsacks, and go over in imagination some of the historic campaigns that we once in reality participated in.

In July, 1862, we enlisted, having at that time arrived at the independent age of 21. A mother's heart was filled with pleasurable grief, sisters wept, and a venerable father counseled and advised, and each and all poured forth a blessing and a God speed as we stepped on board a car, and were whirled towards the seat of war. In due time we arrived in Washington, and as Washington was a great place in our opinion, in fact, the nucleus of our ambition, we thought we ought to look around a little and see the town. At that time men who enlisted were patriots, and they enlisted because they loved their country. There were no bounty-jumpers then, neither were there substitutes bought by patriotic "men of millions," who would tremble at every turn of the terrible "wheel of fortune," but for the fact that each day they realized from Government enough to establish a representative in the army the next.

And so we were allowed a few hours' stroll among the people of Washington city, and we visited the Capitol; and as we went up and down Pennsylvania Avenue, mingling incongruously with Congressmen, Foreign Ministers, Generals, and all grades of notables, and enjoying all the privileges of the masses—but one; they wouldn't sell us any whiskey,—only for that we were as good as the best.

But the time arrived for us to leave all these National scenes and surroundings, for the rough and awful ones of active service, and after 'right-facing to the left,' and 'front-facing to the rear' a few times, we commenced our first march; through the crowded thoroughfares, over the Potomac, via Long Bridge, and for the first time set foot on the soil of Virginia—soil destined to be made immortal by events that have eclipsed all history and surprised a world. An afternoon over dusty roads and under a melting sun, without water, and we reached a point on Arlington Heights, about seven miles out of Washington city, and pitching our tents in an old peach orchard—an old peach orchard that never [illegible]

than a breeze sprung up which gradually increased, until it assumed the proportion and strength of a hurricane, and it shook our frail houses to the very foundations. However, we didn't mind it, but only chatted and smoked the harder, and talked and laughed the merrier, for we had embraced the soldier's motto of 'free and happy always.' Harder the wind blew, and faster the rain fell, until it seemed as if the heavens were let loose with the intent of again deluging the earth, or blowing it away. The last story was told, and drawing our pipe from our mouth, stroked an intrusive rain-drop from our nose, and sank into sweet unconsciousness, to dream of homes, mothers, sweethearts, wives, babies and the like. But our dreams were short, short as they were pleasant, and we awoke. The rain still pelted down, and our tent and clothing were damp and dripping, while underneath us flowed little rivulets. Bedrenched as we were, it was useless to undertake to right matters, and it would have been fool-hardiness to look for new lodgings. So we rolled over, and tried to go to sleep, and tried on till morning, and the final result was, that we did not succeed, but lay awake all night. At the approach of daylight voices were heard without, and attempting to arise, we found many bed-clothes than we could conveniently throw off; but we could crawl out, and did. A pretty spectacle was presented, as we stood and viewed it with laughable astonishment. Of upwards of two hundred tents that had been pitched the night before, a dozen were standing, and the joke was we didn't see anybody stirring. A good many of them couldn't stir. As the morn advanced, things were re-constructed, it was amusing to see the boys as they uncovered, pull themselves out of the spongy mud that had been their beds, stare, wonder, realize and laugh. An old parable was brought to mind, about the wise man that built a house upon a rock, and his neighbor that didn't, and we profited by it.

This was the first introduction of the Regiment to camp life—an introduction calculated to give raw recruits a very fine able impression of life on the tented field, and yet it was experience that we laughed afterwards, when we had gained the coveted and proud title of old soldiers.

The sun rose bright and beautiful, soon ours was a busy and pleasant ground. Clothes were dried, guns and accoutrements cleaned, and we were ordered for [illegible]. No matter about the drill, it was similar to all first drills, and if we didn't know a shoulder shift from 'support,' nor a [illegible] file into line' from a 'right hand,' that was nobody's business, for we knew all about it now. Suffice it that the Colonel dismissed us after two hours of hard labor, not called up again till dress parade. Then a dress parade as it was. We had had two or two dress parades before then, but with muskets and accoutrements, and it is not strange that there should be some incidents of a comical character [illegible]

20 April 1863
New Haven
My Dear Pliny,

I am very sorry not to see you before you go to Baltimore. You must write as soon as you get there and if you want anything let me know and I will send you whatever you want. I can send by the express, give me your address in residence.

In great haste.

Your affectionate grandmother,

Take care of your health and be a good boy, rather than bad company.

7 May 1863
Baltimore Maryland
Dear Steve,

I received Tommy's letter informing me of the death of Grandma, it completely stunned me. You had written to me that she was sick but I had hoped that she would soon be better. If I had known she was so sick I should have gone home at all hazards, but it is best as it is. There is no chance of furloughs here. As things look now have hope that the war will soon be ended as everyone seems to think it will. If you had seen the rebel soldiers that I have I think that you would think so to; ragged and half starved, they look exactly like the pictures that have seen of them with carpets and coverlets and bed quilts for blankets, lean and lanky with long hair hanging over their faces. A person cannot have but respect for them when he sees how they have suffered for their cause. It has stormed here for the past two days and is cloudy and unpleasant today. I have to get me a new cap as I lost mine in the cars when I fell into a dose not having slept for two days and had my head on the edge of window as my cap fell out. Please answer this letter and tell me what Grandma said about me, it will be a great comfort to me to know. Tell Lizzie to write as soon as possible and send me some postage stamps.

P.S. About 2000 beef cattle just passed through in one drove bound south. They were over a half a mile long if you can believe it.

16 June 1863
Dear Steve,

The weather is very hot down here, we have not had any rain for a long while; the top of the earth is baked very hard. We don't have any Sundays down here. The only way I know it is Sunday the Chaplain

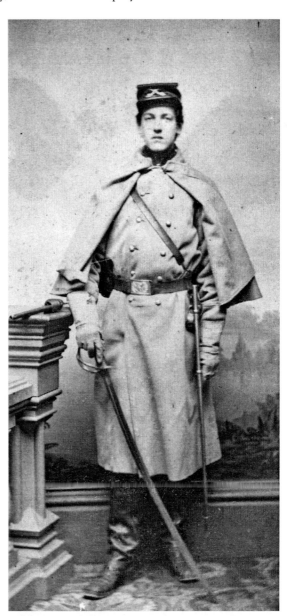

Sergeant Pliny Adams Jewett (Virginia Historical Society).

or Holy Joe as we call him comes in the room and says "Hello boys," and drops three tracks and skedaddles. I always go around after him and collect all I can to clean my tin plate with as cloth, and newspapers are very scarce.

Fifty cars crowded with soldiers have just arrived here from Washington to be transported towards Harrisburg where the rebels are now going. I expect that the rebs will be here in a few days.

An old lady came to the Hospital yesterday and brought preserves I tell you it seemed so good just like home. Two large baggage trains arrived filled with refugees, railroad iron ties and machinery, some refugees left so fast they had no hats on. The last train was loaded with medicine, beds, pillows, tents, blankets and other hospital stores also some wounded soldiers. All this shows that they are advancing. Pickets of our cavalry have been thrown out a distance of six miles from the city.

You would not think meat tough if you had to eat the meat that we do. The fresh meat nearly always has maggots or else stinks. The salt horse and pork stinks like thunder before the ten days rations are up but I have got so that I never think of it. All I do is keep the maggots underneath.

29 June 1863,
Baltimore, Maryland

The city is all excitement now last Saturday the people commenced fortifying this side of the city, all the niggers found in the city were impressed to work on the fort. Every nigger seen by the police was grabbed up no matter where he was. They are throwing up five entrenchments near our camp; they all command the Frederick road. It is fun to go around where they are digging. In the evening you can see large campfires on the different hills where they are at work. They work night and day, the day gang relieved at 7 P.M., and you can hear them singing their evening songs all stretched out on the ground under the huts that they make to sleep in. Some of the nigs are very fancy just taken from barbershops, there is one nigger there not a bit taller than Capt. Glynn but twice as fat, it is fun to see him work. I tell you the grease flies. All the principal entrances to the city have been barricaded and are guarded all the time. Two of the three captured union soldiers were rumored to have been shot. I wish that we had known about it when we had those three rebels in our hands. They would have been dead now but we will not capture any more, we will kill them like dogs. The boys they killed were splendid fellows everyone liked them.

The next three captured soldiers of the opposite side would suffer the same fate as the three dead Union soldiers. The concept of retribution, a life for a life, tooth for tooth, and hand for hand, seems an elemental human trait. The ground rules for war do not change because human nature does not change. Basic communication is by deeds rather than speeches, wishful thinking, or formal conventions. The innocent die and bad things happen.

6 July 1863

I never was healthier in my life than during the week and a half I slept out on the ground in the mud and rain. I hope that you enjoyed yourself on the 4th. I spent mine way up in the woods on picket all day and the night.

24 August 1863
St. Johns College Hospital
Annapolis, Maryland

I have at last got away from the rebs more dead than alive. I have no time to tell you any particulars I am so weak please send me all the New Haven papers. You cannot imagine the misery I have suffered starved all the time we got half a small loaf of bread a day, a pint of water with a few beans in it called soup and 18 pounds of meat (mostly bone) which we had to divide among 100 men. Can you send me a box so that I can get it this week? The men here are getting boxes from home every day. Put in it some good homemade bread cookies, pies and cheese.

How I long to get hold of some good homemade cookies and pies. I wish that you would send it so that I can get it this week if possible. What did you think had become of me? I tell you we had a rough time after we was captured. They made us walk 100 miles in five days. Write and tell me all the news when you send the box you can wrap the different things up in newspapers so that I can get them sent it this week if possible. Write immediately on the receipt of this letter. I was confined in Richmond most of the time that I was prisoner, so I have been to Richmond but I should not wish to make another visit under the same circumstances. I never intend to get taken prisoner again. I would rather die outright than starve to death.

His regiment served in nineteen major battles and ninety skirmishes. There were 57 percent total casualties and 304 prisoners of war, of whom eighty-nine died — most suffering a much longer incarceration than Private Jewett.[2] Getting him an early parole must have been top priority for his uncle.

2 November 1863
Baltimore, Maryland
Dear Steve,

I am guarding a hospital now in Baltimore and had a splendid time for Thanksgiving. I had the whole regiment advising me to go home and not re-enlist. They all told me that I was very foolish. I told them if I left the service I would go out fairly and not sneak out, and on the other hand I like it too well to leave. I arrested a young plug-ugly the other day for cursing the Yankees on purpose to scare him but he acted so ugly that I gave him to a policeman. He had multiple arrests and was sent to jail for 8 years.

10 March 1864
Annapolis Junction
Headquarters Camp, 1st Regiment Connecticut Cavalry

We are encamped halfway between Washington and Baltimore. Last Thursday evening Lt. Gore sent for me and when I went up there he said that Uncle Pliny came through that afternoon and he then handed me a pass for 24 hours to go to Washington. You can believe that I was surprised. I went down the next morning and met Uncle Pliny at Willard's and stayed two days. I had a splendid time. I visited the Capitol and all the other places of note and amongst them the Patent office that beats everything that I ever saw. If a man wanted to examine them closely it would take him over two weeks to look over all the patents. There is a model there of every patent in the US. Among the distinguished officers stopping at the Hotel was Generals Grant, Mead, Burnside, Woolsey, McCook, and Blount. There was a good many other generals that I did not know.

Good old Uncle Pliny was good for a meal ticket, cash, a new hat, maps, books, boots, and whatever else his nephew's heart or soul desired. Willard's was the toniest hotel in town, full of officers resplendent in gold epaulets defending gambling parlors, ladies' virtues or lack thereof, and aging bottles of brandy. Back home Uncle Pliny dealt with political enemies, malingerers, deserters, wounded and terminally ill patients, and their distraught families. For each soldier transferred to the Invalid Corps or given a medical discharge, the replacement would be someone else's son. He must have thought of his beloved nephew in such a setting; this orphaned volunteer risking sickness, crippling injury, and death.

Jan 1864
Winchester, Virginia
Dear Steve,

I am glad to hear that Captain Glynn has at last been married. I have been expecting sometime that he would either commit suicide or get married. We put up a house for winter. The logs are 12 feet by 1 foot in the inside and 5 feet high on the outside. We are to work on the fireplace today. It is occupied by two, the commissary sergeant and me. I want you to send me a cap. I want it made on the plan of Uncle Pliny's, with the fore-piece turned down, and size 7⅛. I want it immediately. I cannot get a cap here for less than double what they are worth and they are good for nothing at that. Order the cap and send it right away, and when you send it can't you make up a box of some sort, all the boys are getting boxes from home, and I can tell you the things taste good. If you send anything send some butter. It is cold now and it will keep good. Write as soon as possible and send the cap, for I need the cap every day for dress parade.

Last Friday I went out and saw a couple of deserters shot. The Chaplain read the funeral service to them and then one of the guards pulled the cap over their heads and told them he thought it rather hard and one of them said "I don't care a damn" and they walked up and sit down on their respective coffin and the guard drew up and fired, one of them rolled off of his coffin dead, and the other lived a little while. The band then struck up "Hail Columbia" and the meeting broke up.

27 March 1864
Headquarters near the Rapidan, Virginia
On other side of Rapidan are rebels within speaking distance but the orders are out to fire at each other. Lt Gore will resign as soon as possible he says that he has served in the army a good many years but he never saw such a regiment before, that he is perfectly disgusted with it.

One of the men was tied up so his company cut him down. We were told to "fall in" and supposed it was for our whiskey rations. We were surrounded by fully armed Company F and Major Blakeslee had a fit demanding to know who cut the prisoner down — no one would speak and he threatened to tie up the entire company ... but the Major cooled down. Many of the regiment wants to hand in sabers but his company told them not to get into trouble for them.

20 May 1864,
Fredericksburg, Virginia
Got letter from Uncle Pliny. Fighting very hard since May 4 and we have driven them over 30 miles from where we commenced fighting. We are confident of victory. There have been over 40,000 killed and wounded on our side. Every house in the city is full of wounded. I helped guard 10,000 rebel prisoners over a week ago. We charged the rebels earth works and were defeated at first but finally took them; the nigs were on our right they fought like devils they kept yelling "Fort Pillow" and took no prisoners and killed nearly all the wounded with their bayonets. It seemed as if the air was full of bullets. I saw one man struck by a shell. There was not a piece left of him as I could see.

We are all perfectly confident of success and every man is of the same opinion as to our General Grant, that he is the best and the greatest General in the world, we almost worship him. We have had one great general.

Ask Uncle Pliny to put in a little money as mine is about gone and we only get 10 crackers and a little sugar and coffee and about a half a ration of beef and some days not that but we do not expect any more when the army is moving. We only get a ration of pork now once in 10 days. Write if possible. Lieutenant Gore left us for good just before the army moved; we did not regret him much. When next I write, I hope to write from Richmond.

20 Oct 1864
Put on steamer Thomas P. Morgan and steered us for Washington. Lucky for me I have money, as they have not given us any rations at all. Meals on boat are $1.00. Provisions were for the boat not the men brought on board

20 October 1864,
At sea on United States Transport America,
Dear Steve,
There were 500 troops on one vessel. It was impossible to move we were so wedged in. Nearly all the guards stood at hatchway with their guns loaded pointed down, bayonets drawn

to keep us down. They called for noncommissioned officers to come on deck, which I did. 100 men came on deck, which eased the crowding. The lieutenants came to me and asked me to take charge of the rations and try to quiet the men. They gave me liberty of the ship and sole charge of the kitchen with two good cooks from their company and liberty to detail as many men as I wished at any time to assist me. I had now to feed 500 men with 1bbl sugar, 1bbl coffee, 3 bbls cooked bacon and 40 boxes of hard bread. These were to last four days. I have a state's room and a Negro detailed for my servant and power to take any number of men for help without asking anyone; in short all the liberty of a commissioned officer.

21 Oct 1864

The men are feeling like dogs, I have to feed them through a hatchway and it would be impossible to carry any thing down, as there is such a rush. About 10 A.M. some were allowed up and kept in the bow of the ship. This pleased them considerably and they behave better. When I feed them coffee they said they wanted nothing to eat but wanted the Lieutenants to kill them.

There were two men said to be dead in the hold as none of the guard dared to go down (it would have been death to them) I searched the boat from stem to stern but found no dead men. But some were very sea sick. The men all mind me; they call me their best friend and say if it had not have been for me they should have died. At noon I fed them bacon through the hatchways. At night I gave them hard tack and some more coffee. The Lieutenants are both very young and totally incompetent to take charge of a set of convalescents. They always say "Do just as you think best Sergeant, everything is in your hands."

23 Oct 1864

Men were all separated and sent to their different army corps. Sheridan men gave us a little to eat and marched us out on a bare spot, put a guard around us and left us to do the best we could. I rolled myself up in my blanket and put my valise under my head and went to sleep.

27 October 1864

There are no rations. Meals are now $2.00. I saw a beautiful bald headed eagle. When near Mount Vernon, three men jumped overboard, they were recruits. A boat was manned by two boat hands, and the steamer turned about and one or two shots brought them too and they were picked up. They were a mile and a half from shore when they jumped. $50 was found on them, $10 was given to the two boatmen. We arrived at Alexandria at 3 P.M. and marched five miles to Camp Distribution where we were put in wards of 100 men each. I was offered the job of ward master of barracks and another position but declined.

I wish you would ask Uncle Pliny to send me a low felt hat, and a pair of warm gloves. I will send my measure you can enclose them in a cigar box. My money won't last long to buy hats with here, they cost so much. It may be a long time before we are paid and my washing cost me considerable.

22 Dec. 1864,

We saddled at 4 A.M. It was extremely cold, the wind blowing very hard we all suffered greatly. When we reached Strasburg I went to a house, they said they had nothing to eat. I told them I would have something by fair means or foul as I was nearly starved and as I had no money I would give them coffee in exchange, The word coffee opened their hearts immediately, they were crazy for it. They immediately set me out a good substantial dinner and when I got through there was no need of washing the platter. We marched 30 miles today and went into camp near our old camp. I now received a letter from Uncle Pliny. The money was a perfect godsend. Went to a farmhouse where I was acquainted and staid all day. I took a good wash and had a good dinner. I thought I must have something besides army rations. I got warmed through for the first time in a week.

25 December 1864

I hope that you all enjoyed happy Christmas. The money was a godsend. We received ten recruits today, they left New Haven 178 men all told, and only 10 men reached here. That is the way the 1st Connecticut Cavalry is recruited. Since I have got my money, I have got along first rate. I bought some tea and sugar of the Commissary and it has done me a good deal of good. I have been using so much coffee. We have been drawing very small rations lately and I have been out several times, but now I can buy from the Commissary. You cannot buy from a Commissary unless an officer certifies it is for his own use. It is a great deal cheaper to buy from a sutler for they sell at Government rates. Tea is $1.40 a pound, sugar 25 cents a pound, ham 29 cents, and bread 8 cents a loaf. It was a poor Christmas but it was one more day towards the three years.

He was living outdoors in the freezing cold with limited rations and mostly hungry, unlike his peers back home.

27 December 1864,
Dear Steve,

Woke at 4 A.M. covered with ice, hailing very fast, my blankets were all frozen stiff, horse broke lose [sic] during the night and not to be found. We started out at 6:30 A.M. in a trot and went five miles. It was cloudy and cold all day. I got some bran and boiled it in water and eaten it and thought that I was living high. I found an old horse and was just saddled when Bang! Bang! Bang! And the rebels were on us, there was mounting in hot haste, myself no exception. The divisions then formed and charged the rebels. We all cheered to let them know we were ready for them. The fight lasted about fifteen minutes. The rebs took all our ambulances at first but we retook them all, killed about 30 rebels and took about 40 prisoners. We did not stop to bury the dead but left them lying where they were shot. We only lost about five killed and about 12 wounded. Some of the men striped [sic] the dead of most everything. We went as far as Woodstock today it was awful, it hailed nearly all day, but when we reached Woodstock we built good fires and thawed out considerably during the day. The captain saw a man riding my horse and returned it to me. The rebels followed us all day and worried us all night.

The chief of staff of Knight U.S. Army General Hospital learned about field life from his intrepid nephew. The noise of battle is deafening. Vision may be blocked by dense clouds of dust. Without coherent sight or sound what is happening before you is maddening chaos enveloped by darkness. The ground trembles, flashes of light signify missiles of death and destruction entering and leaving your small universe striking tree and soil and flesh with thumps, crackles, and whistles. What seems an interminable battle may be seconds or minutes. Men are screaming, crying, moaning, shouting, or silent and dead. There are no speeches, not about politics, religion, or the American way. There are no jokes, puns, or witty sayings to be heard. Faced with life or death, survival requires concentration of thought and action.

Private William Abernathy was twenty years old, orphaned as a toddler, and experienced in the hard life before writing his diary during the war. He describes battlefield experiences in the spring and winter of 1863, having survived a minor wound during the Battle of Suffolk.

A soldier's life indeed is one of dread and fear. Sometimes I get to thinking of the battle with bursting shells, whizzing bullets and mangled bloody corpses borne on the streets lying frozen and stiff. The groans and cries were of those whose limbs were being severed by the surgical knife. There is the dread of these things that came over me and I feel there is no one I can rely except God.

Whiz, whiz are the sounds of bullets. All the men are lying flat. I was so interested in balls and shells going over my head I did not hear the order to lie down. Men began running over the hill below us crying "where is the surgeon." We are getting cut to pieces. A man shot with a bullet looks a great deal more lifelike than one killed in any other way. It does not bleed a lot. The man all healthy and full of blood is not changed as much as one that is sick and dies.

It is the worse [*sic*] of these rifled shells that makes them so dreaded. You can hear them coming to you a mile away. When nearer it means expecting them to burst and not knowing whether a fragment will shatter a leg or break you [*sic*] skull. A bullet comes almost unheard and does its business without any noise.[3]

Private Henry J. Thompson, also of the Fifteenth Regiment, discussed explosives with his wife.[4]

We don't think anything of shooting 5 to 7 miles here. We have heard a gun going off and in less than no time hear an old shell coming like a buzz saw through the air and bang it goes right over our heads and whizt goes all to pieces every way. I have heard 20 of these playthings as some call them. I did not think so when I see the men falling dead and wounded all around me and no way to get away. I stood leaning against a tree seeing the battle, when the first I know whang went a shell close by me and took a piece out of the tree about as big as my head made me dog some, although I had been under fire two days and night before this.

If you can hear it you are safe. It is the missile you do not hear that is to be feared. The *Record* described the predicament that had been faced by many of its readers:

The soldier marches and arrives at the destination. He has a light dinner and gets ready for battle the next day. He can't sleep perhaps. What if he is killed or taken prisoner? Who will care for his family? What if he becomes a prisoner? The next day he falls in. He hears silence, then loud booming noises from musketry and artillery. There is the sharp crack of thousands of rifles, the roar of many cannon, and the groans of dying and wounded. Soon fresh troops are brought up and with a great shout charge. Hundreds are dead and dying strewn on ground. Then there are the shrieks and groans of the wounded. This volunteer has the heart of a lion, is unshakably steadfast, and has the undaunted courage of the constitutionally brave. He is gallant and blessed.

Most critical is the soldier's will to fight and persevere in unflinching manner. The maintenance of that spirit is enhanced by the approval and willingness to sacrifice by society in general. In a poem, around a campfire, three soldiers compare their lives in another *Record* story. One is a drummer boy, the second a young man rejected by his "true" love and the third an old veteran. In this poem both old and young soldiers proclaim, "My country called and I came." Their motives for enlisting ranged from patriotic volunteering, the draft, and escaping life's disappointment. Their home life varied from bare-bones existence to loving children and a devoted wife. Their goals range from survival to victory with glory. All three die in battle. Tombstones of that era often reflected these moral positions. In a cemetery in Grafton, Vermont, a Civil War soldier's tombstone reads "My Country Called and I Obeyed." For some, fire and flag in a sea of fellow bluecoats orchestrated by thundering cannon is a life experience worth dying for. For others war is human sacrifice in a sanctified and glorified package, made mythical by the forces that profit from such conflicts.

In a story titled "My Chum," the narrator describes a friend, a strapping nineteen-year-old soldier of the Fourteenth Connecticut Volunteers. He was the best wrestler and hardest worker, carried the most firewood, participated in every battle, was always helpful to his fellow soldiers, and was out there doing his duty while his friend was home on medical leave. "We tented together, slept together, and ate together, shared dangers of campaign together. We shared all." They did not share death. That his friend did alone. Seeing a "chum" die in battle or from disease has a searing effect. It forces one to focus on the essential, cover yourself and your partner's back and survive. A young man can't learn too early that he is not immortal and that fear can make cowards of us all.

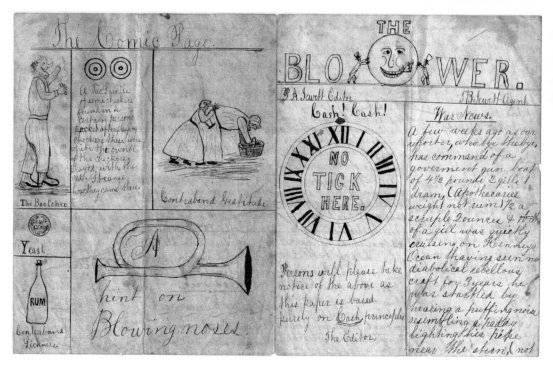

The Blower, regimental newspaper edited by Pliny Adams Jewett, twenty-three-year-old sergeant of First Connecticut Cavalry and nephew of Dr. Jewett (Virginia Historical Society).

27 Dec. 1864
Winchester, Virginia
Dear Lizzie,

It was so cold the morning we fought them that some of the men could not get their carbines to work, the grease in the lock being froze so hard … everything was covered with ice as it hailed part of the days and nearly all the night before. Thursday was the coldest day of all, the wind at times would nearly blow you out of the saddle. The morning we took prisoners, we took one officer who had on a pair of U.S. pants, and Gen Custer rode up to him and asked him where he got them; he said he took them from us. "Take them right off from him" said Custer and off they came. Mr. Rebel Officer walked all the two days on our way back with a pair of drawers on.

Affectionately,
P.A. Jewett Jr.
P.S. Please ask Tommy to send me some *Hospital Record*.

28 Dec. 1864
Dear Uncle Pliny,

I received your letter, with the money enclosed last Thursday evening; it could not have arrived at a better time, for we had just arrived back from a four days raid up the Valley entirely out of rations. Two hundred men were frost bitten and two or three in a regular battery frozen to death, for being regular they were not allowed to dismount and walk. I do not think the men would have suffered so much if they had had rations.

I see by the papers, the people of New Haven and vicinity are making exertions to procure our regiment a New Year's dinner. I wish them success. We have been waiting anxiously for orders to build winter quarters, but it has got so late, that we have almost given up all hope. The prisoners we took last week were dressed in old pieces of carpet and other odds and ends picked up through the country. I wish that you would have someone send me New Haven papers, especially the *Hospital Record*, Connecticut papers are a great treat out here.

Pliny Junior in his spare time was the creator and editor of his regimental newspaper, called the *Blower*. His inspiration was the *Record*, copies of which were mailed from New Haven at his request. The price for his field newspaper was four cents a month, affordable if nothing else. The satirical nature of this experiment was described thusly: "When the clown enters the ring with a bound and a somersault and says 'Here we are,' the audience is immediately put in good humor and prepared to laugh at anything he utters. So we throw ourselves before the public with the greeting of 'here we are,' and respectively ask your kind patronage. This is the end of my tale, as the tadpole said when he turned into a bull frog."[5]

Hometown experiences were thinly camouflaged and the names changed to protect the writer's reception back home. Among the jokes listed

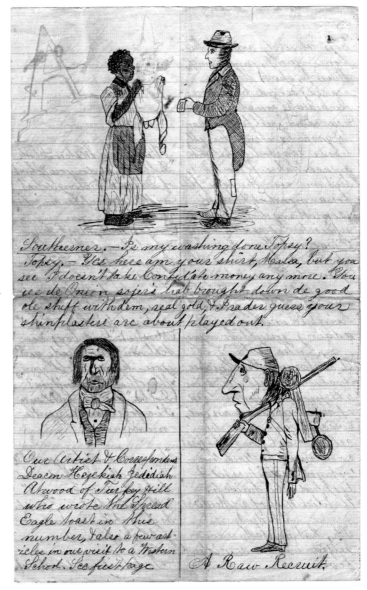

Newspaper sketches: contraband, raw recruit, and deacon (Virginia Historical Society).

in the regimental paper were those inspired by Uncle Pliny and his grandfather, the Reverend Stephen Jewett. "What was a great turnout: when a certain New Haven doctor was upset in Chapel Street." "What is the unfilial wish of a medical student: Oh, that my father was seized with a *remittent* fever." "What blessings children are, said the parish clerk when he took the fee for christening them." "Visit to a Western School: 'Dobbs what do you think of David's killing Goliath?' (Dobbs): 'Well, I don't know what David thought, but I guess Goliath was astonished when he found himself killed by a stone *as such a thing never entered his head before!*"

There is a striking drawing of a "Deacon Hezekiah Jedidiah Atwood" in proper dress with eyes transfixing and uncompromising. "In his manhood, clothed in purple and fine linen, he rides over a continent in cushioned cars, rides over the ocean in palace steamers and sends his thoughts on wings of lightning to the world around." Resemblance to Pliny's grandfather was purely intentional.

The life of this promising young man was coming to an end. He could not know this was his last letter.

> 27 March 1865
> Petersburg, Virginia
> I am all right. We are at White House Landing. We have not had much fighting and have only lost one Lieutenant and four men killed and several taken prisoners. I was paid at White House and received $148.10. We can look right into Petersburg where we are now encamped. It is only a mile and half. Lookout for great fighting now, we are going to try and cut the south side railroad I think. We are close to the front and we can easily see the puffs of smoke from the guns of the pickets, the infantry had heavy fighting here Saturday. Write as often as you can and I shall get the letters sometime. Direct it to Sheridan's Cavalry.

Lee's Army of Northern Virginia was retreating south, rapidly depleted in arms, food, medicines, and soldiers. On April 6, Lee's wagon train near Harper's Farm was attacked but his forces had time to dig in and had forged strong breastworks.[6] General George Armstrong Custer ordered an attack by an undermanned cavalry force, charging directly across an open field. He should have waited for the complete Union force to arrive so that flanking maneuvers could be added, ensuring a quick, certain victory with fewer casualties. Patience and mildly complicated military tactics were not Custer's long suit, consistent with graduating last in his class at West Point. He knew but one military maneuver: plunge straight ahead. At three o'clock in broad daylight, the brigade galloped gallantly forward with only one third of available Union forces being present, only to be terribly repulsed. The results of this "rash order" were that one in five Union men and horses were dropped dead at the Confederate line, a line that held for the last time in the war. Sheridan later called up a larger force, outflanked the rebels, and routed their army. On April 9, Lee surrendered a few miles away at Appomattox Court House.

It was three days too late for Dr. Jewett's beloved orphaned nephew. It was a calamitous "Good Friday" with the death of the nation's leader, a severe leg injury to the surgeon in charge, and a crushing loss for the Jewett family. The young man's death received a special declaration in the *Hospital Record*, between the assassination editorial and description of Jewett's accident, an unusual posting for an enlisted man given the number of soldiers who died without receiving such prominence.

> Sergeant Pliny A. Jewett, of Company E, 1st Connecticut Cavalry, and a nephew of Major Jewett of this city was killed on the 6th. In his death, one more hero is added to the long list of brave men who have freely laid down their lives for our common country.

Uncle Pliny's reaction is not recorded but can be inferred. King David cried out to the heavens about his favorite son sacrificed in the ruthlessness of war and the finality of death: "O my son Absalom, my son, my son Absalom! If only I had died instead of you, O Absalom my son, my son" (2 Samuel 19:1). His cry embodies the nightmare of every father who is unable to protect his child.

In the *Record* was a poem by the Greek poet Cato discussing the loss of a son in battle, a subject of keen interest in hospital wards of soldiers, men who have seen the worst, and whose actions are praised and encouraged by a voice from antiquity.

Thanks to the gods! My boy has done his duty.
Welcome my son! There set him down my friends
Full in my sight, that I may view at leisure
The bloody corpse, and count those glorious wounds,
How beautiful is death when earned by virtue!
Who would not be that youth? What pity 'tis
That we can die but once to save our country!
Why sits this sadness on your brow my friends?
I should have blushed if Cato's house had stood
Secure, and flourished in a civil war.

Clausewitz wrote of war in the nineteenth century that it ought to be advanced only in the interests of a national state and that the entire effort of the nation must be mobilized in service of the military objective. All must participate and all make sacrifices.

Let us not hear of Generals who conquer without bloodshed. If a bloody slaughter is a horrible sight, then that is a ground for paying more respect to war, but not for making the sword we wear blunter and blunter by degrees from feelings of humanity, until someone steps in with one that is sharp and lops off the arm from our body.[7]

The Reverend Stephen Jewett delivered a sermon for a mournful family in 1818 about the death of an army captain from sickness. The sentiments about the hereafter and the consolation of loved ones have an eerie connection to his grandson's death half a century later.[8]

By this we may learn our own frailty. We find that health that greatest of earthly blessings does not always protect us from the shafts of Death. There are various ways, which the brittle threads of our life may be broken asunder. Others by some unforeseen accident are insensibly deprived of life and sent to the world of spirits. And what reason do we have to complain? Shall not the judge of all the earth do right? Surely he who holds the key of hell and death is alone able to determine what is best for us and we may not apprehend how he will provide all justice. In the deaths of others, we may see our own destiny. We may not perhaps die in the same manner but it is sufficient for us that we know we must die and thus we are aspired of in that solemn sentence, "dust thou art and to dust thou shalt thou return." It only remains then for us to live in a state of continual preparation for in what hour we shall be summoned we know not.

☞ Lieut. Pliny A. Jewett, of Co. E, 1st Conn. Cavalry, a nephew of Major Jewett, of this city, was killed on the 6th inst. in action at Burkesville, Va. Lieut. Jewett first entered the service as a private in 1862. He was taken prisoner and remained at Belle Isle for several weeks. He was in the first battles of the Wilderness, where he was prostrated by a sun stroke. He finally recovered from this, and returned to his regiment at Winchester, last winter, and took part in the recent campaigns of Sheridan, and was stricken down while that general was engaged in the pursuit of Lee. In his death one more hero is added to the long list of brave men who have freely laid down their lives for our common country.—*Courier*.

Our cotemporary is mistaken in the rank. He was a Sergeant instead of Lieutenant.—*En. Record*.

☞ We regret to have to record an accident, last Friday afternoon, to Major Jewett. He was riding home in his carriage, and when near the corner of Church and Chapel streets, was run into by a hose cart, his carriage smashed to pieces, and himself somewhat injured about the knee. He, however, manages to get around with the help of a cane, and attends to his duties at this Hospital, as usual.

Knight Hospital Record, April 19, 1865. Description of severe injury to Chief of Staff Jewett and death of his nephew, Sergeant P.A. Jewett (Hartford Medical Society Historical Library, University of Connecticut Health Center, Farmington).

The war was over. Lee's army surrendered under terms proposed by a commanding general who was generous, gracious, and magnanimous in victory. Ulysses S. Grant would allow no victory parade in Virginia. Many families suffered great losses — uncles, cousins, sons, husbands, and nephews — dead or maimed. Many, especially in the South, would lose homes, businesses, and farmlands in addition to their loved ones. Nonetheless, a great joy spread through the North, as reported by the *Record*.

> As soon as the news was received here, our patriotic surgeon in charge, Major Jewett, who is always ready to celebrate victory, ordered the guns, which were stored in the knapsack-room, to be given to the soldiers at the same time sending for a fine new flag and some powder. The men, to the number of fifty or more being provided with guns, were drawn up in line on the parade ground, with the Drum Corps on the right. In the meantime, the powder and flag had arrived. The former was dealt out to the men, and the latter which is a splendid flag, thirty feet by fifteen feet was raised amid the rattling of musketry to the top of the pole. A number of salutes were afterwards fired, the drum Corps at the same time playing patriotic airs.

The roaring cannon accompanied by flags snapping in the breeze brought out all the soldiers: the weak, the infirm, the wheelchair- and bed-bound, all cheering, embracing, and congratulating. The church bells rang and the cannons roared, spewing forth golden-red fire well past midnight. Office and residential windows were soon lit up with candles, accenting the celestial stars with earthly competition. The next morning a procession of seventy-five headed by hospital steward Leicester Carrington and Captain Bullock marched to town. They made a formal stop to see Major Jewett, who in turn gave a small speech expressing gratitude for the victory. Dr. Jewett had to put his personal grief aside and help others rejoice in a great victory. It was time to celebrate, give thanks for the war's end, and reconstruct lives.

CHAPTER FIFTEEN

The Hospital Closes

The guns fell silent and the hemorrhaging stopped. On April 25, 1865, the War Department ordered wholesale patient discharges and the hospitals emptied. The medical staff at Knight U.S. Army General Hospital still had patients with febrile brows and draining wounds, some of whom would be long in healing if ever.

> All soldiers in the hospitals who require no further medical treatment are to be honorably discharged from the service, with immediate payment. All officers and enlisted men who have been prisoners of war and are now on furlough or in parole camps and all recruits in rendezvous except those for regular army will be honorably discharged. Officers whose duty it is to make out rolls and other final papers connected with discharge and payment of soldiers are directed to make them out without delay so that this order may be carried into effect immediately.[1]

Just four days after the signing of the peace treaty at Appomattox, the governor ordered Dr. Coggswell to transfer any patients he could find: "There are 400 vacant beds in the Knight hospital and I am informed that Connecticut soldiers are constantly being sent to hospitals in Philadelphia and Washington instead of New Haven. Can you proceed at once to Washington and to the front if necessary so as to make arrangements to have our sick and wounded men transferred to New Haven?"

For some, the cover of a hospital blanket was preferable to being under a barrage of cannon or minie ball. Exaggerated symptoms and poses might be a ticket for home state bliss and safety. The war's end produced a "miracle" in the hospitals of both the North and the South. It was best described by the matron of Chimborazo Hospital in Richmond, the largest hospital on earth with its 6,000 Confederate patients. Once the cannons were silenced, suddenly the blind could see, the deaf could hear, the once speechless could shout and sing, the crippled could walk, the contracted limbs straightened, back pain and rheumatism were cured, crutches and canes were discarded as the previously sick and wounded walked away miraculously healed, with nary a limp, or a thank you, or a goodbye.[2]

Transfer to a convalescent hospital, especially one in a recruit's home state, was highly desirable from the recruit's point of view. Dr. Roberts Bartholow described this factor in his text on *Recruits* of 1863 and in his essay for the Sanitary Commission in 1867.

The organization of general hospitals in several states for the soldiers of the State was an ill-advised measure, which greatly contributed to producing malingerers. Large numbers feigned disease to be sent to their state hospital. Soldiers feigned those diseases to be nearest their homes.[3]

Henry Gray from Norwalk, a private in the Seventeenth Regiment, enlisted the governor to obtain transfer from a hospital in Maryland April 1863. Assistant Surgeon A. Heger agreed to do so and the sooner the better. "He is sick in this hospital suffering from periodic headaches, complaints of deafness in right ear and a rupture. The rupture does not exist, and the deafness is doubtful. These diseases even if existing would not under the present orders entitle him to a discharge. These circumstances have been still more complicated by a bribe offered to the Surgeon in charge in order to procure his discharge. He has been recommended for transfer to his native state and the order for transfer is looked for daily." Gray received a discharge with disability in October 1864.

Another private from the same regiment and hometown, Charles W. Lounsbury, requested transfer with similar dim cause from a hospital in Baltimore in June 1863. Surgeon C.W. Jones replied as to why not. "The fact that all the male members of the family being in the service is enough to recommend the discharge of any youth who is so poorly able to perform military duty as the one referred, but he being in every way a fit subject for the Invalid Corps to which he is now assigned. Special orders from the war department forbid his discharge."

Knight's Army Hospital had its share of pretenders. Some fabricated their entire condition while others exaggerated real ailments. Some suffered from diseases hard to diagnose, much less treat. One such enigma was Private Lewis Nettleton, of Company E, Fifteenth Connecticut Volunteers. He suffered from rheumatic heart disease, which was little understood. This would affect his views of health care and its providers, as indicated in letters from Portsmouth, Virginia, during the summer of 1863[4]:

21 July 1863
I hope I shall not have to go into the Regimental Hospital for it is a most miserable place for a sick man. Being in the army has proved to me that the doctors don't know half as much as they pretend to. They cannot tell a sick man from one who is well. I could set two men before them, one shall be sick and the other well and I would bet but high, that they could not tell which is the sick one.

25 July 1863
I can hardly say I am sick, but perhaps "played out." I go to the surgeons every morning and get medicine and am excused from duty but those surgeons don't know much. I think on the whole I am gaining slowly and will be on duty before many days. At home I should be all right again.

Nettleton married in 1866, and had five children, but was unable to find gainful employment. He died in 1876 of rheumatic heart disease. Others fared better and were thankful for their life and limbs.

Some facilities did not offer acute care but a permanent home for those who could not care for themselves. The governor of Wisconsin urged converting a military hospital to an "asylum for military invalids." In November 1864 he recommended that federal grounds in Prairie Du Chien be used "for soldiers disabled from wounds and otherwise in the service of their country unable to obtain a livelihood." Amputees and others permanently disabled who were currently in a hospital or already out of the service were increasing in numbers and ought to be provided. Their inadequate pensions forced them to rely on charity, friends or alms from the public.

Political, social, and economic factors were also in play as hospitals were filled with more than malcontents, malingerers, goldbricks, shirkers, and deserters. One third of those sent to state hospitals returned to duty. Some died and some were too ill or wounded to serve again. Sacrifices were made by many, but some were greater than others.

Dr. Silas Weir Mitchell ran a specialty hospital in Philadelphia devoted to neurological conditions. Their experience with the reluctant warrior was extensive and stressed understanding as well as practicality. If there are no obvious findings in a recruit claiming an illness, then malingering was suspected. The benefit of the doubt was extended to the government and not the recruit.

> The great majority of malingerers consist rather of men who exaggerate real maladies of trifling character, or who feign disease outright. Most just exaggerate. There was an increased stimulus for this caused by large bounties. Many conceal symptoms when entering service and exaggerate in order to be discharged only to re-enter for second bounty. Others hoodwink doctors to get hospital ward duty away from picket and other less desirable duty. The surgeon's duty is return the soldier to duty and give the government rather than the man himself the benefit of the doubt. If he was really a well man, no harm is thus done. If he was suffering from diseases, which we have failed to detect, he is pretty sure to find his way into a hospital again. It may be argued that great injury may thus be done but these cases are almost invariably chronic and thus scarcely irreparably injured by simple journey and attempt Malingering is especially rife in general hospitals where their medical officers are not present and field officers alike. If a soldier had a disorder prior to entering service and hid it, they should be made to duty either in hospital, the Veteran Reserve Corps or else in the field.[5]

The ingenuity of the common soldier was not to be underestimated. Swallowing a cork with pins to stimulate bleeding, applying leeches or corrosive solutions to produce angry-looking skin lesions, tying tourniquets around extremities to produce contractures and edema, and inserting animal parts in various orifices were some of the tricks of the trade. Testes of cocks, the combs of turkeys, and the kidneys of hares were a few of the inserted menagerie parts. The diagnostic tools used by the medical staff included espionage, especially when the suspect was off duty. Observing behavior patterns especially in those who don't know they are being watched is often diagnostic. Electric currents were applied to evaluate paralysis, aphonia (loss of speech), or limb contracture. Cautery was applied to the extremity alleged to have no motor or sensory powers and thus could not move or feel. Orifices could be explored with the ophthalmoscope, laryngoscope, and ear speculum. Ether could be administered to see which limbs were truly paralyzed or contracted.

For chronic and obstinate malingerers, discharge was counterproductive as soldiers reenlisted for yet another bonus, behavior both expensive and debilitating for the army. The most effective approach was returning them to duty with a note saying soldier is a malingerer and assigning them the hardest and dirtiest work on police duty. "Loud complaints should be ignored especially allowing one rogue to throw suspicions on a dozen honest men."[6]

The experience on malingering was the same in the Confederacy, as described in Chisolm's *Manual of Military Surgery* of 1862. The reason treatment fails may be absence of disease.

> Ignorant or infatuated is that physician who believes medicine necessary for every temporary indisposition and who adopts the ruse of prescribing drugs for every person who presents himself for treatment. He diminishes effective strength of a command, and squanders medicines

which are only replaced with trouble and expense. A little moral courage on the part of the medical officer to refuse the applicant as a patient and a word to the commanding officer will gain him the trust of the common soldier. Pass judgment only after careful study. Common areas are pain, rheumatism, deafness, and impaired vision. Painful remedies are not objected to in real disease but there is aversion to them when threatened. Use actual cautery, and repeat it if necessary. Pain continues unremitting despite medications. Catechizing in feigned disease leads to inconsistent and contradictory symptoms.[7]

Bartholow discussed in some depth feigning and its harmful side effects. Listed below is his view of the causes in military service[8]:

1. Bounty soldiers.
2. Danger and hardships of service, marches, guard duty.
3. Lack of promotion or professional success, with lack of respect for superiors.
4. Conduct of regimental medical officer. A desire to be popular amongst the men, many of whom are his friends and neighbors, renders the surgeon lenient in his judgment, and disposed rather to gloss over and hide impostures than to expose and bring the offender to punishment.
5. Transfer of sick and wounded to State hospitals with furloughs to sick and wounded.
6. The very large number of medical discharges. The percentage of men discharged for incurable disorders, from which they soon after surprisingly recover, is not small: indeed, in every village there are one or more instances of the expertness or perseverance of the malingerer or carelessness of the surgeon.
7. Leniency of military authorities in treatment of malingering. There is no summary punishment in volunteers, thus there are no fears on part of malingerer. The worst is return to duty.
8. Lacking reason, monomania, and imitation.

State hospitals for some were safe havens allowing release to nearby homes, if even temporarily. Over-friendly regimental surgeons were cited as a cause of feigning. This was not always the case, as Private Judson Abernathy related on January 14, 1863.

Sad news, Charles Stone of Middlebury died, respected and loved by all. Had it not been for the way he was treated, I believe he would be alive today. He had been complaining for some time and tried to get excused by the surgeon but no this unfortunate personage doesn't excuse any one unless he is ready to drop down. Poor Stone would drag himself back then the officers would make him go out on drill. "Have you been excused by the doctor"? "No." "Will you then get your gun and come along." If a man is not excused by the surgeon he must perform all the duties a well man does. No matter how bad he is. I have seen them go inside a tent where a sick man was and take him by the collar drag him into the street by force, and then drill he must. I never said a word against officers before.

In the three years of its existence the Knight hospital treated 9,547 patients. Of these, 3,000 returned to duty, 1,500 were discharged from service, and 206 died (see Table 5). Many of the remaining were transferred to the Veterans Reserve Corps and to other hospitals. A small number had no place to go and remained on campus. The large number of furloughs was in keeping with the reasons behind creating a state hospital for Connecticut citizens. Patients were sent to their individual homes to recuperate. The desertion rate was 13 percent for a year ending in March 1865 and 4.5 percent for the three years of the hospital's existence. Some cases were designated absent without leave, the result of lack of communication, personal emergencies, and faulty recordkeeping. The hospital death rate of 2.3 percent compares quite favorably with hospitals in Washington, where the rates were as high as 18 percent. The badly wounded and the severely ill often did not survive the initial hospital admission. The severity of illness or injury was the prime determinant of the outcome or mortality rate, rather than the geographical location or differences in the quality of medical care. (See Appendix X.)

Statistics reflected the activity of the army at the Battles of the Wilderness, Spotsylvania, Petersburg and so many other campaigns. For the period May 1 through August 20, 1864, there were 854 admissions, 51 discharges, 64 desertions, 201 returned to duty, 22 deaths, and 56 transferred to the Veterans Reserve Corps. Two of the deaths occurred on furlough while at home.

TABLE 5. KNIGHT U.S. ARMY GENERAL HOSPITAL[9]

	1864–65	1862–65
Number admitted	2,887	9,547
Returned to duty	1,036	3,000
Remaining in hospital	0	0
Discharged	363	1,500
Transferred to other hospital	50	640
Deserted	317	410
Died	65	206
Furloughed	25	2,317
Transferred to VRC		137

No stone was left unturned in providing the best in living conditions and medical and surgical care for Connecticut soldiers. Dr. Jewett reported a decade later on their hospital experience:

Eleven of the deaths were accidental. The small percentage of mortality is attributed to location of hospital. It was situated on an elevated plateau. The soil is dry and sandy. The change to such a location in a northern climate from the influences at work on the sick and wounded in a southern climate was very marked. Patients began to improve before a diagnosis was made. Another cause was Connecticut, being in their own state where families and friends could visit them. The buildings were constructed to give perfect ventilation with shaft and roof ventilation. There were 88 cases of typhoid fever of which 14 died. There were no deaths from hospital gangrene, erysipelas, or pyemia. No case of gangrene originated at hospital but several cases were transferred from hospitals at the south. All improved on admission and all recovered. It speaks volume for location of hospital, that such results were attained, when we consider that no sewers were near the hospital with which to connect sinks and water closets. We entirely used cesspools, and for convalescents ordinary privies with shallow vaults. Frequent dry powdered peat was used to keep out offensive odor. As cesspools filled it was cleaned with deodorizers and a new cesspool constructed. The bandages from patients with gangrene were burned. Grounds were kept free from any offensive accumulations. In April 1865, we were ordered by the war department to close the hospital as soon as men under treatment and convalescent could be discharged. This was accomplished by November 1865. In November, hospital property was sold at auction and the buildings turned over to quartermaster department.[10]

Dr. Jewett's rewards had to be spiritual, as there was little public gratitude demonstrated for the personal and professional sacrifices he and other physicians had made. Only one sentence in the *Hospital Record,* July 17, 1865, gave credit to the key player.

In reviewing the history of the past three years, we feel that the Hospital has been a success largely owing to the unwearied efforts and judicious management of the Surgeon in Charge. The whole medical staff has labored in season and out of season for the good of the patients and the interests of the Government. The probability is that as long as any sick or wounded soldiers remain in this military department so long will the Knight Hospital be kept open for their care and protection.

The hospital newspaper published heartfelt formal thanks from Dr. Jewett to those doctors who so generously and ably practiced with him at this hospital:

> The Surgeon commanding desires to publicly express his regret at parting with them; to bear testimony to their high professional attainments and skill to their success in the treatment of the cases under their charge and to their uniform gentlemanly conduct. It is with unfeigned regret that he is forced to close his official relation with them.

Drs. White and Coggswell received their letters of termination on May 17, 1865, and were asked to submit a bill for final payment. The governor added a request of Coggswell indicating a job well done: "The state may require some special service for the benefit of sick soldiers and if so I would like permission to call on you if it may appear to be necessary." Because of illness William Benedict of Plainfield took that role until April 1866.[11]

Colonel Almy continued his work in New York utilizing detectives to protect soldiers from fraudulent mustering out, back pay and claims. He detailed the location of Connecticut regiments and estimated their arrival home. Secretary Stanton was petitioned for discharge by 100 soldiers of the First Connecticut Cavalry on June 14, 1865. "Families dependent upon us for support and our pay as soldiers is barely sufficient to provide them with the necessaries of life. Many have served from the beginnings — hardships and sufferings consequent upon such service are bringing upon us premature old age."[12] The main units of several regiments mustered out, leaving remnants scattered throughout the South.

Almy suggested providing free transportation home at the expense of the state. "While administrative tasks are being done let soldiers be at home. Many have not been paid for many months and are entirely destitute of means to get home. They lay around the various rail roads and [are] subject to much inconvenience in consequence of inability to pay their fare. If the expense appears too great the amount of the same could be deducted from the pay of each soldier with but little additional trouble and I believe this course would be acceptable to the soldiers and gratifying to their friends." Throughout the summer of 1865, the same problem was cited by other agents in all the major cities. "We need to furnish transportation home for members of returning regiments. Many are penniless. They are obliged to get their fares and are humiliated at railroads."[13]

By the fall, agent Benedict in Washington was still having the surgeon general transfer all sick and wounded soldiers to Knight hospital who were not fit for discharge. Because of demand, the Washington office remained open through December and the New York office until January 31, 1866.

Connecticut regiments were mustering out as a unit. Individual soldiers amongst the sick and wounded had to be located separately to receive authorization for discharge. The Fifteenth Regiment suffered a disastrous defeat weeks before the war's end which resulted in a number of casualties and men taken prisoner. George W. Manville was one such soldier and was a patient in Portsmouth Grove Hospital in Rhode Island. The governor wrote the surgeon in charge, advising him the regiment was "out of service," and recommended either direct discharge or transfer to Knight hospital to accomplish the same goal. The advice was promptly followed.

In June 1865 he enlisted the aid of Secretary of War Stanton concerning Private Andrew Hull of the Twelfth Regiment, who was a paroled prisoner of war. Later, in September

1864, he was wounded and then transferred to Knight hospital. "He is a reenlisted veteran but I am of the opinion that the interests of the service would be promoted by his discharge and ask that it may be granted." And it was.

In September 1865 he again sought and got Stanton's support. "There are quite a number of Connecticut soldiers in the Veterans Reserve Corps some of whom were transferred against their wishes and now belong to regiments that have been mustered out of service. About twenty are at Camp Rendezvous in New Haven whom I would like to have discharged at the earliest practicable time."[14]

The winding down of this temporary military hospital would not be without some rancor, as old grievances seemed to linger. While the time had come to start closing this well-worn hospital, it was not done fast enough for some, as indicated in the *Knight Hospital Record* in May 1865.

> The affair of Sunday,
> We merely state the facts. The board fence, the "horse" and a reduction in the number of passes, were what led to the promulgation of the offensive circular found on the Sutler's building. Capt. Barley's reply was not very conciliatory, nor was his course afterwards regarding the muskets, what would be apt to tame them into submission. The "horse" was demolished because the patients considered it too severe a punishment to be inflicted upon men who are crippled and maimed. The fence would have been torn down, not to spite Major Jewett or Captain Barley for it must be remembered that the fence was built during the temporary absence of Major Jewett and before Captain Barley was assigned here. It was torn down because it shuts out entirely the view of the outside world and really does reflect the idea that the men are convicts or prisoners of war. Regarding passes, perhaps there has been an unnecessary curtailing of the number but in that case a petition respectfully worded to Major Jewett direct would have gained all that was asked for, for he is a reasonable man and has a solicitous regard for the men in his charge and in return is very much liked by them.

With the war ending, so had desertion and the need for devices designed to prevent it. The high board fence and "wooden horse" were removed and existing wards made more presentable to the patients and visiting public.

Discharging large numbers of soldiers posed unique problems. The examining board consisted of Acting Assistant Surgeons Wilcoxson, Casey, and Bishop. They held daily sessions and documented with a stable of clerks those men fit for discharge. Reasons for delay were aptly described in the *Record*:

> Five muster-out rolls were made for each man. Our boys must have patience as it takes time to do these things and it is not intended to keep them here any longer than is necessary. When a sufficient number of men are ready the mustering out officer is notified and he will come down and muster them out and pay all money due them. Those entitled to pensions are discharged with Surgeons' certificates of disability while those discharged under recent orders from the War Department will be mustered out at this hospital by the muster-out officer.

By June 250 patients remained. Most wards were closed, and police guards were no longer on patrol. Many of the nurses, doctors, and medical students had been released. "The grounds look neat and clean due to the vigilant efforts of the general ward master Mr. Downs. Patients are all doing well and anxious to get discharged. The necessary papers are being rapidly made out and a squad leaves daily for Hartford to receive their dues."

On June 21, 1865, Jewett received a letter from Paymaster Gosford of the U.S. Army Pay Office in Hartford. Enlisted volunteers were to be mustered out of service "on account of the Government no longer requiring their services, and are entitled the balance of whatever bounty they may be legally running on." No bounty would be paid to those discharged "who were enlisted under the Act of July 4, 1864, and are clearly shown to be discharged from confirmed disability or as pensioners."[15]

The end was bitter for some and bittersweet for others. In thinned regiments, the bronzed heroes began returning with tattered flags and worn blue coats. As the boats landed, men and women, citizens of all ages and strata cheered. Parades were held and speechifying endless, bountiful dinners were served, and bouquets and wreaths strewn before the feet of the victorious soldiers. Connecticut regiments were finally coming home. On July 8, 1865, the Sixteenth and the Eighteenth Connecticut Volunteer Regiments arrived in Hartford and were "handsomely received. The first ship brought home one hundred and thirty men, the next six hundred. The regiments have seen some very hard fighting." Antietam, Fredericksburg, Gettysburg, and Petersburg were just a few of many battles proudly contested.

New Haven's own, the Fifteenth Volunteers, arrived on a Saturday a few days later. Scores were reposed in a cemetery in New Bern, North Carolina, never to return. The rest of the regiment was expected at three o'clock but were late. As the *Record* commented, "We owe it to ourselves and to the country to the memory of those who have fallen and to the widows and orphans whom they have left behind. A bountiful collation should be provided for every regiment on their arrival home and they should be received with the honors due them. It should be shown in some way that we appreciate the services of our nation's heroes." This sentiment was underlined in a popular song:

> The men did cheer, the boys did shout,
> And the ladies they did all turn out,
> And all felt gay,
> *When Johnnie comes marching home.*

The complex jumble of emotions and social reality of a war's end engulfed returning soldiers and their families. Some came home whole and some did not. The survivors were prime topic of thought, reflected in the following poems in the *Record*.

> *The Return*
> Three years! I wonder if she'll know me!
> I limp a little and I left one arm
> At Petersburg, and I am grown as brown
> As the plump chestnuts on my little farm;
> And I am as shaggy as the chestnut burrs,
> But ripe and sweet within and wholly hers.
>
> The darling! How I long to see her!
> My heart outruns this feeble soldier pace;
> But I remember after I had left,
> A little Charlie comes to take my place;
> Ah! How the laughing three year old brown eyes
> (his mother's eyes) will stare with pleased surprise.
>
> Three years — perhaps I am but dreaming,
> For, like the pilgrim of the long ago,
> I've tugged a weary burden at my back
> Through summer's heat and winter's blinding snow
> Till now, I reach my home, my darling's breast.
> There I can roll my burden off and rest.

The Fatal Letter concerns a little blonde girl awaiting with others the return of her father's regiment. A crumpled letter is given to her mother, indicating he would not be among them.

> "They are coming mother, coming! I can hear their merry feet.
> Ringing out upon the pavement, sounding loud upon the street:
> I can hear the drums a-beating and the fifes a-piping loud,
> And the people all are shouting!—such a happy, happy crowd,
> turning out to greet the soldiers back from battle-field and camp
> Can't you hear them cheering, mother? Don't you hear the steady tramp?
> Oh, how tired they are looking, and how worn their suits of blue!
> You are weeping mother, sobbing whereas I'm so very glad
> I could almost shout with rapture, yet you seem to feel so bad!
> Tell me why your tears are falling, and why all the morning pale.
> It is queer you are so silent when the town is mad with joy
> They are all so very happy that the men are home from war
> Ever since you read that letter you have never ceased to cry
> I can guess the reason, mother, why to bitter grief you yield
> Father is not with the soldiers, they have left him on the field!
> Oh tis pitiful, tis dreadful when the town is wild with joy
> We must stifle thoughts of gladness, we must only sob and cry."

The *Register* could not resist publishing a disgruntled letter about the lack of dispatch in discharging patients, stirring up old charges.

1 July 1865
Complaint about Hospital
There is much complaint here among soldiers in the hospital that they cannot get discharged to which they are entitled by reason of disability due to surgeons being interested in keeping up the hospital. Surgeon Barnes considered suspending several hospitals on that account. A gentleman of New Haven with a sick son at the Knight Hospital has written a communication so severe we barely were able to publish it. He says Jewett is interested in keeping soldiers there, refuses to discharge those that could be and the government is paying for such soldiers in the hospital who should be in the field or at work elsewhere being useful. The soldiers themselves complain bitterly.

What is the use in keeping up so large a military force at the hospital now that the war is over? One would suppose that Uncle Sam would be willing to give up even a sick soldier to friends who are willing and release the government of expense and care. It is as hard to get one of them out of the hands of a military doctor as it was to "dodge a draft" during the war!

Those who demanded that the hospital be emptied, savaging Dr. Jewett with charges of keeping patients in the hospital just for economic gain, were not responsible for the soldiers' health and welfare. Some had wounds that did not kill but never healed. Others had diseases and injuries for which there was no cure and only palliative treatment available. Patients with amputations, chronic draining wounds, dysentery, recurrent malaria, and a host of other chronic diseases would have disability, suffering, and pain for decades to come. Mary Livermore, head of the Western Sanitary Commission, noted, "It may not be easy to face death on the battle-field but to lay suffering in a hospital bed for months ... requires more courage."[16]

The last edition of the *Record* was dated July 12, 1865. It printed a belated Valentine card: "To the Surgeon in charge, Major Jewett, the gentlemanly Executive officer and efficient surgeon, L. D. Wilcoxson, Assistant Surgeons and clerks, we return our thanks for their kindly feeling toward us, and for many favors; we shall always cherish a kind feeling for all." There was no parade, no flowers, no collation or speeches for the doctors or nurses, stewards or ward clerks.

The relationship between Major Jewett and the governor remained strong. On August 22, 1865, Jewett offered thanks for a minor financial transaction and intervention on his behalf when arrested in October of the year past. "I have the honor to acknowledge the receipt of the check for $44.60 amount of insurance paid for me and to thank you for the trouble you have taken in the matter. I understand that this hospital is to be continued and used for New England men. Please accept my thanks for your two letters to the Secretary of War."[17] It was the secretary who sprang him from jail.

Returning soldiers were being treated at the state hospital, with the Connecticut Hospital Society sending itemized bills to the governor for approval. For the quarter ending October 1865, the bill was $488.76, or enough for about ten soldiers.

What to do with the pavilion buildings and other structures became the governor's concern. Details never eluded him. "The law does not give expressed authority to dispose of the buildings which were erected by the state upon this hospital ground and yet I think it is advisable to sell them and think I would be willing to adopt any solution that will secure a fair value for them. My first impression is that they should be fully described and advertised."[18] They should be sold "at an advantage" by providing good descriptions of each buildings and their condition.

The governor's recommendation to Dr. Jewett was, "I hope you will remain with others in the hospital and for the present take charge of the sick and wounded. Make inventory of buildings, equipment, supplies and decide what belongs to the state and that of the [federal] government."[19]

By March 1866 he was still sorting out property rights in a trip to Washington, confiding to Jewett, "I am not sure that I can make the sale of the property belonging to the U.S. but I leave for Washington tomorrow and will try to do something with the War Department that will resolve the state belongings connected with that property."[20]

Jewett mustered out on January 4, 1866. He wrote to Surgeon General Barnes on November 30, 1865: "I am on duty and engaged in closing up this Hospital under orders from Medical Director Department." He received certification on June 22, 1865, that as of December 9, 1865, he was "appointed to be colonel by brevet in volunteer Force, Army of the United States for faithful and meritorious services." This promotion prompted by the governor carried a financial bonus that would apply only if a pension were awarded allowing payment at the higher rank. Nevertheless, his enemies were ever vigilant:

New Haven Jan 18, 1966
Hon. Edwin M. Stanton
Secretary of War
Dear Sir,

The War Department has on file a full report of the proceedings of a special commission sent to New Haven in September 1864 to investigate charges against Surgeon Jewett of the Knight Hospital in that City. A large number of witnesses were examined. Immediately after the transmission of the report, Dr. Jewett was removed from office. It was understood that in accordance with the usual course in such cases, a court martial would soon follow finally to decide the case. But some months afterward, General Dix restored Surgeon Jewett without trial to his former position, then commanding the Department of the East. The proceeding as far as can be ascertained was entirely arbitrary reversing without evidence the preliminary decision which the department at Washington had made on abundant testimony. The whole matter must have escaped the attention of the authorities at Washington or it would never have been tolerated.

The politician who instigated it felt that they could best accomplish their object by avoiding the War Department where the subject was understood thus inducing General Dix to act on his own authority. The undersigned was at the time out of the country or he would then have entered his most earnest protest against General Dix's course.

I learn by a recent letter that Surgeon Jewett has been honorably discharged and is further recommended for a brevet colonelcy. The object of this letter is simply but earnestly to request that before any such honor be conferred the report referred to be consulted.

Honors to Dr. Jewett are imputations of dishonor and perjury to the witnesses who appeared against him and too innumerable others of our citizens who approved of the finding of the original commission.

John A. Porter
Late professor Organic Chemistry in Yale College[21]

We learn that the investigation was instigated by a politician, nameless but no doubt of the opposition party. The investigatory commission consisted of one person. No witnesses ever presented evidence because no trial was ever held. No evidence was ever published in any newspaper or heard in any courtroom. Jewett's fiduciary responsibility was to ensure that the bills were paid and medical care provided. The doctor did more than his duty and was instrumental in the care of the Union's soldiers, saving lives and limbs, making sacrifices personal, professional, and financial with nary a thanks, only continued unfounded criticisms. His financial reward was the monthly salary of a major. The professor was out of country in 1864, did not serve nor was inconvenienced by the war.

The "Patriots," the "Johnnies" of this war came home by the thousands. One million men returned "from the public udder to obtain sustenance elsewhere. It is an immense accession of dependents and labor seekers to a country—and will be seriously felt in all departments of trade and business." After the parades concluded and the band stopped playing, would they have a seat at the table? Justice demanded well-earned job opportunities for returning veterans. One of the lecturers Dr. Jewett brought in was New Yorker George W. Bungay. He assured soldiers that there would be plenty of jobs for them, that they would not have to beg, and that "those who stayed home should be replaced by soldiers."

As the war came to an end, the *Record* reproduced a Washington newspaper editorial of June 1865 on the plight of veterans. The stark reality of returning volunteers was certain to strike a resonant chord in its readers.

> The tramp of soldiers can still [be] heard here, but how changed from a few brief months ago. Then they marched to the front. Now they tread to be mustered out, paymaster in their eye, and home and wife and children and parents and loved ones in their hearts. Surely there is but one national debt we cannot pay and that is to the brave men whose breasts have stood a wall of resistless fire to stop the rolling waves of treason. Let not the people's gratitude find its only expression in words. These men need work-employment. Their life in the field has greatly interrupted their opportunities and facilities for falling into remunerative occupation. Let every good citizen do what he can to ensure these bronzed veterans permanent and profitable employment. Far better this than noisy reception or festival recognition, all well and proper in their way.

This prescription surely should have applied to Dr. Jewett, who was a veteran faced with stark reality. Following the death of Dr. Knight, a new chief of surgery had been appointed; his name should have been Jewett, but it was Bacon. The rare and invaluable experience of running a thousand-bed hospital was over. Would this achievement go to waste? The prospects of returning to the private practice of medicine and the demands of being a surgeon may not have been appealing to a fifty-year-old man with a gimpy knee holding up a 230-pound body. He no longer had a junior partner or an active practice waiting. All those young doctors he had helped train were returning from the war and would double the number of doctors competing for patients in New Haven. Was there another option that could maximize his unique experience and natural talents?

A short story in the *Record* tells of a physician trying to get home in a fierce storm. He struggles in a violent downpour to get his reluctant horse, Don Juan, to cross a bridge over a raging river in the pitch blackness of night. After a successful crossing, he learns from the innkeeper that a miracle had occurred: the bridge had been knocked down hours *before* his crossing. The doctor was so grateful that the horse never worked again and went on to outlive his master, residing in a barn made of mahogany. The doctor's will made provisions for the horse to be buried in the family plot, with the remains in a luxurious coffin.

The Union soldier was the reluctant horse. He carried a frightened passenger, his country, to safe ground in the darkest hour across a raging and violent torrent. The horse was entitled to attention and care from grateful nation.

"How many lives has the war cost," was a cry from the *Register*. The Union estimate alone was 270,000, with an additional 20,000 predicted to die soon after the war was over. Some of the returning veterans came home in a box. Some never came home. They were someone's son, husband, father, uncle, nephew, or brother. They would hear no band playing, nor receive warm hugs or kisses. The "unreturning brave" left bones bleaching in battlefields, in hollow skulls with eyeless sockets, lying in shallow graves. They left "desolate homesteads, mourning friends, and tearful wives with … prattling babes." They left loathsome prisons. Some were maimed and diseased, lingering in hospitals until death mercifully intervened. Sometimes it is not death that is so terrible but the dying. Some New England homes were filled with rejoicing, while others were filled with tears of sorrow and desolation.

The war was two months ended, yet the list of dead got longer and was dutifully posted in the *Record* matter-of-factly, wedged between local, national and hospital news. Two hospital fatalities were recorded for June 1865.

> Died in this Hospital, June 8th, of congestion of the brain, Private Wm. Riley Company B, Thirteenth Regiment Connecticut Volunteers. [He had enlisted December 17, 1861, and served in Virginia and North Carolina through May 1865.]

> The remains of Sergeant Harrison B. Grant, who died in this Hospital on Sunday last, of dropsy, were escorted to the depot by a detachment of the Veterans Reserve Corps, there to be placed aboard the train for South Coventry, where his wife resides.

The governor's final address to the state legislature was in May 1866. A final accounting was made. The 37th Congress paid the state $1.5 million for expenses in "enrolling, enlisting, clothing, arming, equipping, paying and transporting its troop." The costs for hospital buildings were $22,216.91 and for supplies for sick and wounded soldiers at the Knight hospital $5,777.71. "Many of the buildings erected by the State have been enlarged and sealed by the government and are owned jointly by the State and by the United States. If sold in the usual manner the loss might be a large percentage on the cost." Supplies would not be reimbursed. The governor recommended that "all claims for supplies be relinquished on condition that government take the buildings and pay all bills incurred in their erection. War department gave reasonable hope of an early settlement." Claims made for expenditures after January 1863 were disallowed. Other claims disallowed were charges of interest, costs for arresting deserters, damages to property, transportation and subsistence of men who rendezvoused but were not mustered into the service, advertising, telegraphing, claims made for chaplains and second assistant surgeons, the appointment of such officers and all charges for the payment of officers from commissioning to discharge.[22]

The State General Assembly of 1861 appropriated $3001 for payment of personal expenses incurred by the governor in the discharge of his official duties. He declined the money and ordered it used for public purposes. The hospital addition costing $10,597.25 was the result of "a number of highly respected and influential citizens of the state memorializing the executive to enlarge the hospital buildings." The decision to reimburse was up to the legislature based on "the importance of the object attained" and not that it was already done. The new beds were not utilized much, although all knew how they was financed and no payments were forthcoming to the benefactor.[23]

Connecticut fielded 54,882 men of whom 5,690 (10 percent) died. Of the 5,506 wounded, 1,980 succumbed, along with 2,801 to disease. 4,206 were captured and 689 (16 percent) died from prison life. Discharged with disability were 4,824.

CHAPTER SIXTEEN

To South Carolina and Back

Aiken, South Carolina, had two virtues. The town was located in the cooler western part of the state providing a refuge from the hot and fever-ridden summers indigenous to the South. Of equal importance was its spring water, said to heal all manner of maladies and considered beneficial to the sense of well-being. Cotton mills were established in 1845, followed a decade later by mining of kaolin, used in porcelain manufacturing. The longest railroad in the world was the South Carolina Canal and Railroad Company, which connected Aiken and Charleston, at the time the richest city in the world. Fortunes had been made from plantations growing cotton, tobacco, sugarcane, and rice. Residents of Charleston built mansions, rode horses, and basked in mineral waters during the summer months. Providing the wealthy with a cool and disease-free summer seemed to guarantee success. As a local poet proclaimed,

> You'll find the smile of Dixie,
> In Aiken's hills and dells.
> If you are aching, come to Aiken.
> Have an ache, come to Aiken.
> Stop your achin, come to Aiken.
> Aching, not in Aiken.

In February 1865, General William Tecumseh Sherman sent a detachment of Fifth U.S. Cavalry under Judson Kilpatrick to destroy the cotton mills in Graniteville, South Carolina. It was a feint, as the main Union force was sent up the center of the state into North Carolina. Charleston was bypassed but the city of Columbia was not. It was essentially burnt to the ground, consistent with the scorched-earth policy intended to end the war. Fences, posts, buildings, barns, stores, train depots, and anything standing was knocked down, destroyed, or bent permanently out of shape. The treasonous insurrection started and would end there, said Sherman.[1]

Waiting in Aiken were General Joe Wheeler and 2,000 Confederates. The collision was brief: "A crush of horses, flashing of sword blades, five or ten minutes of blind confusion and then those who have not been knocked out of their saddles by their neighbor's horses, and have not cut off their own horses' heads instead of their enemies, find themselves, they know not how, either running away or being run away from."[2] Kilpatrick escaped, admitting to a loss of thirty-one troops and his hat. The western side of the state saw no further action and suffered none of the devastation visited elsewhere.

B.P. Chatfield of Waterbury, Connecticut, was an entrepreneur who wanted to build a grand hotel and sanitarium in Aiken right after the war. This health unit would have 1,000 beds under the charge of P.A. Jewett. His experience in New Haven running a state-of-the-art health care facility assured medical and administrative know-how. The hotel eventually was successful, though a catastrophic fire a decade later led to its demise. The sanitarium closed in two years. Jewett had invested heavily in this enterprise and lost it all.

Jewett, a Connecticut Yankee, chose to relocate in a Confederate state once considered a mortal enemy that had its center cauterized by the Union army, leaving it and the rest of the South bankrupt. Once-wealthy plantation owners had little to no money to spend, could not afford the taxes and were losing their homes. Were northerners likely to visit the charred remnants of a community that some considered traitors, and whose inhabitants were understandably resentful of damn Yankees?

The Jewetts returned home, residing at 340 Chapel Street, not far from their previous house on Wooster Street. This would also be Jewett's office address in a new career. Years before, half the family fortune had been donated outright to the church and Trinity College. The generosity of the Reverend Stephen Jewett viewed fifty years later must have seemed profligate to the surviving Jewetts. The prodigal son was no longer on the staff at Yale Medical School nor would he ever be reinstated. In his two-year absence his patients had been absorbed by doctors who were younger, eager, and available. By 1871 there were ninety-eight physicians in New Haven County and fifty in the city of New Haven. Of the latter group, forty were graduates of Yale Medical School and thus trained by Dr. Jewett.

He was a consultant called in for the "difficult" cases. "Difficult" is often defined as the hopeless or inexplicable cases, patients who are often without financial resources. Jewett's personality lent itself to the medical-legal world. He made an excellent witness, able to endure questioning on the facts of the case and the science of medicine, and he was certain in his opinions. He understood the complexity of questions and was not afraid to employ wit, charm, ridicule, or scorn.

His large graying presence was reassuring and authoritative to a jury. Murder cases, railroad accidents, and insurance company liability cases became Jewett's strong suit. He was consulted on a prominent murder case in East Rock where, with his delicate touch and ability with wounds, he deduced that the blunt scalp wounds were caused by a knife. He found a speck of steel, which was later matched to the knife of the perpetrator, thus solving the crime.

A veteran suffered from severe tooth decay and necrosis of the lower jaw, likely the result of heavy doses of calomel. He had difficulty eating and became desperately ill and unemployable. Jewett told the patient and his wife in clear, unequivocal terms, "If I can tone him up, three weeks hence I will remove the whole jaw." The procedure was accomplished with the tongue anchored to available tissues. Jewett advised, "He may die but he won't swallow his tongue." The surgeon conscientiously performed the post-operative care. This resulted in a patient whose health and ability to function in society was restored. A life could begin anew. He had created a "useful membranous substitute for a jaw." The bill for this success was, "Go to a dentist and get him to provide you with a good set of teeth and then come and show yourself for I think you will be a handsomer man than ever before."[3] A reconstructive surgical procedure was pioneered by America's first plastic surgeon, Dr. Gurdon Buck of New York, to specifically deal with this complication. Flaps of local skin were created in a multistage surgical procedure to rebuild the face. Vulcanized rubber implants replaced absent structures such as the mandible. To the sufferers from this calamitous and debilitating condition, the reconstructive surgery truly was a miracle. The patient regained his strength and returned to his old job at a match factory.

When Jewett was a visiting dignitary at a clinic where a thigh amputation was performed, he was asked to comment privately. He replied, "Yes it was well done only you should have amputated just below his ears, for the patient is not toned up to live and the stump will never heal." He was proved correct. The notion of "toning up" patients so that they would survive surgery, especially for prospective amputations, was stressed in all authoritative texts. Patients suffering from malnutrition, significant blood loss, infection, or dehydration often died after surgery.

As a surgeon Jewett was in advance of the times, skillful and exceedingly benevolent, often performing formidable operations without charge. After the war he would do for a poor soldier whatever service his profession was capable of without reference to compensation. A sailor with nonunion of radius and ulna of long standing was successfully treated. The bill for operation and subsequent care was receipted in full "by the satisfaction of making a good arm."[4]

Jewett continued as a director and consultant to the General Hospital Society of Connecticut, having relinquished the secretary position in 1864 after twenty years of service. He held several positions with the Connecticut Medical Society (CMS), including vice president in 1874 and president the following year. His presidential address concerned the testimony of medical experts in cases of alleged insanity in criminal trials, an area in which he was now expert, having testified in several New England states and Pennsylvania. He was one of a committee of three on a bill before the state legislature concerning licensure of doctors and credentialing, including oral and written examinations. His experience as a member of the medical board during the war was critical. A seven-part resolution was introduced and then tabled. He realized that it was political poison and could not be pressed on his reluctant colleagues. Jewett was president of the State Pharmacy Commission (founded in 1881), was a fellow of the New York and New Haven Medical Societies, and was still considered the New England area's most prominent surgeon and medical-legal authority.

As their numbers escalated, the sick and wounded soldiers and thousands of amputees became more conspicuous to the public, the government, and profiteers. How to support these soldiers along with their dependent families was a critical concern. War offers the enterprising and unscrupulous entrepreneur limitless opportunities. That a profit could be made from the fighting man's pension and bounty became clear. The following ad was published in 1864 in the *Knight Hospital Record*, the *Palladium*, and the *Register*.

Wounded Soldiers
S. B. Gilbert
Notary Public, General Claim Agent (Duly licensed by the United States)
Applies For United States Pensions, Bounties and Back Pay
For families of Deceased Soldiers, also for Discharged Soldiers

$100 Bounty due soldiers discharged on account of wounds received in battle, promptly collected.

Claims against the State of Connecticut due Soldiers' families, and claims of every description promptly attended to.

Parties from out of the City can have their business done by mail.

Mr. Gilbert did provide a service. He wrote to Regimental Surgeon Hubert Vincent Holcombe of the Fifteenth Connecticut Volunteers in February 1865: "I am collecting the pension for M. Clark Company E. He had a disease called 'congestive fever.' Send me a form filled out. No postage is required on your letter to the department." A month later, he writes on the same subject, "I wrote you 3 February for certification for widow of Theodore M. Clark. You state his disease [heart disease] existed before his enlistment. His wife says such is not the case and she can prove he was sound and healthy when he enlisted. A certificate such as you speak would be of no benefit unless they were to prove him in good health at enlistment. Would you give any different certificate from what you stated?"[5] The soldier was discharged from the army on February 4, 1863, having served six months, and despite the facts of the case the widow received a pension. Gilbert thus earned his fee. Having ailments certified as service-connected was a stock with both growth and value components.

The revolving door of employment in Washington, D.C., where government employees became entrepreneurs in a closely related private sector, was in full swing even then. Negotiating in the government's corridors of power could be lucrative. A former soldier, J. Lawrence Jr., worked in an auditor's office of a New York regiment. He formed his own company, advertising as a claims agent in Washington, D.C.:

> Having been in the Government Department at Washington City D.C. for more than a year, we take leave to call your attention to the fact, that we have a thorough knowledge of all Government accounts, and consequently can prepare and prosecute claims of any and all description with dispatch and to the entire satisfaction to the claimant. Particular attention paid to army officers' claims. Quartermasters' vouchers cashed. Back pay, Bounty, Pensions of discharged and deceased officers and soldiers procured. Our motto is, "pay when the work is satisfactorily done." The average price for collecting is $25, though we attend to some cases for $5. Should you wish us to do your work, fill the blank Power of Attorney here attached.[6]

A local provost marshal described the lot of Emile de Speyer, a substitute private from Bridgeport who spoke poor English. "He fell into the hands of a broker in New York City whom he claims he can identify who swindled him of both his private and substitute money." Obtaining a proper pension was of great importance, but there were hurdles to overcome besides just being eligible. Detailed warnings were posted in several newspapers, including the *Record*. "Exorbitant fees are charged for collecting bounties and pensions due soldier's widows. Not more than ten dollars is justified for service or a $300 fine or imprisonment for two years. C.G. Werbe in Indianapolis was found guilty of charging a widow $100." In New York City there were "numerous arrests of recruiting officers, mustering officer, substitute brokers, internal revenue assessors and others connected with the enlisting business."

The governor saw theft for what it was, advising Secretary Stanton on necessary punishment for this criminal enterprise in February 1864.

> There have been great frauds committed against the government by men who have acted as substitute brokers and who have induced men to enlist for the purpose of obtaining the bounties and then aided in their desertion. It is reported and believed that they have gone so far as to color the hair and obtain false teeth from old men and thus deceive government officials. I am of the opinion that a special agent appointed by the war department could arrest and convict so many of them as to lead the people to have a higher regard for authority of the government and I recommend William H. Riley.

In June 1865 the *Record* continued educating its readers about "The Sharpers and the Discharged Soldiers." Paymasters were instructed to make payments only to the soldier who could properly sign. No checks were to be sent to agents, notary public or lawyer.

We would caution all our soldiers who are being discharged, to be on the lookout for the sharpers who infest every city in the Union, and who under the garb of friends and pretended claim agents and government officials and the like, worm themselves into the confidence of the soldier and rob and cheat you out of your hard earned money. Many instances have come to light, where soldiers have lost all they had by these scoundrels, and it is worthwhile for every soldier to be on his guard against the villains.

"Swindlers and irresponsible claim agents" were taking advantage of the vulnerable and expectant soldier. A *Hartford Daily Courant* editorial warned the unwary of the dangers in losing well-earned benefits. The newspaper decried self-appointed "substitute brokers" as well as recruiting and pension agencies that contained "a good many shysters." In the next edition, the paper then corrected itself to appease advertisers, claiming they "did not mean to reflect on honorable Hartford brokers, referring to out of Towner's only." New Haven papers also reported "exorbitant charges by claims agents for collecting bounties and pensions due soldier's widows."

The U.S. Sanitary Commission then offered the same service at no charge in a bureau of employment for disabled and discharged soldiers and sailors. Its secretary, Frederick Law Olmstead, had warned the governor to appoint "suitable trustees for the men of each regiment. The moneys should be distributed among the honest people of Connecticut rather than among the camp followers or the liquor dealers in the enemy's country. It would appear that each regiment may be easily induced to return to the state $100,000 per annum."

> The soldiers aid society of New Haven under instructions from parent society are prepared to procure free of charge Pensions, Bounties and Back-pay. Invalid soldiers, and seamen, widows, minor children, dependent mothers and orphan sisters in the order named are entitled to pensions and soldiers and seamen discharged on account of wounds received; those who have served two years and more; widows of soldiers and seamen and their children, fathers, and mothers, brothers and sisters in the order named. If residents of the United States, they are entitled to Bounties.[7]

The requirements for pension applications were two witnesses confirming identity of the applicant and facts of the claim. Also required was a post office address in the county applied to and a fee of twenty-five dollars payable only if a pension was issued. The pension could not be attached for liability or debts owed.

In June 1879, Dr. Jewett, age sixty-three, applied for a disability pension based on the knee injury which occurred on Good Friday, April 14, 1865, while on duty at the hospital. A New Haven Fire Department vehicle collided with his carriage and severely injured his knee. Months later he filed a suit for $5,000 and was awarded $750. The facts of the injury were published in the *Knight Hospital Record* days after the accident.

> We regret to have to record an accident, last Friday afternoon, to Major Jewett. He was riding home in his carriage, and when near the corner of State and Chapel streets, was run into by a hose cart, his carriage smashed to pieces, and himself somewhat injured about the knee. He, however, managed to get around with the help of a cane, and attends to his duties at this Hospital, as usual.

His affidavit of August 1882 for pension application follows.

> While on duty as Surgeon in charge of Knight Hospital I was proceeding from the hospital to office of assistant quartermaster on official business. A hose cart driver at a rapid rate came violently in contact with my carriage crushing the wheels upon the left side of the carriage and throwing me to the pavement. My whole might and force of the blow was received upon my left knee with the result of disabling me from the active performance of my duties in the hospi-

tal although I did ride to the hospital daily and attended to the office duties but was entirely unable from the time until the closing of the hospital to make any of the usual inspections of the buildings and grounds. My knee was badly swollen and painful and remains so up to the present time. My injury has resulted in disabling me to such an extent that I have had to forego practice as a physician to a great extent, where I would have to ascend and descend stairs.[8]

He indicated that he treated himself and listed four doctors who could confirm the facts of the injury and treatment. T.B. Townsend, his former junior partner, was living at the Union League Club in New York City, having retired from private practice at age thirty-seven. His at-large family still lived in New Haven but was absent from the proceedings. Also failing to testify was Jewett's executive officer, L.D. Wilcoxson, who lived just up the street from him at 537 Chapel Street. Dr. David L. Daggett was still practicing in New Haven, and according to the examining commissioner, "Daggett could say neither more nor less than Dr. Lindsley had testified to and being pressed for time by professional engagements, I did not detain him for a deposition."[9] Daggett found time to be a pallbearer at Jewett's funeral and was one of several who gave a eulogy.

The only physician who testified was Dr. Charles Lindsley. He had known Jewett for thirty years both professionally and personally, lived across the street and served under him at the Knight hospital. He admitted he did not see the alleged knee injury but convincingly described the pain and difficulty Jewett suffered for the next thirty years. He described Jewett as being completely unable to perform manual work as a result of the injury. "I know that since an accident he received in 1865 (I did not see the accident) he has been more or less lame. I believe the lameness is due to that accident which was the overturning of his carriage. I have been associated with him frequently in professional capacity and have met him weekly and sometimes daily since that time." When asked how it incapacitated Jewett from performance of manual labor, he answered, "almost entirely." When pressed on the subject, Lindsley added, "It states facts to my knowledge that I have no qualification to make except that I do not wish to be understood that I had personal knowledge of the accident. I was not an eye witness of it." He added that he had examined Jewett's knee condition on a few occasions but that it was self-treated, "the claimant being himself a surgeon." He added that there was no preexisting knee condition, and that "he cannot walk without pain, aggravated by even moderate exercise. Hence he has been disabled to a great extent from pursuing the active duties of his profession."[10]

Dexter R. Wright, Colonel of the Fifteenth Connecticut Volunteers, fully supported Dr. Jewett's affidavit. He noted that Jewett was blameless for the accident and that it occurred en route to a meeting with the assistant quartermaster about hospital matters. This attorney goes on to say, "He is still suffering from said injury, is lame and will probably never recover from said injury." In other words, the injury was service connected, the patient permanently disabled and all that was left was to determine the disability rating.

Dr. E. Bissell recorded an independent examination of Jewett's leg in August 1882, including a sketch with descriptive writings. This physician graduated from Yale Medical School in 1860, was assistant surgeon of the Fifth Connecticut Volunteers approved by Major Jewett, and practiced in New Haven for many years afterwards. He was a prisoner of war, spending time at Libby prison before being exchanged, and also served at the Battles of Chancellorsville, Gettysburg, and Kennesaw Mountain. He diagnosed Jewett's condition as "chronic synovitis from an injury," and described a man six feet, two inches, tall and weighing 260 pounds.

Knee somewhat enlarged, joint is stiff and painful on forcible flexion, slight fluctuation around inner condyle extending in front of patella. Skin is glossy and edematous. There is a cicatrix below the patella. Claimant expresses intense pain when compelled to keep limb in an extended position. There is impaired power of locomotion compelling claimant to use a cane. Circumference of affected knee is 17¾ inches, the unaffected 17 inches. He walks with a limp. He *states* that the exertion of walking any distance or going up any lengthy flight of stairs causing him intense pain for a long period of time. Claimant has extensive varicose veins, which no doubt is traceable to the injury in question.[11]

Physical exam showing a stiff and chronically swollen knee was consistent with traumatic arthritis. A letter from the War Department concerning his military records, however, indicated "no record of disability." He was basically self-treated and no other recorded medical evidence existed. The petition was denied. He applied to the pension board in Hartford County, and again was denied because he did not have a Hartford address. The case was sent to special commissioner George Paschal in Southington, Connecticut, in August 1882. His report follows:

Dr. Charles Lindsley indicates that the pensioner has been totally incapacitated for the performance of manual labor. Dr. Lindsley is a physician of the highest character and standing and I believe unbiased and without interest. I had interviewed a gentleman who is inimical to the pensioner and from whom I expected to get some data to guide me in ascertaining the real merit or demerit of the original claim. While he would not himself testify in the matter it appeared to me that he sought to convey the impression to my mind that the claim has no merit and the pensioner no disability and I was referred to Dr. Daggett as one knowing the facts. Several of the physicians in New Haven were surgeons attached to Knight General Hospital under the pensioner, among them Doctors Daggett and Lindsley and one other who wished that neither his name nor anything he might say to me was to be divulged under any circumstances. I informed him that I could not receive in confidence that which would affect only the right of the party to a pension. But as nothing bearing upon that point on implicating the party criminally was communicated, I presumed that I am bound to regard as sacredly confidential what was communicated. The impression left upon my mind is that a good deal of the old hospital medico-military bickering, personal feeling and politics are mixed up somewhere against the pensioner, who is conceded to stand professionally in the front rank of Connecticut physicians and surgeons.[12]

He concluded, "Pliny Jewett is totally incapacitated for obtaining his subsistence by manual labor from the cause above stated. Judging from his present condition and from the evidence before us it is our belief that the said disability did originate in the service in the line of duty. The disability is permanent." The commissioner allowed accrued monies to be collected from the date of discharge from the service. Jewett had served honorably and ably for three long years, but it took just as long with multiple hearings before his pension was approved. Even soldiers with self-inflicted wounds and documented malingerers received pensions. The government spent on veteran's benefits four times the cost of fighting the war. By 1890 Civil War pensions made up 50 percent of the federal budget. When one considers Dr. Jewett's service record, a monthly pension of twenty-five dollars seems like a bargain for the taxpayer and at least a financial and moral victory for his family. The first pension check was cut for the Jewett family in the summer of 1882. Less than two years later Dr. Jewett was dead.

He was called as an expert witness in a manslaughter trial of defendant Charles Skuce in Providence, Rhode Island, and stayed at the Narragansett Hotel, arriving on a Saturday and soon began having fever and chills. Despite this illness, he performed his role as witness for two days with eyes undimmed and vigor unabated. By the next Sunday, he was "completely prostrated from pneumonia" and was seen by a series of four doctors as his condition worsened. His son Dr. Thomas Jewett was at the bedside, having arrived earlier in the week, his wife too ill to travel. A deathwatch was maintained, with both New Haven newspapers giving the latest bulletins on Dr. Jewett's status in bold print, on the front page and above the day's headline. The *Register* reported on April 9, 1884, on the very top of page one this headline:

Critically Ill
Reports from bedside last night gave little hope for recovery.
At 2 P.M. a telegraph by son read "No change, chances for recovery slight."
At 8:30 P.M. "No change, prepare for the worst."
The interpretation is that Dr. Jewett is already dead.

This was the same newspaper that trumpeted the "necessary" arrest of this man some years earlier and decried his early release from incarceration and lack of subsequent prosecution. They then reminded the public six months later of this injustice, reaccusing him of the same charges. The tune now sung was "When people start saying nice things about you, it means you are dead." The *Register* gushed on.

During the war, he was remarkable, and able and successful. Many veteran soldiers who are alive today can bear witness to Jewett's kindness and skillful attention. It was largely due to his ability and zeal that this hospital succeeded. Dr. Jewett is a man of massive physical proportions and a noticeable figure in the streets. No doctor in New Haven had wider personal acquaintance or received more friendly greetings in his rides and walks. He had a genial character, a ready wit, and was courteous.

It was another Good Friday, April 10, 1884, at 7:40 A.M. when Pliny Adams Jewett finished his earthly tour of duty and had his final mustering out. Pneumonia with cardiac complications was thought to be the cause of death.[13] The governor commented, "The city seemed gloomy after the telegraph announced his death, everybody that heard it felt a great man had died." An anonymous veteran wrote his tribute, "Many veterans of the late war from wounds or disease were like other inmates at the Knight General Hospital. We have profound regret on the death of Dr. Jewett. He was a Good Samaritan of that institution. So long as we live we shall hold him in tender and grateful remembrance for his skill and fatherly care. To him, very many of us under God owe our lives."

Funeral services were held at St. Paul's Church. The casket was covered with plain broadcloth; in accordance with the family's wishes, no flowers were present. Dr. Charles Lindsley served as master of ceremonies as Drs. Hubbard, White, Daggett, and Bartlett gave eulogies. Seventeen physicians attended, mostly from New Haven. Among the pallbearers were Drs. Ives, Daggett, and Wilcoxson. Dignitaries, political figures, and newspaper reporters helped fill the church to overflowing. Dr. Hubbard, another Knight hospital staff member, described him as "the light of the medical school in 1846," and said that he considered him a "genial friend and honorable counselor."

If ninety percent of life is just showing up, Dr. Lindsley was valedictorian of his class. He alone testified for Jewett at the pension hearing. It was Lindsley who gave an oil portrait of Jewett to the school of medicine. He pronounced his friend and colleague "destined by his dexterous surgical skill, devotion to calling and rare mental abilities to inherit the mantle of his companion and teacher, the pre-eminent and unexcelled Dr. Knight." He reminded the audience that Jewett had "sacrificed his fortune in a venture that brought him no reward but profit to others. He died poor in this world's goods but rich in esteem of our profession."

Jewett was the preeminent star of the world of surgery and medical school in the prewar era. He was "a genial friend, an honorable counselor, the necessary assistant of Knight, and the ablest surgeon in the state."

His old nemesis, the *Register*, placed his name in bold letters on April 17, 1884, getting the day he died and a few other particulars wrong but still offering an olive branch, albeit a bit late for the dead surgeon to appreciate. Included was the doctor's arrest twenty years earlier, in case their older readers had forgotten and the new ones did not know.

> Dr. Pliny A. Jewett died Thursday. Few professional men of New Haven have in the past thirty years been so universally known at home or have earned themselves as widely extended reputation abroad. Of strikingly commanding personal appearance and signatory frank and courteous in bearing he had long professional life of talents of the highest order, inspired confidence and personal friendship to an extent seldom equaled in life of a single individual. At the start of the war he had a very extensive surgical practice (in rank next to Knight and Hooker). The Doctor's arrest upon charges, which on full examination failed to justify, and he was fully exonerated and reinstated. His duties at the hospital with as many as 900 patients in all stages of disability from wounds and disease compelled the entire relinquishment of the private practice which went to T. B. Townsend who had been a student of Jewett.

The governor wrote "A Personal Tribute" in the same issue. Jewett is described as "a rare success," of "strong body and mind," and a man who "followed the impulse of his nature." There was no case or situation too formidable. He was an "unselfish man who never valued money as equivalent for service rendered and who rendered much professional service for free and as much as for pay."

The *Palladium* simply quoted the New Haven Medical Society, whose special meeting at the home of Dr. Beckwith memorialized the passing with the following tribute:

> Dr. Knight many years his senior had Jewett as an assistant. He refused for years to longer rely on himself without aid and support of Dr. Jewett. There was enormous gratitude for difficult and critical professional service for which he neither asked for nor expected reward. He did not care for money nor did he let it stand in the way when he could relieve suffering and save life. He rendered service without fee and paid for prescriptions and mechanical devices out of his own shallow pocket. Dr. Jewett was unselfish, generous and liberal to a fault, to the point of impoverishing himself and his family. He made himself at all times agreeable and accessible to high and low, rich and poor. He performed formidable operations without charge. After the war, he rendered service to soldiers free.

All had a Pliny story to tell. This was a large man in many ways, almost bigger than life. They talked about his sound judgment in diagnosis, his comforting and encouraging presence, and his rare operative skill during surgery. Two formal obituary columns were written. One appeared in the *Medical and Surgical Reporter*: "During the war he relinquished everything else and devoted himself to the care of the wounded and disabled soldiers placed under his treatment at Knight Military Hospital." The relationship with the past chief of surgery was underlined. "Knight had no son of his own, so the two got along well. Knight seldom undertook an operation unless Jewett was with him." He was "Knight's adopted son." The arrest was mentioned and dismissed: "He was briefly held at Fort Lafayette prison although the cause was unknown. This was possibly because he did his duties 'without going through channels.' But he was fully exonerated and reinstated losing neither rank nor pay, but upset having to bless his enemy." It was in matters of money that he was not a success. Not only was he prodigal, he was convivial.

The second obituary was published in the *Proceedings of the CMS*: "None was more

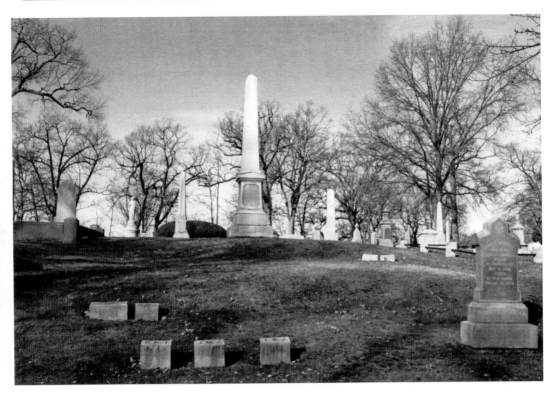

Jewett family plot in Evergreen Cemetery, New Haven, Connecticut (author's collection).

ambitious for professional usefulness and distinction. None was more zealous in guarding the integrity and honor of its members, no one more relentless to its ever-seeming foes." Mention is made of an autocratic father and the son inheriting the same disposition. His "quick and able intellect" combined with a physical presence that fitted perfectly a command position. He was "a man positive in his opinions, forcible in their expression, vehement in their defense, contravening opposite opinions with a curious intermingling of facts, ridicule, reasoning and sarcasm." In surgery he achieved the highest reputation, visiting most of the towns of the state. He was often fearless, successfully operating where other surgeons had deemed an operation impracticable.

The Jewett family plot lies in the Evergreen Cemetery in New Haven. It is populated by the bluebloods and the well-to-do of bygone eras. At the top of a small hill is the main monument, a white four-sided spire that extends upward nine feet. On one surface are engraved the names of the Reverend Jewett and his wife, dead at age seventy-eight and seventy-four, respectively. On another surface are the names of Pliny Jewett, his wife, and eldest son, dead at age sixty-eight, sixty, and thirty-four, respectively. On the third side appear the names of Pliny's younger brother and his wife, both aged twenty-seven at death; it was their son who was killed at Appomattox. On the fourth side are engraved the names of Pliny's son who died in 1902 in Seattle and an adopted daughter of the clergyman.

The land slopes down and away from the monument. Just off the road are two small white tombstones or markers. They are engraved with the letters P. A. J. on one and T. B. J. on another. One marker represents the namesake and nephew of Dr. Jewett and the other his beloved firstborn son, Timothy, who became a physician and died just a few years after his father from infection. These small monuments are proof that a living, breathing person once lived and then died. This was not a blood-soaked field of battle but one of eternal rest where all participants are covered with the same blanket of earth. Here Pliny was gathered with his kin. Biblical lore says it is he who brings up, not he who begets, who is the true father. By that reckoning, is it not fitting and proper for Dr. Jewett to oversee the final resting place of his surrogate and natural born sons, each of whom died so young? In times of peace, it is the sons who bury the fathers but in times of war, it is the fathers who bury the sons.

Epilogue

One out of 12 soldiers died. Americans died from disease at twice the rate from wounds, in the Mexican War seven times and in the Crimean four. (See Appendix XI.)[1]

The level of scientific development determines whether limb and life can be saved. Today an effective and scientifically based treatment is available for most of the 152 diagnostic categories listed in the monthly regimental reports. Knowing the causes of disease and having the means to influence their natural course greatly improves morbidity and mortality. The time from injury to treatment was reduced from days to minutes due to the helicopter, which, combined with truly effective treatments, dramatically affects patient outcomes. The wounded patients in a Civil War hospital had a mortality rate of 13.8%, compared to 1.5% in the Vietnam War, and 0.5% in the Iraq conflict. The comparison of combat medical experience in past wars reflects advancing technology. (See Appendix XII.) Certain numbers do not change. The commonest cause of death on the battlefield is still exsanguination. As the severity of wounds produced by modern weapons increases, the ability to repair becomes more difficult, if not impossible.[2]

How one proceeds from forty hospital beds to 136,894, from no general hospitals to 202, from 107 medical officers to over 11,000, and from a yearly medical expense of $115,000 to $1,594,650 is a journey worthy of study. For $3.50 a week, each soldier was furnished with rations, quarters, medications, and round-the-clock availability of doctors and nursing staff. The program was run and financed primarily but not exclusively by the federal government. This was a successful experiment in the delivery of universal health care in a mostly single-payer system. To be sure, the State of Connecticut, the City of New Haven, Yale College, private citizens and especially Governor Buckingham contributed in financial and other ways.

The federal government clearly had partners willing and able to do whatever was necessary. In this model all health care providers were on salary, paid for by Washington. Some doctors supplemented this with fee-for-service private practice. The land upon which the hospital sat, the eggs and bread patients ate, the beds and sheets they slept on, the drugs and medical equipment they were treated with, the post office and police department — all were paid for by Uncle Sam. It demonstrated an unprecedented effort to provide state-of-the-art health care to millions of soldiers in the midst of an enormously destructive civil war. The political, economic, religious and social fabric of this society provided the framework from which the doctors, nurses, and other personnel provided health care at this newly created institution.

How would today's medical establishment provide treatment for 1.1 million new cases of any disease thrust on an already taxed medical system? How would we provide care for the 23,000 casualties sustained in one day at the Battle of Antietam or the 52,000 casualties in three days at the Battle of Gettysburg? These were not atomized patients but people still whole who required all the health care available. Are there enough ambulances in the world today to evacuate in a timely fashion such a large number of casualties, much less provide appropriate and definitive treatment? Amputations can be consummated in minutes. Modern limb-saving surgery takes hours. Head, chest and abdominal surgeries now possible are also extensive users of time and personnel. Can we learn from the past, build on it, and provide our own template for the future?

Medicine is both art and science, which makes its measurements all the more difficult. The science involved may be incidental to policies that are actually followed. As Oliver Wendell Holmes noted in 1860, "The truth is that medicine, professedly founded on observation, is as sensitive to outside influences, political, religious, philosophical, imaginative, as is the barometer to the changes of atmospheric density." Looking through the prism of history, we need to understand what happened and learn from the triumphs and the mistakes. What is considered a good or even acceptable result from treatment varies with time and place. A leg healed and viable from injury but somewhat shortened and not quite straight was a gift from God in the 1860s but today might be a source for litigation.

The ruling class was white, male, protestant, and Anglo-Saxon. They were sons of physicians, clergymen, lawyers, and businessmen who would lead and make whatever sacrifices were required. Some sacrifices are rewarded, some are voluntary and some mandatory. The pagan ritual of individual human sacrifice has been replaced by mass deaths in a process called war. The consequence of responding to the country's call to duty determines who makes the sacrifices. Who shall serve, you or me, your son or mine?

Each generation must struggle with these changing definitions and parameters. Ethics, morals, religious beliefs, national values, and ethnic background may each play a role. In 1862 Governor Buckingham asked his citizens to leave their businesses, farms, homes and family to fight, risking loss of limb and life. The response was overwhelming. One hundred and thirty years later another Connecticut governor, facing financial calamity, proposed 4.5% income taxes, resulting in the largest crowd in state history surrounding the capital, with spasms of rioting and burning in effigy.

What are the reasons to ask a citizen to risk life and limb? Are they duty, honor, and country? The apocalyptic horses of war gallop on and do so with a casual but gruesome regularity. The country's existence and our way of life are at stake. Your duty is to preserve and protect your country. This will end all wars. People are suffering and dying, we must go and save them. Let us bring freedom and liberty and make the world safe for democracy.

Henry Ingersoll Bowditch, an abolitionist physician and pro-war, sacrificed his son Nathaniel to the guns to put down the rebellion. He remarked to his medical students, "The profession of medicine is man's noblest work, and the physician God's vice regent on earth." One of Dr. Bowditch's pallbearers extolled his nobility and lifelong studiousness and hard work. "Youth should kindle its torch at the funeral pyre of the best and the noblest past." Dr. Benjamin Spock in the 1960s risked his career and imprisonment opposing war that he saw as at odds with his conscience and life's work.

War has been a most valuable school for surgery where exposure to the charnel houses of death from the battlefield or from disease is the doctor's fate. The soldier may be stricken with fear and panic but the physician must persevere and face the onslaught without flinching or hesitation. Self-sacrifice is required to face these horrors.

Dealing with ignorance, prejudice, superstition, dogma and fanaticism requires a surgeon with principle and a reservoir of stamina. Repetition is the hallmark of education, but of facts, not baseless opinion. What works rather than what was traditionally done must be the goal. It is better to admit not knowing than give useless or dangerous advice. Too often authority trumps facts as the basis for treatment.

The results of the Civil War generation's efforts were impressive and inspiring, considering where they started and the distance traveled. The intricacies, difficulties and frustrations that were overcome would bedevil the angels. Creating an all-inclusive health care system for several million soldiers was achieved amidst the direst of circumstances. Their accomplishments allowed a great nation to emerge onto the world stage and demonstrate what a free society is capable of. Those of us fortunate enough to represent the latest generation of this heritage, a millennia-long union of physicians, nurses, and other health care providers, can look back with pride and admiration in the hope that we can continue this proud advance with efficiency, excellence and courage. Our challenge was proclaimed in Lincoln's Second Inaugural Address: "To bind up the nation's wounds, to care for him who shall have borne the battle and for his widow and his orphan."

Appendices

I. Townsend's Charges

Procedure	Fee	Procedure	Fee
Visit (long wharf)	$1.00	Dislocated radius reduction	$4.00
Visit	$0.50	Dislocation shoulder	$2.00
Out of town visit	$4.00	Broken arm	$3.00
Out of town visit	$2.00	Fracture dislocation radius	$1.00
Autopsy (state of Ct.)	$30.00	Dislocation elbow	$1.00
Recruits, bill lieutenant	$10.00	Amputation arm	$25.00
Recruits examination	$50.00	Broken leg	$25.00
Soldier certificates (29)	$29.00	Broken leg	$25.00
Prescription	$0.50	Hip fracture	$15.00
Cupping	$2.00	Fracture thigh	$15.00
Vaccination	$0.25	Amputated toe	$5.00
Examining lungs	$2.00	Strapped testicle	$1.00
Inject morphine	$1.00	Hydrocele (officer 15 Ct. V.)	$30.00
Rupture	$2.00	Spermatorrhea	$2.00
Excise tumor	$2.00	Spermatorrhea Paris student	$25.00
Remove foreign body from eye	$1.00	Stricture	$5.00
Injury eye	$1.00	Introducing bladder catheter	$2.00
Cataract	$50.00	Amenorrhea	$2.00
Opacity of cornea (In House)	$0.50	Delivery of placenta	$10.00
Bruise on eye of child	$0.25	Open abscess of mammae	$1.00
Pulling tooth	$0.25	Hemorrhoids	$10.00
Palatine excision	$2.00	Pass bougie	$2.00
Fracture jaw	$3.00	Extirpate testicle	$25.00
Bullet in neck	$2.00	Syphilis	$2.00
Opening of abscess	$0.50	Syphilis	$2.00

Dressing scalp wound	$2.00	Bubo	$2.00
Dressing hand (dog bite)	$1.00	Gonorrhea	$2.00
Hand injury, dressing	$13.00	Irishman (clap)	$5.00
Dressing cut leg	$2.00	Dressing Irishman's hand	$1.00
Opening felon	$0.50	Bill Mitchells Irishman	$1.00
Sprain	$0.50	John York's Irish girl, sprain	$3.00
Amputation finger	$3.00	(three visits)	
Amputation fingers	$5.00	Operation on hand	$8.00
Amputation fingers	$13.00	Excision of bones	$3.00
Amputate hand	$75.00	Wound of radius, artery	$2.50
Thumb dislocation	$2.00		

II. Surgical Cases of Timothy Beers Townsend Reported in *Medical and Surgical History of the War of the Rebellion (MSHWR)*

(1) D. McCarthy, Private, Company C, Second Massachusetts Volunteers. Twenty-two-year-old wounded on August 9, 1862, underwent surgery on September 15, 1862. The original wound was in the right popliteal space (behind the knee joint), and the leg was successfully "amputated through the right thigh by Acting Assistant Surgeon, T. B. Townsend." The patient was discharged on April 26, 1865.

(2) D. A. Johnson, Private, Company E, Forty-third New York Volunteers. Thirty-seven-year-old wounded on November 7, 1863, underwent tibia excision on the day of injury. On July 2, 1864, Acting Assistant Surgeon T. B. Townsend performed circular amputation through the thigh. The patient died of gangrene on August 6, 1864.

(3) H. Nason, Sergeant, Company F, Twenty-eighth Massachusetts Volunteers. Shot wound May 16, 1864, with secondary gangrene. On August 9, 1864, "acting assistant surgeon T. B. Townsend performed secondary amputation at the shoulder joint." The patient died on August 12, 1864. (Secondary amputations, especially in the face of infection, were often fatal.)

(4) B. Heath, Private, Company A, Sixth Connecticut Volunteers. Wounded on May 20, 1864, underwent secondary amputation of his left arm where "bone was sawn off at surgical neck with flap closure," on March 26, 1865. He was discharged on May 23, 1865, and then pensioned.

(5) R. Brown, Private, Company G, Twenty-third Massachusetts Volunteers. Wounded on May 16, 1864, underwent a secondary right circular amputation on September 19, 1864, by Townsend. The same patient had undergone a forearm amputation on the left arm on June 9, 1864. He was discharged on February 7, 1865, and then pensioned.

(6) W. Dexter, Private, Sixth Connecticut Volunteers. Thirty-five-year-old sustained a gunshot wound in Virginia on May 20, 1864, and was admitted to Knight U.S. Army General Hospital on June 13, 1864. The entrance wound was under the spine of the left scapula and extended toward the vicinity of his chest. There was "gangrene of the wound the size of an orange extending deeply into the tissues and in addition there was secondary hemorrhage from branches of axillary artery." On June 18, 1864, to stop the bleeding, the outer third of the sub-clavian artery was ligated. (This vessel runs under the clavicle, becoming the axillary artery in the armpit.) By June 20 there were chills, followed by symptoms of pyaemia. "He was treated by administration of morphia and whiskey and bromine was applied to gangrenous parts." He died on June 24, 1864. A woodcut of the specimen was published in the *MSHWR* with the caption "contributed with history of case by acting assistant Surgeon T. B. Townsend."

Desperate conditions often require desperate solutions. The extensiveness and location of this wound with the spreading of infection would likely be fatal even today. In 1863 Surgeon Goldsmith demonstrated bromine to be of value in treating gangrenous wounds. He recommended debriding (removing dead tissue with a scissor or knife) and then applying bromine to cauterize the wound.[1] Townsend's efforts were state-of-the-art treatment for infected and gangrenous wounds.

(7) J. Jackson, Private, Company K, Ninth Massachusetts Volunteers. He sustained injury to his left leg from a train derailing while being transported from Knight U.S. Army General Hospital to a facility in Massachusetts on October 15, 1864. He had a flap amputation of the left leg two days later and died on October 19, 1864.

III. Graduates of Yale Medical School Dying in Service

Name and Position	Class	Place of Death	Date of Death
M. Leavonworth Asst. Surg., 12th Ct. Vol.	1817	New Orleans, LA	Nov. 1862
Dewitt Lathrop Asst. Surg., 8th Ct. Vol.	1846	New Bern, NC	Apr. 1862
Renson Lyon Surgeon, 28th Ct. Vol.	1853	Port Hudson, LA	Aug. 1863
Lewis Alling Asst. Surg., Hampton Hosp.	1860	Smithville Flats, NY	Sept. 1864
John Welch Asst. Surg., 12th Ct. Vol.	1860	New Orleans, LA	Feb. 1862
Nathanial French Asst. Surg., 50th MA Inf.	1862	Baton Rouge, LA	Apr. 1863

There were three other fatalities of Yale medical graduates. Francis Miller McClellan, a surgeon of the Thirteenth New York Artillery, died in Maspeth, Long Island, in November 1863. Henry Hadley worked for the Sanitary Commission and died in Washington, D.C., in August 1864. On the Confederate side was Samuel Maverick Van Wyck, surgeon of Forrest's Cavalry, who was killed near Princeton, Kentucky, in November 1861.[2]

IV. Surgical Cases of Dr. Charles Lindsley Reported in *MSHWR*

(1) Under the category "Amputation of leg for shot flesh wounds" is listed eighteen-year-old G. Brown, Private, Company C, Ninety-seventh Pennsylvania Volunteers. He was wounded at Petersburg, Virginia, in June 1864. He was admitted to the hospital at Fort Monroe two days later, where Assistant Surgeon E. McClellan noted a gunshot wound to the flesh of the right foot. Private Brown was transferred to Knight hospital, where an amputation was performed. He was then transferred to McDougall Hospital in New York in January 1865. Surgeon Clements noted that a Minié ball had passed through the metatarsus, entering the dorsum of

the foot. Mortification supervened, and the constitutional condition of the patient was feeble. On July 11, Acting Assistant Surgeon C. Lindsley performed the original circular amputation just above the ankle at Knight hospital. Two ligatures were applied, and ether was used as an anesthetic. Healing progressed well for three weeks, after which point the stump sloughed; that was arrested in four or five days. The leg was reamputated in April 1865 on account of "a sloughing ulcer and a cold and blue condition of the stump." The stump healed five weeks after the final operation, and the patient was supplied with an artificial leg about two months afterwards. He was discharged in August 1865 and pensioned. In 1875 the patient noted that the stump was in good condition.

Amputating at the proper level requires experience and skill. Initially not enough bone was removed to allow a viable soft tissue envelope long enough to cover the bone ends. The end result, however, was an ambulatory patient with a useful extremity.

(2) The second case is listed under category "Summary of 347 successful intermediary amputations in forearm for shot injury." Twenty-year-old P. Flansburgh, Private, Company E, Forty-third New York Volunteers, was wounded on May 5, 1864. On May 28 he underwent a circular amputation of his left arm. He was discharged on June 1, 1865.

(3) Under the same category was thirty-seven-year-old B.F. Wyer, Corporal, Company H, Fifty-eighth Massachusetts Volunteers. He was wounded on May 13, 1864, and on May 21 underwent a flap amputation of his left arm by Acting Assistant Surgeon Lindsley. He was discharged on October 18, 1864.

V. Surgical Case of Dr. Timothy H. Bishop Listed in *MSHWR*

1. Listed under the category "Summary of 127 cases of recovery after secondary amputation in middle third of shaft of humerus." Twenty-six-year-old S. Davis, Private, Company B, Sixth Connecticut Volunteers, was wounded on June 17, 1864, and underwent a flap amputation of the left arm by Acting Assistant Surgeon T. H. Bishop on July 26, 1864. He was discharged on April 13, 1865, and received a pension. He was maintained on staff through July 1865.

VI. Surgical Cases of Dr. William B. Casey Listed in *MSHWR*

(1) Under the category "Summary of amputations of leg for complicated shot injuries unattended by fracture" was twenty-six-year-old E. Maguire, Private, Company I, Eighth Connecticut Volunteers, who was wounded in September 1864. In March 1865, Acting Assistant Surgeon W. B. Casey performed amputation of his right leg, which was "gangrenous due to ulceration of the anterior tibial artery." The patient was discharged November 1865.

(2) Under the category "Secondary amputation in lower third of femur for shot fracture" is eighteen-year-old F. Jacobson, Private, Company C, Eleventh Connecticut Volunteers. He was wounded on June 18, 1864, and developed gangrene of his left leg. Dr. Casey performed a circular amputation on August 20, 1864. The patient died on August 26, 1864.

(3) Under the category "Summary of 94 cases of recovery after intermediary amputation in lower third of shaft of humerus" is twenty-five-year-old N. Hinds, Private, Third Vermont Volunteers. He sustained injury on May 5, 1864, and underwent amputation by Dr. Casey on May 27, 1864. He was discharged on February 22, 1865 and received a pension.

The final case was submitted by Dr. Jewett, but Dr. W. B. Casey performed the autopsy.

(4) Thirty-five-year-old L. Stearns, Private, Fourteenth Connecticut Volunteers, was admitted as a transfer patient from Washington, D.C., in February 1865 due to chronic diarrhea. He originally was treated in Washington in September 1863 for acute diarrhea, having been treated in three previous hospitals and been sick six months. He was much emaciated and very feeble, with four to eight thin stools daily. The treatment was with astringents, opiates, tonics, nourishing diet, and stimulants. He gradually sank and died in March 1865. At autopsy, Dr. Casey noted numerous nearly circular patches of ulceration with a deposit of pseudo-membrane in the cecum and ascending colon.

VII. Surgical Cases of Dr. Henry Pierpont Listed in *MSHWR*

(1) Under the category "Excision of testis for shot injuries" was twenty-two-year-old W. N. C., Corporal, Tenth Vermont Volunteers. He was wounded on November 29, 1863, by a gunshot to the right testicle. The ball was cut out, the testicle removed, and the patient transferred to Brattleboro Hospital. A note by Pierpont in 1873 describes the resultant wound ten years later: "The ball entered through adductor longus muscle and thru the gluteus minimus. Wound of exit opens occasionally and also abscesses in inner portion of thigh near the perineum. He is most troubled during warm weather, and was paid a pension September 1873."

(2) Under the category "Shot fractures of the shaft of the humerus" is listed thirty-two-year-old J. Sheffery, Corporal, Fifth New York Volunteers. He was wounded in June 1862 and taken prisoner. He sustained a gunshot wound to the middle third of the left humerus. Prior to his admission, fragments of bone were excised through an incision on the outer side of the arm. He was left with a superficial ulcer and no bony union. He was discharged September 1862 with a pension. In July of 1867, Examiner H. Pierpont of New Haven reported, "Wound upper third of left arm resulting from excision of two thirds of the upper humerus and subsequent necrosis and slough of soft parts. At the present time hand and arm are of no use whatever. The flexors of the hand and fingers are contracted with flexion of wrist to a right angle and the fingers flexed with loss of power to extend either fingers or wrist." The pensioner died in March 1872.

Resecting comminuted fractures, or excising the wound, was thought to be a means of diminishing the chances of infection and promoting wound healing. Small and medium-sized bone fragments were removed, effectively excising the fracture. As the war progressed, this procedure was practiced less and less. It left chronic draining wounds with unstable extremities that were rendered useless, especially so in this case where the radial nerve damage added to the difficulty.

(3) Under category "Intermediary excisions at elbow" is twenty-six-year-old P. Warner, Private, Seventh Ohio Volunteers. He sustained a self-inflicted gunshot wound while loading his gun in March 1862. On April 6, 1862, excision was performed. The surgeon submitted a long report. He noted abscesses and old hemorrhages and fractures of radial head and lateral humeral condyle, "Some difficulty was experienced in dividing the internal ligaments and after the restricted portion had been divided by blunt-pointed bistouries, which by slipping cut my left index finger used as a guide, it was thought by some of the assistants that the nerve had been severed. Whether the bundle divided was the nerve, was not then ascertained. He complains of numbness in little and ring fingers having had he states, sensation in them prior to the operation. The unavoidable inference is that the nerve was injured. On August 1, 1862 he wrote to me that

his arm is doing very well, that the ulcers had healed, that strength in arm was increasing and motion of articulation very perfect. Also that sensation in the little finger was still absent though motion exists." In April 1863, Examiner H. Pierpont of New Haven certified that "[Warner] was wounded through the left elbow joint, resulting in resection of the joint, but has an arm reflecting much credit upon the operating surgeon." In 1873 another surgeon, Rawson of Iowa, noted that "the limb is two and half inches shorter than the right, is one inch smaller below the joint and two and half inches less around the humerus. [The patient] can flex his forearm and carry it to the head but has no power of extension. Can rotate forearm on arm. Circulation is good except tendency in two lesser fingers to coldness."

Intra-operative complications occur, especially in a month-old infected fracture in which anatomy is distorted by edema and scarring. Additional surgery is more difficult because anatomical landmarks are distorted. The candor of the surgeon is refreshing, and his report instructive. Surgeons rarely if ever acknowledge cutting their own fingers as well as intact nerves during a procedure no matter the degree of difficulty or under these circumstances expect thanks for a job well done. He had injured the ulna nerve that runs on the inside of the elbow near the "funny" bone. It supplies sensation to the small and ring finger and muscle power to the hand involving grip and pinch strength, both of which would be greatly diminished. A soldier shooting himself to escape the war might remove a toe or finger, thus allowing discharge with minor pain, disability, or deformity. The acrobatics required to shoot one's own elbow with a long rifle must have been challenging. There were no hard feelings from this patient as his goal was achieved, namely removal from the battlefield and a pension following him home.

(4) Under the category "Fractures of ulna treated by expectation" is listed thirty-one-year-old A. Wilcox, Private, Sixth Connecticut Volunteers. In October 1862, he received a gunshot wound of the ulna just above olecranon. Two days later he underwent surgery by Surgeon Bontecou: "Considerable tumefaction of whole arm induced me to relieve tension of fascia by the knife and lay the arm on a simple straight splint applied to palmer side with ice bag over thin poultice to wound. There was some discharge through December but the bone united." In August 1863, Examiner H. Pierpont of New Haven noted that "[Wilcox] was wounded by a piece of shell in right arm about three inches below elbow joint crushing ulna. The bones are not yet firmly united. The extensors of fingers and hand are contracted so as to prevent the shutting of it." In 1873 another surgeon noted that there was "no motion of the forearm. The hand can only be partly closed on account of adhesion of muscles and skin to the bones."

Increasing pressure in a closed compartment can cause death of muscle, nerve, and other tissues. New York surgeon Bontecou basically performed a pressure-releasing fasciotomy, very rare for that period, as compartment syndrome was unknown. To be effective the procedure need be done within twenty-four hours or sooner to avoid a poorly functioning hand. Nonetheless he had performed a very modern and correct procedure ahead of its time. This surgeon documented many of his cases with albumin print photographs, a new method of medical illustration for research and teaching purposes.

(5) Under the category "Gunshot wound of the skull" appears twenty-five-year-old W. Whitelaw, Private, Second Connecticut Volunteers. On September 19, 1864, at the Battle of Winchester, he sustained a bullet wound that perforated and depressed the frontal bone in the median line. Missile and fragments of bone had been removed before his October 12, 1864, admission to Frederick Hospital. On November 20, 1864, a circular disc of bone the size of a bullet came out of the orifice and was removed by the patient. On October 28, 1864, a surgeon removed two pieces of jagged bone an inch long and one-third of an inch wide. Pension examiner H. Pierpont reported the man incapable of active exertion due to the severe headache and roaring in the ears ensuing upon slight exercise.

Most patients with open head wounds involving skull fracture died due to infection, or cerebritis, an inflammatory process caused by bone fragments embedded in the brain. The roaring noise Whitelaw experienced might have been due to a traumatic arterio-venous aneurysm.

VIII. Surgical Cases of Frederick Levi Dibble Listed in *MSHWR*

(1) Under the category "Summary of 1,157 cases of primary amputations in middle third of femur for shot fracture" is listed twenty-one-year-old A. Grogan, Lieutenant, Company G, Sixth Connecticut Volunteers. He was shot on June 29, 1864, and underwent a left-sided amputation with anterior and posterior flaps. The patient was discharged on November 26, 1864.

(2) Under the category "Summary of 1,029 cases of primary amputations in upper third of leg for shot injuries" appears A. Smith, Private, Third Rhode Island Artillery, who was wounded April 9, 1863. He underwent amputation of the left leg with flap the same day. On July 10, 1863, his right leg was amputated. He was discharged on August 25, 1864.

(3) Under the category "Summary of 151 cases of fatal primary amputations in middle third of bones of leg" is eighteen-year-old R. Valley, Private, Third Rhode Island Artillery. He was wounded in April 1863 when the magazine of a gunboat near Beaufort, South Carolina, exploded. The left tibia fracture was treated with amputation, but the thigh continued to swell, and the stump looked poor. It was reamputated two days after the injury, but the patient later succumbed. He also had an ulna fracture, a fracture of the mid-shaft of the right femur, and fractures of the right tibia and fibula as well. (Infection post amputation, in a multiply injured patient, did not bode well for survival in the absence of intravenous fluids, blood or antibiotics.)

(4) Under the category "172 Cases of double amputation" is listed twenty-three-year-old A. Smith, Private, Third Rhode Island Artillery. He sustained fracture of both legs on April 8, 1863, due to the explosion of the magazine steamer *George Washington*. The following day a flap amputation of the upper third of the left leg was performed. The patient was discharged on August 26, 1864.

(5) Under the category "Shot fractures of scapula" is C. D. S., Corporal, Company H, One-hundredth New York Volunteers. While on picket duty on April 10, 1863, he was wounded and taken prisoner. Surgeon Dibble of the Sixth Connecticut reported, "As his wound was severe he was left by the enemy on the field and was taken to the regimental camp three hours afterward. On April 11, he was removed to a hospital steamer by Surgeon Kittenger who then examined the wounds. Due to a conical rifle ball, the scapula was extensively fractured. He was also shot in ankle and was amputated just above the malleoli. Both wounds became infected, and he died April 30, 1863."

(6) Under the category "Summary of 250 cases of recovery after primary excision at elbow joint for shot injury" is listed thirty-seven-year-old J. Speidel, Lieutenant Colonel, Sixth Connecticut Volunteers. On October 22, 1862 he was hit by canister shot and sustained fracture of the articular surfaces of the right humerus, radius, and ulna. Surgery was performed on October 24, 1862, where Dibble excised "the entire right elbow joint and portion of shaft of humerus through an H incision." It was felt that the procedure might result in a useful arm. The patient was discharged on July 11, 1864, with a pension. Dibble then concluded, "The wound was open and amputation will be necessary eventually." A flail arm with a draining infected wound signifies a painful, useless extremity that could lead to sepsis and death. Thus, Dibble's conclusion was correct as to the poor prognosis for the arm and even the life of this soldier.

IX. Reports from Hospital Steward

1. Register of patients.
2. Prescription and diet book.
3. Case book.
4. Meteorological register.
5. Copies of his registrations, annual returns.
6. Surgeon's Morning Report.
7. Quarterly reports of sick and wounded.
8. Order and letter book.
9. Muster and pay rolls of medical cadets, hospital steward, female nurses and matrons, and of all soldiers on hospital or sick leave and rolls of cooks and nurse for extra-duty pay.
10. Return of Hospital Stores, Furniture, Provisions and Medicine.
11. Requisitions for Medical and Hospital Supplies.
12. Requisitions for Forage, Straw and Fuel.

X. Knight U.S. Army General Hospital Statistics 1863–65

1863	*April*	*May*	*June–July*	*Aug*	*Sept*
Admitted	78	72	245	215	168
Discharged	0	10	2	0	2
Desertions	0	1	2	13	5
Returned to duty	0	0	0	0	11
Transferred	0	0	0	5	0
Died	0	0	0	0	2

1863-64	*Oct*	*Nov*	*Dec*	*Jan '64*	*Feb '64*
Admitted	25	22	28	99	123
Discharged	2	17	13	1	7
Desertions	4	6	7	1	11
Returned to duty	14	93	16	6	16
Transferred	62	0	0	0	0
Died	3	0	0	4	9

1864	*March*	*April*	*May 1–Aug 20*	*Aug 21–31*
Admitted	114	199	854	71
Discharged	5	1	51	0
Desertions	10	16	64	16
Returned to duty	124	3	201	76
Transferred	0	7	56	5
Died	7	7	22	3

1864-65	Sept	Oct	Nov	Dec	Jan
Admitted	341	95	67	85	75
Discharged	47	63	37	35	30
Inpatients	1,083	969	537	432	438
Desertions	34	90	18	21	20
Returned to duty	48	134	77	82	25
Transferred	62	395	8	37	26
Died	4	4	3	2	3
Furloughed	0	0	500	0	0

1865	Feb	March	April	May	June
Admitted	226	75	152	225	79
Discharged	16	30	25	231	340
Remaining in hosp.	563	205	547	484	207
Desertions	15	23	5	11	7
Returned to duty	45	2	72	44	1
Transferred	11	5	50	7	8
Died	3	4	4	3	2

XI. Union Mortalities by Means and Race

Means of Mortality	White	Colored	Total
Killed in battle	42,724	1,514	44,238
Died of wounds	47,914	1,817	49,731
Died of disease	157,004	29,212	186,216
Died of unknown cause	23,347	837	24,184
TOTAL	270,989	33,380	304,369

XII. Mortality Statistics in Five Military Conflicts

	Civil War	World War I	World War II	Korea	Vietnam
No. Serving	3,214,000	4,744,000	16,354,000	5,765,000	3,744,000
Total Casualties	647,000	321,000	1,078,000	158,000	211,000
Deaths: Total	365,000	117,000	407,000	54,000	59,000
During Battle	141,000	54,000	292,000	34,000	47,000
Annual Death Rate/1,000					
Overall	109.5	34.3	12.9	5.5	
During Battle	40.1	14.0	8.6	3.4	
Disease	62.0	16.5	0.6	0.5	
Ratio Killed/Wounded	1/4.7	1/4.2	1/4.1	1/4.1	1/5.6
Rx Time	hrs. to days	>12 hrs.	9.8 hrs.	2.75 hrs.	65 min
Dying of Wounds (Hospital)	13.8%	8.1%	4.5%	2.5%	1.5%

Notes

Prologue

1. George Washington Adams. *Doctors in Blue: The Medical History of the Union Army in the Civil War.* New York: Henry Schuman, 1952.

2. *MSHWR.* Vol. 2, Part 3, Medical Volume, p. 896.

3. Thomas Longmore. *A Treatise on Gunshot Wounds.* Philadelphia: Lippincott, 1862, p. 132.

4. *Knight Hospital Record.* Bound newspaper. October 1864–July 1865. Hartford Medical Society, Farmington, CT.

Chapter One

1. Samuel D. Gross. *A Manual of Military Surgery: Hints on Emergencies of Field, Camp, and Hospital Practice.* Philadelphia: Lippincott, 1861.

2. R. La Roche. *Yellow Fever Considered in Its Historical, Pathological, Etiological, and Therapeutic Relations.* Volumes I and II. Philadelphia, 1855.

3. Ibid.

4. James Paget. *Lectures on Surgical Pathology.* Philadelphia, 1853.

5. John Riddell. "On Yellow Fever." *New Orleans Medical and Surgical Journal* 10 (May 1854): 813–814.

6. Daniel Drake. *A Systematic Treatise Historical, Etiological and Practical of the Principal Diseases of the Interior Valley of North America as They Appear in the Caucasian, African, Indian, and Esquimaux Varieties of Its Populations.* Cincinnati: Winthrop B. Smith & Co., 1850.

7. R. La Roche. *Yellow Fever.*

8. Toby Appel. "The Thomsonian Movement, the Regular Profession, and the State in Antebellum Connecticut: A Case Study of the Repeal of Early Medical Licensing Laws." *Journal of the History of Medicine and Allied Sciences* 65, no. 2 (2010): 153–185.

9. Oliver Wendell Holmes. "Currents and Countercurrents in Medical Science." *MedicalCommunications of the Massachusetts Medical Society*, 2nd ser., 9 (1860): 305–343.

10. U.S. Sanitary Commission. *A Report to the Secretary of War of the Operations of the Sanitary Commission and upon the Sanitary Condition of the Volunteer Army, Its Medical Staff, Hospitals and Hospital Supplies.* December 1861.

11. Ibid.

12. Henry Peck. Letters. Yale University, New Haven, CT.

13. Robert Bartholow. *A Manual of Instructions for Enlisting and Discharging Soldiers.* Philadelphia: Lippincott, 1863.

14. A Physician. *Liquor and Lincoln.* Pamphlet, 1862. Abernathy Papers. U.S. Military History Institute. Carlisle Barracks, PA.

15. *MSHWR.* Vol. 1, Part 3, Medical Volume. Washington, DC: GPO, 1888, p. 890.

16. L. Walker. "Surgery at Yale in 1843: Professor Jonathan Knight's Lectures." *Yale Journal of Biology and Medicine* 74 (2001): 111–137.

17. Hartford Medical Society. Minutes, 1860–1866. Hartford Medical Society, Farmington, CT.

18. George Winston Smith. *Medicines for the Union Army.* Madison, WI: American Institute of the History of Pharmacy, 1962.

19. *MSHWR.* Vol. 3, Part 3, p. 788.

20. Thomas Wentworth Higginson, ed. "Robert Ware," *Harvard Memorial Biographies.* Vol. 1. Cambridge: Sever & Francis, 1866.

21. Lewis J. Nettleton. Diary, Nettleton-Baldwin Family Papers, Department of Manuscripts and Archives, Yale University Library, New Haven, CT.

22. William J. Abernathy. Letters and diaries, 1862–65. Fifteenth Connecticut Volunteers Regiment. U.S. Military History Institute, Carlisle Barracks, PA.

23. Walter Osborne. Letters. New Haven Historical Society, New Haven, CT.

24. Alfred Holcomb. Military Records. National Archives, Washington, DC.

25. Alfred Holcomb. Letters. Twenty-seventh Massachusetts Volunteers. Carlisle Barracks, U.S. Army Archives, Carlisle, PA.

26. Henry Thompson Papers. Duke University Library Special Collections, Durham, NC.

27. George H. B. Maclead. *Notes on the Surgery of the War in the Crimea* Philadelphia: Lippincott, 1862.

28. William H. Van Buren. *Rules for Preserving the Health of the Soldier,* U.S. Sanitary Commission, 1861.

29. Joseph Jones. *Quinine as a Prophylactic against Malarial Fever,* Report to Surgeon General of C.S.A., August 1864.

30. Samuel Gross. *A Manual of Military Surgery: Hints on Emergencies of Field, Camp, and Hospital Practice.* Philadelphia: Lippincott, 1861.

31. Ibid.

32. Oliver Case. Letters. Archives of Simsbury Historical Society, Simsbury, CT.

33. Charles Tripler, George C. Blackman. *Hand-book for the Military Surgeon.* Cincinnati: Robert Clarke, 1861.

34. *New Haven Daily Palladium,* September 12, 1864.

35. Frederick Dibble. "Hygienic Teachings of the Late War," *Proceedings of the Connecticut State Medical Society* (1866).

36. Personal communication.

37. Dibble.

Chapter Two

1. Harold Burr. "Jonathan Knight and the Founding of the Yale School of Medicine." *Yale Journal of Biology and Medicine* 1, no. 6. (1929): 327–343.

2. Samuel Harvey. Surgery of the Past in Connecticut. The Heritage of Connecticut Medicine. New Haven. 1942, p. 180.

3. Ibid.

4. Worthington Hooker. "Biographical Sketch of Jonathan Knight." *Proceedings of the Connecticut Medical Society* (1864): 147–151.

5. Samuel Harvey.

6. *Benham's New Haven Directory, 1863–1864,* New Haven, CT: New Haven Colony Historical Society.

7. Jonathan Knight. "Lectures." *Yale Journal of Biology and Medicine* 74 (2001), pp 111–137.

8. Obituary of Pliny Jewett. *The Medical and Surgical Reporter* (May 1887).

9. Jewett Family Records. Connecticut Historical Society, Hartford.

10. Discourse on the Life of Stephen Jewett. Manuscript, New Haven Historical Society, New Haven, CT.

11. Ibid.

12. Ibid.

13. Ibid.

14. *New Haven Daily Palladium,* September 1839.

15. Pliny A. Jewett. Letters, Manuscript Section, Sterling Library, Yale University, New Haven, CT.

16. Ibid.

17. Samuel Morton. *Illustrations of Pulmonary Consumption, Its Anatomical Characters, Causes, Symptoms and Treatment.* Philadelphia, 1837.

18. A.P. Louis. *Pathological Researches On Phthisis.* Translated from the French with introduction, notes, additions and an essay on treatment by Charles Cowan M.D. (Edinburgh). Revised and altered by Henry I. Bowditch, M.D., 1836.

19. William Osler. "Influence of Louis on American Medicine." *Bulletin of the Johns Hopkins Hospital* 8, nos. 77–78 (August-September 1897): 161–167.

20. *MSHWR.* Vol. 3, Part 3, p. 818.

21. Samuel Morton. *Illustrations of Pulmonary Consumption, Its Anatomical Characters, Causes, Symptoms, and Treatment.* Philadelphia: Key & Biddle, 1837.

22. Carl Ives. "Prophylaxis of Phthisis Pulmonalis." *Proceedings of the Connecticut State Medical Society.* (May 1866).

23. Frederick L. Dibble. "Hygienic Teachings of the Late War," *Proceedings of the Connecticut State Medical Society* (October 1866).

24. *New Haven Daily Palladium,* October 1864.

25. Hannah Barsky, *Guillame Dupuytren: A Surgeon in His Place and Time.* New York: Vantage Press, 1984.

26. Pliny A. Jewett. Jewett family records, Connecticut Historical Society, Hartford.

27. Pliny Jewett Archives. Manuscripts. Sterling Library. Yale University.

28. Medical student dissertations of 1863, Harvey Cushing/John Hay Whitney Medical Library, Medical Historical Library. Yale University, New Haven, CT.

29. Charles S. Tripler and George C. Blackman. *Hand-book for the Military Surgeon.* Cincinnati: Robert Clarke, 1861, pp. 23–29.

Chapter Three

1. Doris Townshend. *Townshend Heritage.* New Haven: New Haven Colony Historical Society, 1971.

2. Personal collection. Surgical set owned by author.

3. Townshend. *Townsend Heritage.*

4. William A. Hammond. *Treatise on Hygiene with Special Reference to the Military Service* (Philadelphia: Lippincott, 1863).

5. William Hammond. Lectures on Venereal Diseases. Philadelphia: Lippincott, 1864, p. 289.

6. *MSHWR.* Part 3, Medical Volume, p. 893.

7. S.C. Gordon. "Reminiscences of the Civil War from a Surgeon's Point of View," in *War Papers Read before the Commandery of the State of Maine.* Vol.1. Portland: Thurston, 1898, pp. 129–144.

8. *MSHWR.* Part 3, Medical Volume, p. 893.

9. Townsend's office ledger and account books.

10. George Rosen. "Fees and Fee Bills: Some Economic Aspects of Medical Practice in Nineteenth-Century America," *Supplements to the Bulletin of the History of Medicine* 6. Baltimore: Johns Hopkins University Press, 1946.

11. Beckwith, Josiah. "Medical Progress." Presidential address, Connecticut State Medical Society, May 29, 1862.

12. Obituary of T.B. Townsend. *New Haven Daily Courier,* April 1, 1893.

Chapter Four

1. Frederick Clayton Waite. *The First Medical College in Vermont: Castleton 1818–1862.* Montpelier: Vermont Historical Society, 1949.

2. Annual Announcement, Cincinnati College of Medicine and Surgery, Session 1861–1862; catalogue, Medical Department, University of Vermont, June 1864; catalogue and circular, Albany Medical College,

December 1865; catalogue, University of Nashville Medical Department, session 1857–1858.

3. Paul Starr. *The Social Transformation of American Medicine*. New York: Basic Books, 1982.

4. Bartlett, Charles. "Medical Licensure in Connecticut." In *The Heritage of Connecticut Medicine*, Herbert Thoms, editor, 126–135. New Haven: [Printed by the Whaples-Bullis company], 1942.

5. Toby Appel. "The Thomsonian Movement, the Regular Profession, and the State in Antebellum Connecticut: A Case Study of the Repeal of Early Medical Licensing Laws." *Journal of the History of Medicine and Allied Sciences* 65, no. 2 (2010): 153–185.

6. William Frederick Norwood. *Medical Education in the United States before the Civil War*. Philadelphia: University of Pennsylvania Press, 1944, pp. 380–386.

7. Frederick Kilgour. *The Library of the Medical Institution of Yale College and Its Catalogue of 1865*. New Haven: Yale University Press, pp. 7–21.

8. Oliver Wendell Holmes. "Currents and Countercurrents in Medical Science." *Medical Communications of the Massachusetts Medical Society* 9, no. 6 (1860): 305–343.

9. Austin Flint. *A Treatise on the Principles and Practice of Medicine*. Philadelphia: Henry C. Lea, 1866.

10. Henry Ingraham Bowditch. The Young Stethoscopist or the Student's Aid to Auscultation. New York, Boston, 1846.

11. Frederick Clayton Waite. *The First Medical College in Vermont: Castleton, 1818–1862*. Montpelier: Vermont Historical Society, 1949.

12. Catalogue of University of Vermont Medical School.

13. Medical student letters to the dean of the Medical Institution of Yale College, 1860s, Harvey Cushing/John Hay Whitney Medical Library, Medical Historical Library, Yale University, New Haven, CT.

14. Medical student dissertations, 1863, Harvey Cushing/John Hay Whitney Medical Library, Medical Historical Library, Yale University, New Haven, CT.

15. Yale Medical School. *Memorial of the Centennial of the Yale Medical School*. New Haven: Yale University Press, 1915.

16. William Henry Welch. "The Relation of Yale to Medicine," *Yale Medical Journal* 8 (1901).

17. Beckwith. *Medical Progress*.

18. Charles Lee. Professor, Material Medica and General Pathology. Address to the Graduating Class of Geneva Medical College. June 22, 1852.

19. Frank Hamilton. *A Treatise on Military Surgery and Hygiene*. New York: Balliere Brothers, 1865.

20. Frederick Law Olmsted, *Hospital Transports: A Memoir of the Embarkation of the Sick and Wounded from the Peninsula of Virginia in the Summer of 1862*. Boston: Ticknor & Fields, 1963, p. 36.

21. *MSHWR*. Part 3, Medical Volume. p. 896.

Chapter Five

1. W. Buckingham. *Memorial Addresses*. Washington; Government Printing Office, 1975, pp. 8, 9.

2. Ibid.

3. Buckingham family correspondence, 1831–1875. Connecticut Historical Society.

4. Nathaniel Hayward papers, 1846–1877. Connecticut Historical Society.

5. Nutmeg. "The Outside Column," *Hartford Courant*, September 4, 1947.

6. Rev. Samuel G. Buckingham. *The Life of William A. Buckingham, The War Governor of Connecticut*. Springfield, MA, 1894.

7. Mike Woshner. *India-Rubber and Gutta-Percha in the Civil War Era*. Alexandria, VA: O'Donnell Publications, 1999, pp. 121–142.

8. Proclamations, 1858–1866. Connecticut Historical Society.

9. Ibid.

10. W.A. Buckingham. Message to Legislature. May 1862.

11. Ibid.

12. W.A. Buckingham. Message to Legislature. May 1863.

13. W.A. Buckingham. Governor's correspondence. Incoming letters October–January 1865. RG 005. Box 25.

14. W.A. Buckingham. Address to Legislature. May 1862.

15. U.S. Sanitary Commission. *A Report to the Secretary of War of the Operations of the Sanitary Commission and upon the Sanitary Condition of the Volunteer Army, Its Medical Staff, Hospitals and Hospital Supplies*. Washington, DC, 1861.

16. W.A. Buckingham. Incoming letters. October 1861–1862. RG 5. Box 86. Connecticut State Library.

17. T.L. Almy. Letter to Secretary Stanton, March 1862. Letters received by secretary of war. Series March 1862–June 1862. National Archives.

18. Buckingham family correspondence 1831–1875. Connecticut Historical Society.

19. Reports from state agents to the governor. Governor's correspondence, Incoming letters. Box 92.

20. Ibid.

21. Ibid.

22. *Hartford Courant*, September 25, 1862.

23. Report to Legislature on State Agents. January 1863.

24. State agents reports. Governor's correspondence. Incoming letters. Box 92.

25. William H. Coggswell, M.D. and William M. White, M.D. Report as special agents to visit Connecticut sick and wounded soldiers in the U.S. General Hospitals. May 1863.

26. Official letter book of Governor Buckingham. July 1863–June 1864. Connecticut State Library.

27. W.A. Buckingham. Military correspondence. Part 2. State agents' reports. RG 005. Box 92.

28. Senator Ferry. Memorial to Buckingham. 1875.

29. John B. Lewis. "Reminiscences of a Civil War Surgeon." Edited by Stanley Weld and David Soskis. *Journal of the History of Medicine and Allied Sciences* 21 (1966): 47–58.

30. W.A. Buckingham. Outgoing letters. Volume 4. RG 005. Connecticut State Library.

31. W.A. Buckingham. Outgoing letters. Volume 5. April–October 1864. RG 005. Connecticut State Library.

32. Ibid.

33. Ibid.

34. William Coggswell, M.D., and William White,

M.D. Report as special agents to visit Connecticut Sick and Wounded soldiers in the U.S. General Hospitals.1864. Ct. State Library.

35. W.A. Buckingham. Office of the Governor. Military correspondence. Medical Board reports 1861–1864. RG 005. Box 93.

36. W.A. Buckingham. Governor's correspondence. Incoming letters July–September 1864. Box 24.

37. Ibid.

38. Ibid.

39. Ibid.

40. W.A. Buckingham. Governor's correspondence. Incoming letters October–January 1865. Box 25.

41. W.A. Buckingham. Governor's correspondence. Incoming letters. Box 24.

42. W.A. Buckingham. Governor's correspondence. Incoming letters October–January 1865. Box 25.

43. W.A. Buckingham. Governor's correspondence. Incoming letters July–September 1864. RG 005. Series 4. Box 24.

44. Ibid.

45. W.A. Buckingham. Outgoing letters. Volume 5.

46. W.A. Buckingham. Incoming letters July–September 1864. Box 24.

47. W.A. Buckingham. Incoming letters October–January 1865. Box 25.

48. W.A. Buckingham. Incoming letters January 1864–November 1864. Box 87.

49. W.A. Buckingham. Incoming letters October–January 1865. RG 005. Box 25.

50. W.A. Buckingham. Incoming letters. Box 24.

51. W.A. Buckingham. Incoming letters. RG 005. Box 24.

52. Ibid.

53. Ibid.

54. Letters received by Secretary of War. National Archives Microfilm Publications Microscopy No. 221.

55. Ibid.

Chapter Six

1. A.J. Phelps. "On the Causation of Disease." U.S. Sanitary Commission. Documents of the United States Sanitary Commission. Vol. 1. New York, 1866.

2. W.A. Buckingham. Governor's correspondence. Incoming letters August 1861. RG 005. Box 13.

3. U.S. Sanitary Commission. *A Report to the Secretary of War of the Operations of the Sanitary Commission and upon the Sanitary Condition of the Volunteer Army, Its Medical Staff, Hospitals and Hospital Supplies.* Washington, DC, December 1861.

4. Connecticut Medical Society. Records and Correspondence, 1861–1865, Connecticut State Library, Hartford, Connecticut.

5. Ibid.

6. Ibid.

7. *Proceedings of Connecticut State Medical Society,* 1957.

8. Letter to C.A. Lindsley. Yale Medical History Library.

9. Obituary of Gurdon Russell. *Proceedings of the Connecticut Medical Society* (1909).

10. Ibid.

11. Stanley Weld. *Connecticut Physicians in the*

12. Ashbel Woodward. "Life and Medical Ethics." *Proceedings of the Connecticut Medical Society* (May 1860): 4–19.

13. Ashbel Woodward. "Vindication of Army Surgeons," *Proceedings of the Connecticut Medical Society* (1863): 256–264.

14. W.A. Buckingham. Medical Board reports 1861–1864. RG 005. Box 93. Connecticut State Library.

15. W.A. Buckingham. Office of Governor's Records. Applications of surgeons. Series 6. Box 62.

16. Ibid.

17. Ibid.

18. Ibid.

19. Ibid.

20. Connecticut Medical Society. Records and Correspondence, 1861–1865. Connecticut State Library. Archives. RG 138.

21. Obituary of M. Leavonworth. *Proceedings of the Connecticut Medical Society* (1866): 269.

22. W.A. Buckingham. Governor's correspondence. Incoming letters June 1859–September 1861. RG 005. Box 85.

23. W.A. Buckingham. Governor's correspondence. Incoming letters October 1861–1862. Box 86.

24. W.A. Buckingham. Applications for surgeons. RG 005. Box 6.

25. Ibid.

26. Connecticut Medical Society Records and Correspondence, 1861–1865. Archive RG 138. Connecticut State Library.

27. Ibid.

28. W.A. Croffut and John M. Morris. *The Military and Civil History of Connecticut during the War of 1861–1865.* New York: Ledyard Bill, 1869.

29. W.A. Buckingham. Incoming letters July–September 1864. Box 24.

30. Applications of surgeons. Office of governor's records. Series 6. Box 62.

31. Ibid.

32. W.A. Buckingham. Military correspondence. Medical Board reports 1861–1864. RG 005. Box 93.

33. Ibid.

34. W.A. Buckingham. Military correspondence. Incoming letters January 1864–November 1864.

35. W.A. Buckingham. Applications of surgeons. Series 6. Box 62.

36. Nathan Mayer. Military and pension files, RG 15, National Archives, Washington, DC.

37. Ibid.

38. Hubert V. Holcombe. Military and pension files, RG 15, National Archives, Washington, DC.

39. Ibid.

40. Connecticut Medical Society Records and Correspondence (1861–1865). RG 138. Connecticut State Library.

41. Frank Hamilton. Letter to army general. Undated, author's collection.

42. Ashbel Woodward. "Vindication of Army Surgeons." *Proceedings of the Connecticut State Medical Society* (May 1863): 256–264.

43. Silas Weir Mitchell. "Some Personal Recollections of the Civil War." *Transactions of the College of Physicians,* 3d series, 27 (1905): 87–94.

44. Ashbel Woodward, "Vindication of Army Surgeons."

45. Walt Whitman. *Specimen Days*. Philadelphia, 1892, p. 35.

Chapter Seven

1. Elliot, S.H. *The Attractions of New Haven, Connecticut; A Guide to the City*. New York, Tibbals & Co. 1869.

2. Ibid.

3. Ibid.

4. Benham's New Haven Directory, 1863–1864.

5. Ibid.

6. Ibid.

Chapter Eight

1. *MSHWR*. Vol. 2, Part 3, pp. 896–965.

2. W.A. Buckingham. Office of Governor's Records. RG 005. Series 6. Box 62.

3. Pliny Jewett. *Semi-Centennial History of the General Hospital Society of Connecticut*. New Haven: Tuttle, Morehouse & Taylor, 1876.

4. Ibid.

5. Ibid.

6. Message of His Excellency to the legislature, May 1860.

7. Governor's correspondence. Incoming letters. June 1859–September 1861. Box 85.

8. Ibid.

9. W.A. Buckingham. Office of Governor's Records. Applications of surgeons. Series 6. Box 62.

10. U.S. Sanitary Commission. *A Report to the Secretary of War of the Operations of the Sanitary Commission and upon the Sanitary Condition of the Volunteer Army, Its Medical Staff, Hospitals and Hospital Supplies*. Washington, DC. December 1861.

11. *MSHWR*. Vol. 1, Part 3, pp. 896–965.

12. Bonnie Ellen Blustein. *Preserve Your Love for Science: Life of William A. Hammond, American Neurologist*. Cambridge: Cambridge University Press, 1991, pp. 66–67.

13. Pliny A. Jewett. Medical Officer File, 1862–1866, RG 94, National Archives, Washington, DC.

14. W.A. Buckingham. Military correspondence. Medical Board reports 1861–1864. RG 005. Box 93. Connecticut State Library.

15. W.A. Buckingham. Applications of surgeons. RG 005. Series 6. Box 62. Connecticut State Library.

16. Pliny A. Jewett. Military records. General and Staff Officer File. National Archives, Washington, DC. RG 94.

17. Ibid.

18. Jewett. *Semi-Centennial History*.

19. Jewett. Military Records. National Archives.

20. *MSHWR*. Vol. 2, Part 3, p. 896.

21. Ibid.

22. *Hartford Daily Courant*, June 12, 1863.

23. Ibid.

24. "The Funeral of Lieut. Col Merwin." *New Haven Palladium*, July 9, 1863.

25. W.A. Buckingham. Incoming letters January–November 1864. Box 87.

26. W.A. Buckingham. Incoming letters July–September 1864. Box 24.

27. Ibid.

28. W.A. Buckingham. Outgoing letters. Volume 5. October 1864–July 1865. RG 005.

29. Ibid.

30. W.A. Buckingham. Incoming letters. RG 005. Box 88.

31. Ibid.

32. W.A. Buckingham. Outgoing letters. October 1864–July 1865. RG 005.

33. Ibid.

34. W.A. Buckingham. Military correspondence. Incoming letters. RG 005. Box 88.

35. *Knight Hospital Record*, 1864–1865, Hartford Medical Society, Farmington, CT.

36. *Knight Hospital Record*, March 1865.

37. Ibid.

38. J.B. Ripley. *Six Soundings*. Philadelphia: James Callen & Son, 1860. p. 155.

39. Oliver Wendell Holmes Jr. *Touched with Fire: Civil War Letters and Diary*. Cambridge, MA: Harvard University Press, 1946.

40. Ichabod Simmons. Funeral Service of Captain Joseph Toy, Simsbury, CT. July 1862. Sterling Library, Manuscripts. Yale University, New Haven, CT.

41. *MSHWR*.

42. Secretary of War. Letters received. National Archives. Microfilm Publications. Roll 228. April–September 1863.

43. Knight General Hospital, reports 1863–1865.

Chapter Nine

1. Thomas Jewett, "Temperaments." MD thesis, Medical Institution of Yale College, 1879.

2. Hubert V. C. Holcombe Collection, Register of Sick and Wounded, Prescription Books, Letters, Connecticut Historical Society, Hartford.

3. U.S. Sanitary Commission, *A Report to the Secretary of War*.

4. U.S. Army Medical Department. Orders and letters. Hospital Department. Fifteenth Connecticut Regiment. RG 13, Box 229.

5. Obituary of Charles A. Lindsley, *Proceedings of the Connecticut Medical Society* (1906).

6. Charles A. Lindsley, "Puerperal Convulsions," *Proceedings of the Connecticut Medical Society* (1858): 71–83.

7. William Carmalt. Obituary of Charles A. Lindsley, M.D. *Proceedings of the Connecticut Medical Society*. Vol. 114 (1906): 292–297.

8. Charles A. Lindlsey, letters, Yale Medical Historical Library, Yale University, New Haven, CT.

9. Henry J. Thompson. Letters and correspondence. Duke University Library Special Collections, Durham, NC.

10. William C. Minor, Acting Assistant Surgeon, post-mortem exams made at the Knight U.S. Army General Hospital, 1864, Harvey Cushing/John Hay Whitney Medical Library, Medical Historical Library, Yale University, New Haven, CT.

11. John Henry Burnham. Military and Pension Records, Sixteenth Connecticut Regiment, National Archives, Washington, DC.

12. Simon Winchester. *The Professor and the Madman.* New York: HarperCollins, 1998.

13. Obituary of William B. Casey. *Proceedings of the Connecticut Medical Society* (1870).

14. William B. Casey. "Essay on Some Diseases of the Cervix Uteri," *Proceedings of the Connecticut Medical Society* (1854): 61–83.

15. Hartford Medical Society, minutes, 1865, Farmington, CT.

16. Casey. "Essay on Some Diseases of the Cervix Uteri."

17. Ibid.

18. E.B. Nye. "Memoir of William B. Casey, M.D." *Proceedings of the Connecticut Medical Society* Vol. III (1870): 403.

19. Obituary of Worthington Hooker. *Proceedings of the Connecticut State Medical Society* (1870).

20. Henry Bronson, "Profess. Charles Hooker, M.D." *Proceedings and Medical Communications of the Connecticut Medical Society* (1867): 144–145.

21. Worthington Hooker. "Dissertation on the Respect Due to the Medical Profession and the Reasons That It Is Not Awarded by the Community." *Proceedings of the Connecticut Medical Society* (1844): 4–48.

22. Worthington Hooker. *Homeopathy, Examination of Its Doctrine and Evidences.* New York: Scribner, 1851.

23. Worthington Hooker. "The Treatment Due from the Medical Profession to Physicians Who Become Homeopathic Practitioners," *Proceedings of the Connecticut Medical Society* (1852).

24. Oliver Wendell Holmes. "Currents and Countercurrents in Medical Science." *Medical Communications of the Massachusetts Medical Society,* 2nd ser., 9 (1860): 305–343.

25. *Journal of Bone and Joint Surgery* (June 2004).

26. Obituary of Henry Pierpont, M.D., *Proceedings of the Connecticut Medical Society* (1892).

27. Obituary of Frederick L. Dibble, M.D. *Proceedings of the Connecticut Medical Society* (1898).

28. Charles Cadwell, *The Old Sixth Regiment* (New Haven: Tuttle, Morehouse & Taylor, 1875).

29. Fred Dibble. Military Records, National Archives, Washington DC.

Chapter Ten

1. J.J. Woodward. *Hospital Steward's Manual.* Philadelphia: Lippincott, 1863, pp. 43–47.

2. Stanley B. Weld. *Connecticut Physicians in the Civil War.* Hartford: Connecticut Civil War Centennial Commission, 1965, p. 45.

3. Letters of application to the Medical Department, microfilm roll 1064, National Archives, Washington DC.

4. Ibid.

5. George Bronson. Hospital Steward letters, Eleventh Connecticut Regiment, U.S. Military History Institute, Carlisle Barracks, PA.

6. J.J. Woodward. *Hospital Steward's Manual.*

7. Frank Bond, court-martial file, RG 153, National Archives, Washington, DC.

8. Charles Morris, court-martial file, RG 153, National Archives, Washington, DC.

9. Surgeon Ferris Jacobs. Third New York Cavalry. Letters of application to the Medical Department, microfilm roll 1064, National Archives, Washington DC.

10. Ibid.

11. Assistant Surgeon Committee to Investigate Charges against the Taking of Illegal Fees. *Journal of Connecticut House of Representatives* (1862).

Chapter Eleven

1. Pliny Adams Jewett. *Semi-Centennial History of the General Hospital Society of Connecticut.* New Haven: Tuttle, Morehouse & Taylor, 1876.

2. Frederick Law Olmsted. *Hospital Transports,* p. 84.

3. Charles S. Tripler and George C. Blackman. *Hand-book for the Military Surgeon.* Cincinnati: Robert Clarke, 1861.

4. Provost Marshal. Letters. RG 110, Draft Registration Records, National Archives, Waltham, MA.

5. Pliny A. Jewett. "Regulations of General Hospital Society of Connecticut," in *Semi-Centennial History of the General Hospital Society of Connecticut.*

6. W.A. Buckingham. Incoming letters. October–January 1865. RG 005. Box 25. Connecticut State Library.

7. Thomas Wentworth Higginson, ed., "Robert Ware," *Harvard Memorial Biographies,* Vol. 1. Cambridge: Sever & Francis, 1866, pp. 238–252.

8. Silas Weir Mitchell. "The Medical Department in the Civil War." *Journal of the American Medical Association* 62 (1914), pp. 1445–1550.

9. Patricia Spain Ward. *Simon Baruch, Rebel in the Ranks of Medicine, 1840–1921.* Tuscaloosa: University of Alabama Press, 1994, p. 47.

10. Letters received by Secretary of War. April–September 1863. National Archives. Microfilm Publications. Roll 228.

11. Edwin L. Bennett vs. Pliny A. Jewett. Habeas Corpus before Judge Dutton of the Supreme Court of Errors. *Hartford Courant,* July 11, 1863.

Chapter Twelve

1. Civil War Draft Registration Records for New England. Medical Register of Men Examined by Surgeon for Exemption. December 1864–April 1865. National Archives, Waltham, MA. RG 110.

2. Ibid.

3. Bartholow, *A Manual of Instructions for Enlisting and Discharging Soldiers,* p.71.

4. Ibid. p. 64.

5. "The Captain of the Provost (A Parody)," Civil War Sheet Music, Library of Congress.

6. Bartholow. *A Manual of Instructions for Enlisting and Discharging Soldiers.*

7. Provost Marshal. Draft Registration Records.

8. Ibid.

9. "How Are You exempt?" Civil War Sheet Music, Library of Congress.

10. Letters sent to Knight General Hospital, 1863–1865, RG 13:45, Box 115, Connecticut State Library, Hartford.

11. John Henry Burnham. Letters. Connecticut State Library.

12. Governor's correspondence. State agents' reports. Box 92. RG 005.

13. Ibid.

14. Ibid.

15. Official letters book of Governor William Buckingham. Volume 1. April 1863–January 1864. RG005. Series 4. Connecticut State Library.

16. Letters received by Secretary of War. National Archives. Microfilm Publications. October 1864.

17. Ibid.

18. Ibid.

19. Provost Marshal. National Archives, Waltham, MA.

20. Ibid.

21. Henry J. Thompson letters, Company B, Fifteenth Connecticut Volunteers, Special Collections Department, Duke University, Durham, NC.

22. Knight Army Hospital, Letters received. Draft Registration Records, National Archives, Waltham, MA.

23. Knight Army Hospital, Letters to Provost Marshal. Draft Registration Records. National Archives, Waltham MA.

24. Knight Army Hospital, letters sent to and received from military commanders relating to sick soldiers, January 1864–March 1865. Civil War Draft Registration Records, National Archives, Waltham, MA.

25. Knight Army Hospital, reports, 1863–1865, Connecticut State Library, Hartford.

26. Knight Army Hospital to the Department of the Provost Marshal, 1863–1865. National Archives, Waltham, MA.

27. Knight Army Hospital. Letters received. Waltham, MA.

28. Knight Army Hospital. Letters sent to and received from military commanders. Waltham, MA.

29. Ibid.

30. Roberts Bartholow. *Sanitary Memoirs of the War of the Rebellion*. New York: U.S. Sanitary Commission, 1867, pp. 3–7.

31. Rev. Samuel G. Buckingham. *The Life of William A. Buckingham, The War Governor of Connecticut.* Springfield, MA, 1894.

32. W.A. Buckingham. Outgoing letters. Volume 5. Connecticut State Library.

33. Knight Army Hospital. Letters received, Draft Registration Records 1863–1865. Waltham, MA.

34. Knight Army Hospital. Letters received. Connecticut State Library.

35. Ibid.

36. Knight Army Hospital, Letters sent to and received from military commanders. Connecticut State Library.

Chapter Thirteen

1. State agents reports. March 1864.

2. Letters of Charles Foote. Fifteenth Regiment. 1862–1865. Connecticut State Library.

3. Letters of Major Eli Osborne. Fifteenth Volunteers. New Haven Historical Society.

4. Letters to Secretary of War. October 1864.

5. Letters received by the Secretary of War. National Archives. Microfilm Publications. October 1864.

6. Ibid.

7. *Knight Hospital Record.* December 1864.

8. Governor's correspondence. Incoming letters July–September 1864. Box 24.

9. W.A. Buckingham. Governor's correspondence. Incoming letters July–September 1864. Box 24.

10. Ibid.

11. W.A. Buckingham. Outgoing letters. Volume 5. October 1864–July 1865. RG 005.

12. Pliny A. Jewett. Letters. Sterling Library, Yale University, New Haven, CT.

13. Walter Ralph Steiner. "The Evolution of Medicine in Connecticut, with the Foundation of the Yale Medical School as Its Notable Achievement." In Yale University, *Memorial of the Centennial of the Yale Medical School.* New Haven: Yale University Press, 1915, pp. 10–33.

14. Prospectus of the "Knight" Medical School. Manuscript. Medical Historical Library, Yale University.

15. Francis Bacon. Register no. 94. Entry 561 Medical officer staff file. National Archives, Washington DC.

16. Ibid.

17. Samuel Harvey. *Surgery of the Past in Connecticut.* The Heritage of Connecticut Medicine. New Haven, 1942, p. 180.

18. William Bigelow. Letters. Seventh Connecticut Volunteers. Simsbury Historical Society, Simsbury, CT.

19. *New Haven Daily Palladium,* July 1864.

20. Blustein. *Preserve Your Love for Science,* pp. 86–87.

21. William A. Hammond. *Defense of Brigadier General William A. Hammond, Surgeon-General, U.S. Army, with His Statement of the Causes Which Led to His Dismissal.* Washington, DC: privately printed, 1864, pp. 8–9.

22. Henry Bowditch. *A Brief Plea for an Ambulance System for the Army of the United States.* Boston: Ticknor & Fields, 1863, pp. 5–8.

23. Governor's correspondence. Incoming letters. Box 88A. RG 005.

24. Ibid.

25. William A. Hammond. *A Defense of Brigadier General Hammond.*

26. W.A. Buckingham. Office of the Governor. Military correspondence. Incoming letters January 1864–November 1864. Connecticut State Library.

27. F.S. Treadway. "A Dissertation on Yellow Fever." M.D. thesis, the Medical Institution of Yale College, 1863. Medical History Library, Yale University.

28. *Columbian Weekly Register,* September 3, 1864.

29. *Columbian Weekly Register,* October 1, 1864.

30. "Grand Torchlight Procession." *Hartford Courant,* November 4, 1864.

31. *Columbian Weekly Register,* November 19, 1864.

32. Pliny A. Jewett. Medical Officers File, 1862–1866, RG 94, National Archives, Washington, DC.

33. Ibid.

34. Ibid.

35. Joseph Vail. Letter, U.S. Army Archives, Carlisle Barracks, Carlisle, PA.

36. Knight General Hospital, endorsements sent and received by surgeons, September 1963–July 1864, Vol. 1, No. 57, RG 110, Draft Registration Records, National Archives, Waltham, MA.

37. Civil War sheet music, Library of Congress.

38. Francis Bacon. Register no. 94. Entry 561. Medical officer staff file. National Archives, Washington DC.

39. Hubert Holcombe Collection, Register of Sick and Wounded, Prescription Books, Letters, Connecticut Historical Society, Hartford.

40. George Page. *Sanitary Commission Bulletin* 1 (1863–1864).

41. William J. Abernathy. Diary 1862–1865, Fifteenth Connecticut Regiment, U.S. Military History Institute, Carlisle Barracks, PA.

42. Ibid.

Chapter Fourteen

1. Pliny A. Jewett, Company E, First Connecticut Cavalry Regiment, Jewett Family Papers, Virginia Historical Society, Richmond.

2. Connecticut Adjutant General's Office, *Record of Service of Connecticut Men in the Army and Navy of the United States during the War of the Rebellion.* Hartford: Case, Lockwood, Brainard, 1889.

3. William Abernathy. Diary 1862–1865.

4. Henry Thompson Papers. Duke University Library Special Collections, Durham, NC.

5. Pliny A. Jewett, Company E, First Connecticut Cavalry Regiment, Jewett Family Papers, Virginia Historical Society, Richmond.

6. Regimental History, First Connecticut Cavalry Volunteers in the War of the Rebellion, 1861–1865, 1889. Connecticut State Library.

7. Carl von Clausewitz. *On War.* Edited and translated by Michael Howard and Peter Parent. Princeton, NJ: Princeton University Press, 1993.

8. Pliny A. Jewett, Company E, First Connecticut Cavalry Regiment, Jewett Family Papers, Virginia Historical Society, Richmond.

Chapter Fifteen

1. *Knight Hospital Record*, April 16, 1865.

2. Phoebe Yates Pember. *A Southern Woman's Story: Life in Confederate Richmond.* New York: G. W. Carleton, 1879, p. 137.

3. Roberts Bartholow. *A Manual of Instructions for Enlisting and Discharging Soldiers*, pp. 88–91.

4. Lewis J. Nettleton, diary, Nettleton-Baldwin Family Papers, Department of Manuscripts and Archives, Yale University Library, New Haven, CT.

5. William W. Keen, Silas Weir Mitchell, and George R. Morehouse, "On Malingering, Especially in Regard to Simulation of Diseases of the Nervous System," *American Journal of Medical Sciences* 48 (1864): 367–372.

6. Ibid.

7. Chisolm, *A Manual of Military Surgery*, pp. 438–446.

8. Bartholow, *A Manual of Instructions for Enlisting and Discharging Soldiers*, pp. 88–91.

9. Knight General Hospital, reports, 1863–1865, RG 13:45, Box 115, Connecticut State Library, Hartford.

10. Pliny A. Jewett, *Semi-Centennial History.*

11. W.A. Buckingham. Outgoing letters.

12. Governor's correspondence. State agents' reports. Box 93. 1865.

13. Ibid.

14. W.A. Buckingham. Official letter book. May 1865–April 1866.

15. Pliny A. Jewett. Letters. Sterling Archives. Yale University, New Haven, CT.

16. Mary Livermore, *My Story of the War: A Woman's Narrative of Four Years of Personal Experience.* Hartford, CT: A.D. Worthington, 1889, p. 286.

17. Governor's correspondence. Incoming letters. Box 88. RG 005.

18. W.A. Buckingham. Official letter book. May 1865–April 1866.

19. Ibid.

20. Ibid.

21. Pliny A. Jewett. Medical Officers File. National Archives, Washington DC.

22. "Governor's Message to Senate and House." *Hartford Courant*, May 1866.

23. Ibid.

Chapter Sixteen

1. Lloyd Lewis. *Sherman: Fighting Prophet.* Lincoln: University of Nebraska Press, 1993.

2. Ibid

3. Obituary of Pliny A. Jewett. *Proceedings of the Connecticut Medical Society* (1887): 169.

4. Ibid.

5. U.S. Army Medical Department, Hospital Department orders and letters to the Fifteenth Connecticut Regiment, RG 13, box 229, Connecticut State Library, Hartford.

6. Lawrence & Co. Claim Agents. Form for Pensions, bounty or back pay. Personal collection.

7. *Knight Hospital Record*, March 1865.

8. Pliny A. Jewett, Medical Officers File. 1862–1866. National Archives, Washington, DC. RG 94.

9. Ibid.

10. Ibid.

11. Ibid.

12. Ibid.

13. *New Haven Daily Palladium*, April 1884.

Epilogue

1. *MSHWR*, Vol. 3, Part 1.

2. Ralph Bellamy, "Combat Trauma Overview," in *Textbook of Military Medicine, Vol. 4: Anesthesia and Perioperative Care of Combat Casualty*, ed. R. Zajtchuck and C. M. Grande. Washington, DC: TMM Publications, 1995, pp. 1–42.

Appendices

1. Middleton Goldsmith, *A Report on Hospital Gangrene, Erysipelas and Pyemia.* Louisville: Bradley & Gilbert, 1863, p. 94.

2. Eliot Ellsworth. *Yale in the Civil War.* New Haven: Yale University Press, 1932.

Bibliography

Abernathy, William J. Letters and diaries 1862–1865. 15th Connecticut Volunteers Regiment. U.S. Military History Institute, Carlisle Barracks, PA.

Adams, George W. *Doctors in Blue: The Medical History of the Union Army in the Civil War*. New York: Henry Schuman, 1952.

Albany Medical College. Catalogue and circular, December 1865.

Andrew, John. An Address to the Graduating Class of the Medical School in the University at Cambridge. Harvard. March 1864.

Appel, Toby. "The Thomsonian Movement, the Regular Profession, and the State in Antebellum Connecticut: A Case Study of the Repeal of Early Medical Licensing Laws." *Journal of the History of Medicine and Allied Sciences* 65, no. 2 (2010): 153–185.

Bacon, Francis. Registry No. 94. Entry 561. Medical officer staff file. National Archives, Washington, DC.

Barsky, Hannah. *Guillame Dupuytren: A Surgeon in His Place and Time*. New York: Vantage Press, 1984.

Bartholow, Roberts. *A Manual of Instructions for Enlisting and Discharging Soldiers: With Special Reference to the Medical Examination of Recruits, and the Detection of Disqualifying and Feigned Diseases*. Philadelphia: J.B. Lippincott, 1863.

_____. *Sanitary Memoirs of the War of the Rebellion*. New York: U.S. Sanitary Commission, 1867. pp. 3–7.

Bartlett, Charles. "Medical Licensure in Connecticut." In *The Heritage of Connecticut Medicine*, Herbert Thoms, editor, 126–135. New Haven: [Printed by the Whaples-Bullis company], 1942.

Bartlett, Elisha. *The History, Diagnosis and Treatment of the Fevers of the United States*. 4th ed. Philadelphia: Lea & Blanchard, 1856.

Beckwith, Josiah. "Medical Progress." Presidential address, Connecticut Medical Society, May 29, 1862.

Bellamy, Ralph F. "Combat Trauma Overview." In *Textbook of Military Medicine*, Vol. 4: *Anesthesia and Perioperative Care of Combat Casualty*, edited by R. Zajtchuck and C. M. Grande, 1–42. Washington, DC: TMM Publications, 1995.

Benham's New Haven Directory 1863–64. New Haven, CT: New Haven Historical Society.

Bigelow, William. Letters. Seventh Connecticut Volunteers. Simsbury Historical Society.

Bishop, Ebenezer, M.D. Obituary. *Proceedings of the Connecticut Medical Society* (1891): 302.

Blustein, Bonnie Ellen. *Preserve Your Love for Science: Life of William A. Hammond, American Neurologist*. Cambridge: Cambridge University Press, 1991.

Bowditch, Henry. *A Brief Plea for an Ambulance System for the Army of the United States*. Boston: Ticknor & Fields, 1863.

_____. *The Young Stethoscopist, or the Student's Aid to Auscultation*. New York, Boston, 1846.

Bronson, George. Hospital Steward Letters. Eleventh Connecticut Regiment. U.S. Military History Institute, Carlisle Barracks, PA.

_____. Pension Records. RG 15. National Archives, Washington, DC.

Buckingham, Rev. Samuel G. *The Life of William A. Buckingham, The War Governor of Connecticut*. Springfield, MA, 1894.

Buckingham, W.A. Memorial Addresses on the Life and Character of William A. Buckingham delivered in the Senate and House of Representatives. Washington, DC: Government Printing Office, 1875.

_____. Message of His Excellency, Governor of Connecticut, to the Legislature. May 1860. New Haven: Carrington and Hotchkiss, State Printers.

_____. Message of His Excellency, Governor of Connecticut, to the Legislature. May 1862. New Haven: Babcock and Sizer, State Printers.

_____. Message of His Excellency, Governor of Connecticut, to the Legislature. December 1862. New Haven: Babcock and Sizer, State Printers.

_____. Military correspondence. Part II. State agents' reports. RG 005. Box 92. Connecticut State Library.

_____. Office of Governor's Records. Applications for Surgeons, 1862–1864. RG 005, Series 6, Box 6. Connecticut State Library.

_____. Office of Governor's Records. Incoming letters. RG 005, Series 4, Boxes 24, 25. Connecticut State Library.

_____. Office of Governor's Records. Military correspondence. Incoming letters. RG 005. Boxes 86, 87A, 88, 94. Connecticut State Library.

_____. Office of Governor's Records. Outgoing Letters. Volumes 2–6. RG 005, Series 4. Connecticut State Library.

_____. Official letter books of governor. 1861–1866. Connecticut State Library.

_____. Proclamations, 1858–1866. Connecticut Historical Society.

Buckingham Family Correspondence, 1831–1875. MS 80401. Connecticut Historical Society.

Burnham, J.H. Military and Pension Records. 16th Connecticut Regiment. RG 15. National Archives, Washington, DC.

Burnham, John Henry. Letters to his mother, Sarah, 1862–1865. Sixteenth Connecticut Regiment. Connecticut State Library, Hartford.

Burr, Harold. "Jonathan Knight and the Founding of the Yale School of Medicine." *Yale Journal of Biology and Medicine* 1, no. 6 (1929): 327–343.

Butler, Benjamin F. *Private and Official Correspondence during the Period of the Civil War.* Norwood, MA: Plimpton Press, 1917.

Cadwell, Charles. *The Old Sixth Regiment.* New Haven: Tuttle, Morehouse & Taylor, 1875.

Cartwright, James. Letters. Forty-fourth Massachusetts Regiment. U.S. Military History Institute, Carlisle Barracks, PA.

Case, O.C. Letters October 20, 1861–August 7, 1862. Eighth Connecticut Volunteer Regiment. Archives of Simsbury Historical Society. Simsbury, CT.

Carey, William B. "Essay on Some Diseases of the Cervix Uteri." *Proceedings of the Connecticut Medical Society* (1854): 61–83.

_____. *Military Proceedings of the Connecticut Medical Society* (1870): 403.

Chisolm, John Julian. *Manual of Military Surgery for the Use of Surgeons in the Confederate States Army, with an Appendix of the Rules and Regulations of the Medical Department of the Confederate Army.* Richmond, VA: West and Johnson, 1861.

Churchman, John W. "The Use of Quinine during the Civil War." *Johns Hopkins Hospital Bulletin* 17 (1906): 175–181.

Cincinnati College of Medicine and Surgery. Annual Announcement, Session 1861–1862.

Civil War Draft Registration Records for New England. Letters sent to and received from military commanders relating to sick soldiers. January 1864–March 1865. RG 110. National Archives, Waltham, MA.

Civil War Draft Registration Records for New England. Medical register of men examined by surgeon for exemption. December 1864–April 1865. RG 110. National Archives, Waltham, MA.

Civil War sheet music. Library of Congress. Washington, DC. http://lcweb2.loc.gov/ihas/loc.music.sm1850.471570

Clausewitz, Carl von. *On War.* Edited and translated by Michael Howard and Peter Parent. Princeton, NJ: Princeton University Press, 1993.

Coggswell, William, M.D., and William White, M.D. Report as special agents to visit Connecticut Sick and Wounded soldiers in the U.S. General Hospitals. J.M. Scofield & Co. State Printers, 1863.

Columbian Weekly Register [New Haven], 1862–1865.

Connecticut Adjutant General's Office. *Record of Service of Connecticut Men in the Army and Navy of the United States during the War of the Rebellion.* Hartford: Case, Lockwood, Brainard, 1889.

Connecticut Medical Society Records and Correspondence, 1861–1870. Connecticut State Library, Hartford.

Croffut, W.A., and John M. Morris. *The Military and Civil History of Connecticut during the War of 1861–1865.* New York: Ledyard Bill, 1869.

Dibble, Frederick L. "Hygienic Teachings of the Late War." *Proceedings of the Connecticut Medical Society* (1867), pp. 300–310.

Dibble, Frederick L., M.D. Obituary. *Proceedings of the Connecticut Medical Society* (1898): 354.

Drake, Daniel. *A Systematic Treatise Historical, Etiological and Practical of the Principal Diseases of the Interior Valley of North America as They Appear in the Caucasian, African, Indian, and Esquimaux Varieties of Its Populations.* Cincinnati: Winthrop B. Smith, 1850.

Elliot, S.H. *The Attractions of New Haven, Connecticut; A Guide to the City.* New York: Tibbals & Co., 1869.

Ellsworth, Eliot. *Yale in the Civil War.* New Haven: Yale University Press, 1932.

Emerson, L.O. "We Are Coming Father Abra'am," Civil War song sheets, Library of Congress.

Fishbein, M. *Doctors at War.* New York: Dutton, 1945.

Flint, Austin. *A Treatise on the Principles and Practice of Medicine.* Philadelphia: Henry C. Lea, 1866.

_____, ed. *Contributions Relating to the Causation and Prevention of Disease and to Camp Diseases:*

Sanitary Memoirs of the War of the Rebellion. New York: Hurd & Houghton, 1867.

Fulton, John F. "The Library of Jonathan Knight, 1789–1864." *Yale Journal of Biology and Medicine* (1953): 468–76.

Goldsmith, Middleton. *A Report on Hospital Gangrene, Erysipelas and Pyemia.* Louisville: Bradley & Gilbert, 1863, p. 94.

Gordon, S.C. "Reminiscences of the Civil War from a Surgeon's Point of View," in *War Papers Read before the Commander of the State of Maine.* Vol. 1. Portland: Thurston, 1898, pp. 129–144.

Greenleaf, Charles R. *A Manual for the Medical Officers of the United States Army.* Philadelphia: J.B. Lippincott, 1864.

Gross, Samuel D. *A Manual of Military Surgery: Hints on Emergencies of Field, Camp, and Hospital Practice.* Philadelphia: J.B. Lippincott, 1861.

Hamilton, Frank. *A Treatise on Military Surgery and Hygiene.* New York: Balliere Brothers, 1865.

Hammond, W.A. *Treatise on Hygiene with Special Reference to the Military Service.* Philadelphia: Lippincott, 1863.

Hammond, William A. *Defense of Brigadier General William A. Hammond, Surgeon-General, U.S. Army with His Statement of the Causes Which Led to His Dismissal.* Washington, DC: privately printed, 1864.

_____, ed. *Military Medical and Surgical Essays, Prepared for the United States Sanitary Commission.* Philadelphia: Lippincott, 1864.

Hart, Albert Gaillard. "The Surgeon and the Hospital in the Civil War." *Military Historical Society of Massachusetts Papers* 13 (1913): 229–286.

Hartford Daily Courant. 1862–1865.

Hartford Daily Times. 1862–1865.

Hartford Medical Society. Minutes of meetings. 1860–1866. University of Connecticut Health Center. Farmington, CT.

Harvey, Samuel. *Surgery of the Past in Connecticut. The Heritage of Connecticut Medicine.* New Haven. 1942, p. 180.

Hayward, Nathaniel. Account Books, 1861–1863. Colchester. Connecticut Historical Society.

_____. Papers, 1846–1877. Colchester. Connecticut Historical Society.

Higginson, Thomas Wentworth, ed. "Robert Ware," in *Harvard Memorial Biographies.* Vol. 1. Cambridge: Sever & Francis, 1866.

Holcomb, Alfred. Letters. 27th Massachusetts Volunteers. U.S. Military History Institute, Carlisle Barracks, Carlisle, PA.

Holcombe, Hubert Vincent. Obituary. *Proceedings of the Connecticut Medical Society* 4 (1875): 441–442.

Holcombe, Hubert Vincent. Pension Files. Military Record Files. RG 15. Veterans Administration. National Archives, Washington, DC.

Holmes, Oliver Wendell. "Currents and Counter-currents in Medical Science." *Medical Communications of the Massachusetts Medical Society* 9, no. 6 (1860): 305–343.

_____. "On Intermittent Fevers in New England." In *The Boyleston Prize Dissertations for the Years 1836 and 1837.* Boston: Charles C. Little & James Brown, 1838.

Holmes, Oliver Wendell, Jr. *Touched with Fire: Civil War Letters and Diary.* Cambridge, MA: Harvard University Press, 1946.

Hooker, Worthington. "Biographical Sketch of Jonathan Knight." *Proceedings of the Connecticut Medical Society* (1865): 147–151.

_____. "Dissertation on the Respect Due to the Medical Profession and the Reasons That It Is Not Awarded by the Community." *Proceedings of the Connecticut Medical Society* (1844): 4–48.

_____. *Homeopathy: Examination of its Doctrine and Evidences.* New York: Scribner, 1851.

_____. Obituary. *Proceedings of the Connecticut Medical Society* (1870): 397.

_____. "The Treatment Due from the Medical Profession to Physicians Who Become Homeopathic Practitioners." *Proceedings of the Connecticut Medical Society* (1852): 1–11.

Hubert V.C. Holcombe Collection. Register of Sick and Wounded, Prescription Books, Letters. Hartford. Connecticut Historical Society.

Ives, Carl. "Prophylaxis of Phthisis Pulmonalis." *Proceedings of the Connecticut Medical Society* (1866): 185.

Jacobs, Ferris. Surgeon, Third New York Cavalry. Letters of application to the Medical Department, microfilm roll 1064, National Archives. Washington DC.

Jewett family records, Connecticut Historical Society, Hartford.

Jewett, Pliny Adams. Committee meetings. *Proceedings of the Connecticut Medical Society* (1857, 1861).

_____. Letters. Manuscript Section. Sterling Library, Yale University, New Haven, CT.

_____. Letters 1862–1865. First Connecticut Cavalry Regiment. Virginia Historical Society, Richmond.

_____. Medical Officers File. 1862–1866. RG 94. National Archives, Washington, DC.

_____. Military and Pension Records. Medical Officer File RG 94, entry 561. Microfilm 1064, roll 100. National Archives, Washington, DC.

_____. Military Records. General and Staff Officer File. National Archives, Washington, DC.

_____. Obituary. *Medical and Surgical Reporter* 18 (1887): 544.

_____. Obituary. *Proceedings of the Connecticut Medical Society* (1887): 169–172.

_____. *Semi-Centennial History of the General Hospital Society of Connecticut.* New Haven: Tuttle, Morehouse & Taylor, 1876.

Jewett, Stephen. Discourse on the Life of the Reverend. Manuscript. New Haven Historical Society. New Haven, CT.

Jones, Joseph. *Quinine as a Prophylactic against Malarial Fever.* Nashville, TN: University Medical Press, 1867.

Keen, William W., Silas Weir Mitchell, and George R. Morehouse. "On Malingering, Especially in Regard to Simulation of Diseases of the Nervous System." *American Journal of Medical Sciences* 48 (1864): 367–394.

Kilgour, Frederick. *The Library of the Medical Institution of Yale College and Its Catalogue of 1865.* New Haven: Yale University Press, 1960.

Knight, Jonathan. "Lectures." *Yale Journal of Biology and Medicine* 74 (2001): 111–137.

Knight Army Hospital. Endorsements sent and received by surgeons. September 1863–July 1864. RG 110. Civil War Draft Registration Records. National Archives, Waltham, MA.

_____. Letters from the department to the provost marshal. 1863–65. RG 110. Civil War Draft Registration Records. National Archives, Waltham, MA.

_____. Letters sent to and received from military commanders relating to the registration records. Civil War Draft Registration Records. National Archives, Waltham, MA.

_____. Reports. 1863–1865. RG 13:45. Box 115. Connecticut State Library, Hartford.

Knight Hospital Record. Bound newspaper. October 1864–July 1865. Hartford Medical Society, University of Connecticut Health Center, Farmington, CT.

Knight Medical School Prospectus. Knight General Hospital. Harvey Cushing/John Hay Whitney Medical Library, Medical Historical Library. Yale University, New Haven, CT.

La Roche, R. *Yellow Fever Considered in Its Historical, Pathological, Etiological, and Therapeutic Relations.* Volumes I and II. Philadelphia, 1855.

Leavonworth, M. Obituary. *Proceedings of the Connecticut Medical Society* (1866): 269.

Lee, Charles A., Professor, Material Medica and General Pathology. Address to the graduating class of Geneva Medical College at the annual commencement. June 22, 1852.

Lewis, John B. "Reminiscences of a Civil War Surgeon." Edited by Stanley Weld and David Soskis. *Journal of the History of Medicine and Allied Sciences* 21 (1966): 47–58.

Lewis, Lloyd. *Sherman: Fighting Prophet.* Lincoln: University of Nebraska Press, 1993.

Lindsley, C.A. Letters. Harvey Cushing/John Hay Whitney Medical Library, Medical Historical Library. Yale University, New Haven.

_____. Obituary. *Proceedings of the Connecticut Medical Society* (1906).

_____. "Puerperal Convulsions." *Proceedings of the Connecticut Medical Society* (1858): 71–83.

Livermore, Mary. *My Story of the War: A Woman's Narrative of Four Years of Personal Experience as a Nurse in the Union Army.* Hartford, CT: A.D. Worthington, 1887.

Longmore, Thomas. *A Treatise on Gunshot Wounds.* Philadelphia: Lippincott, 1862.

Lonn, Ella. *Desertion during the Civil War.* Gloucester, MA: Peter Smith, 1928.

Louis, A.P. "Pathological Researches on Phthisis." Translated from the French with introduction, notes, additions and an essay on treatment by Charles Cowan, M.D. (Edinburgh). Revised and altered by Henry I. Bowditch, M.D., 1836.

Macleod, George H.B. *Notes on the Surgery of the War in the Crimea.* Philadelphia: Lippincott, 1862.

Maher, Sister Mary Denis. *To Bind Up the Wounds: Catholic Sister Nurses in the U.S. Civil War.* New York: Greenwood Press, 1989.

Maxwell, William Quentin. *Lincoln's Fifth Wheel: The Political History of the United States Sanitary Commission.* New York: Longmans, Green, 1956.

Mayer, Nathan. Collection. Hartford Medical Society, University of Connecticut Health Center. Farmington, CT.

_____. Obituary. *Hartford Times,* July 11, 1912.

_____. Pension and Military Record Files. RG 15. Veterans Administration. National Archives, Washington, DC.

Medical student dissertations of 1863, Harvey Cushing Medical History Library, Yale University, New Haven, CT.

Medical student letters to the dean of the Medical Institution of Yale College, 1860s. Harvey Cushing Medical Historical Library, Yale University, New Haven, CT.

Minor, William C. Acting Assistant Surgeon. Postmortem exams made at the Knight U.S. Army General Hospital, 1864. Harvey Cushing Medical Historical Library, Yale University, New Haven, CT.

Mitchell, Silas Weir. "The Medical Department in the Civil War." *The Journal of the American Medical Association* 62, no. 19 (May 9, 1914): 1445–1550.

_____. "Some Personal Recollections of the Civil War." *Transactions of the College of Physicians of Philadelphia* 27 (1905): 87–94.

Morris, Charles. Court-martial file. Records of Judge Advocate. RG 153. National Archives, Washington, D.C.

Morton, Samuel. *Illustrations of Pulmonary Consumption, Its Anatomical Characters, Causes, Symptoms, and Treatment.* Philadelphia: Key & Biddle, 1837.

Nettleton, Lewis J. Diary. Nettleton-Baldwin Family Papers. Civil War Manuscript Collection. Yale University Library Department of Manuscripts and Archives, New Haven, CT.

_____. Pension files. RG 15. Veterans Administration. National Archives, Washington, DC.

Nettleton-Baldwin Family Papers. Duke University Library Special Collections, Durham, NC.

Newhall, Horatio. Letters. Forty-fourth Massachusetts Regiment. U.S. Military History Institute, Carlisle Barracks, PA.

Norwood, William Frederick. *Medical Education in the United States before the Civil War.* Philadelphia: University of Pennsylvania Press, 1944.

Nutmeg. "The Outside Column," *Hartford Courant,* September 4, 1947.

Olmsted, Frederick Law. *Hospital Transports: A Memoir of the Embarkation of the Sick and Wounded from the Peninsula of Virginia in the Summer of 1862.* Boston: Ticknor & Fields, 1863.

Ordronaux, John. *Manual of Instructions for Military Surgeons on the Examination of Recruits and Discharge of Soldiers.* New York: D. Van Nostrand, 1863.

Osborne, E.W. Letters. E.W. Osborne Manuscripts, no. 77, Box 2. New Haven Colony Historical Society.

_____. Letters. Manuscripts, no. 77, Box 2. New Haven Historical Society. New Haven, CT.

Osler, William. "Influence of Louis on American Medicine." *Bulletin of the Johns Hopkins Hospital* 8, nos. 77–78 (August-September 1897): 161–167.

Paget, James. Lectures on Surgical Pathology. Philadelphia, 1853.

Peck, Henry. Letters. Sterling Library. Yale University, New Haven, CT.

Pember, Phoebe Yates. *A Southern Woman's Story: Life in Confederate Richmond.* New York: G. W. Carleton, 1879.

Phelps, A.J. "On the Causation of Disease." U.S. Sanitary Commission. Documents of the United States Sanitary Commission. Vol. 1. New York, 1866.

Pierpont, Henry, M.D. Obituary. *Proceedings of the Connecticut Medical Society* (1893): 244.

"The Primary Cause of the Great Mortality in Our Large Cities." *Medical and Surgical Reporter* 13 (August 1865).

Provost Marshal. Letters. Draft Registration Records. RG 110. National Archives, Waltham, MA.

Regimental History, First Connecticut Cavalry Volunteers in the War of the Rebellion, 1861–1865, 1889. Connecticut State Library.

Ripley, J.B. *Six Soundings.* Philadelphia: James Callen & Son, 1860.

Rosen, George. *Fees and Fee Bills: Some Economic Aspects of Medical Practice in Nineteenth-century America.* Supplements to *Bulletin of the History of Medicine* 6. Baltimore: Johns Hopkins University Press, 1946.

Rothstein, William. *American Physicians in the Nineteenth Century: From Sects to Science.* Baltimore: Johns Hopkins University Press, 1972.

Russell, Gurdon. Obituary. *Proceedings of the Connecticut Medical Society* (1909): 380.

Smith, George Winston. *Medicines for the Union Army.* Madison, WI: American Institute of the History of Pharmacy, 1962.

Starr, Paul. *The Social Transformation of American Medicine.* New York: Basic Books, 1982.

Steiner, Walter Ralph. "The Evolution of Medicine in Connecticut, with the Foundation of the Yale Medical School as Its Notable Achievement." In Yale University, *Memorial of the Centennial of the Yale Medical School.* 10–33. New Haven: Yale University Press, 1915.

Thompson, Henry J.H. Letters. Duke University Library Special Collections, Durham, NC.

Thorpe, Sheldon B. *The History of the Fifteenth Connecticut Volunteers in the War for the Defense of the Union, 1861–1865.* New Haven: Price, Lee & Adkins, 1893.

Townsend, Timothy B. Obituary. *New Haven Daily Courier,* April 1, 1893.

Townsend, Timothy B., MD. Office ledger and account books. 1860–1872. Harvey Cushing/John Hay Whitney Medical Library, Medical Historical Library. Yale University, New Haven, CT.

Townshend, Doris. *Townshend Heritage.* New Haven: New Haven Colony Historical Society, 1971.

Treadway, F.S. "A Dissertation on Yellow Fever." Graduation thesis, the Medical Institution of Yale College, 1863. Harvey Cushing Medical Historical Library. Yale University, New Haven, CT.

Tripler, Charles S., and George C. Blackman. *Handbook for the Military Surgeon.* Cincinnati, OH: Robert Clarke and Co., 1861.

U.S. Army Draft Rendezvous Hospital. Correspondence. Connecticut State Library, Hartford.

_____. Letters sent in care of Acting Assistant Surgeon E. W. Blake. Connecticut State Library, Hartford.

U.S. Army Medical Department. *General Medicine and Infectious Diseases.* Vol. 2, *Internal Medicine in Vietnam,* edited by Andre Ognibene and O'Neill Barrett. Washington, DC: GPO, 1982.

_____. Hospital Department. Fifteenth Connecticut Volunteers. Orders and Letters. RG 13. Box 229. Connecticut State Library, Hartford.

U.S. Sanitary Commission. *Documents of the United States Sanitary Commission.* Vol. 1. New York, 1866.

_____. Hints for the Control and Prevention of Infectious Diseases, in Camps, Transports, and Hospitals. New York: W. Bryant & Co., 1863.

_____. *A Report to the Secretary of War of the Operations of the Sanitary Commission and upon the Sanitary Condition of the Volunteer Army, Its Medical Staff, Hospitals and Hospital Supplies.* Washington, DC, December 1861.

_____. *Sanitary Memoirs of the War of the Rebellion.* New York: Hurd & Houghton, 1867.

_____. *United States Sanitary Commission Bulletin.* Vol. 1 (1863–1864).

_____. *Value of Vaccination in Armies.* 3rd edition. U.S. Sanitary Commission, 1865.

U.S. Secretary of War. Letters received. Microscopy No. 221. Main series, 1801–1870. National Archives Microfilm Publications.

U.S. Surgeon General's Office. *The Medical and Surgical History of the War of the Rebellion.* Washington, DC: Government Printing office, 1875–1885.

U.S. War Department. *Regulations for the Medical Department of the Army.* Washington, DC: A.O.P. Nicholson, 1856.

University of Nashville Medical Department. Catalogue, session 1857–1858.

University of Vermont Medical Department. Catalogue, June 1864.

Vaill, Joseph. Letter. November 1864. Eighth Connecticut Regiment. Knight Army Hospital. U.S. Army Military Institute. Carlisle Barracks, PA.

Van Buren, William H. *Rules for Preserving the Health of the Soldier.* Washington, DC: United States Sanitary Commission, 1861.

_____. "The Use of Quinine as a Prophylactic against Malarious Diseases." In *Military Medical and Surgical Essays, Prepared for the United States Sanitary Commission,* edited by William A. Hammond, 93–115. Philadelphia: Lippincott, 1864.

Waite, Frederick Clayton. *The First Medical College in Vermont: Castleton, 1818–1862.* Montpelier: Vermont Historical Society, 1949.

Walker, L.G., Jr. "Surgery at Yale in 1843: Professor Jonathan Knight's Lectures." *Yale Journal of Biology and Medicine* 74 (2001): 111–137.

Ward, Patricia Spain. *Simon Baruch, Rebel in the Ranks of Medicine, 1840–1921.* Tuscaloosa: University of Alabama Press, 1994.

Warren, Edward. *An Epitome of Practical Surgery for Field and Hospital.* Surgeon General of North Carolina, 1863.

Welch, William Henry. "The Relation of Yale to Medicine." *Science* 14 (1901): 825–840.

Weld, Stanley B. *Connecticut Physicians in the Civil War.* Hartford: Connecticut Civil War Centennial Commission, 1965.

Wheeler, George. Lecture, 1915. Medical Reunion Mollus, Vol. 3. U.S. Army Military History Institute. Carlisle Barracks, PA.

Whitman, Walt. *Specimen Days.* Philadelphia. 1892. p. 35.

_____. *The Wound Dresser: A Series of Letters Written from the Hospitals in Washington during the War of the Rebellion.* Boston: Small, Maynard, 1898.

Wilbur, Joshua. Letters. 18th Massachusetts Regiment Volunteers. U.S. Military History Institute. Carlisle Barracks, PA.

Winchester, Simon. *The Professor and the Madman.* New York: HarperCollins, 1998.

Woodward, Ashbel. "Biographical Notice of Dewitt Clinton Lathrop, MD." *Proceedings of the Connecticut Medical Society* (1861): 64–65.

_____. "Life and Medical Ethics." *Proceedings of the Connecticut Medical Society* (May 1860): 4–35.

_____. "On Specialism in Medicine." *Proceedings of the Connecticut Medical Society* (1866): 264.

_____. "Vindication of Army Surgeons." *Proceedings of the Connecticut Medical Society* (May 1863): 256–264.

Woodward, Joseph Janvier. *Hospital Steward's Manual.* Philadelphia: J.B. Lippincott, 1863.

Woshner, Mike. *India-Rubber and Gutta-Percha in the Civil War Era.* Alexandria, VA: O'Donnell Publications, 1999.

Yale Medical School. *Memorial of the Centennial of the Yale Medical School.* New Haven: Yale University Press, 1915.

Index

Numbers in **bold italics** indicate pages with photographs.